Nano- and Biomaterials

Nano- and Biomaterials

Compounds, Properties, Characterization, and Applications

Zhypargul Abdullaeva

WILEY-VCH

Author

Prof. Zhypargul Abdullaeva
Kumamoto University
Materials Science & Engineering
2-39-1 Kurokami
Engineering Research Bldg.
860-8555 Kumamoto
Japan

Cover

Fullerene - fotolia_©ogwen
nanotube - fotolia_©daniel700 and
cell - fotolia_©Garry DeLong.

Library of Congress Card No.: applied for

British Library Cataloguing-in-Publication Data
A catalogue record for this book is available from the British Library.

Bibliographic information published by the Deutsche Nationalbibliothek
The Deutsche Nationalbibliothek lists this publication in the Deutsche Nationalbibliografie; detailed bibliographic data are available on the Internet at <http://dnb.d-nb.de>.

Print ISBN: 978-3-527-34270-9
ePDF ISBN: 978-3-527-80705-5
ePub ISBN: 978-3-527-80703-1
Mobi ISBN: 978-3-527-80704-8
oBook ISBN: 978-3-527-80702-4

Cover Design Adam-Design, Weinheim, Germany
Typesetting SPi Global, Chennai, India
Printing and Binding Markono Print Media Pte Ltd, Singapore

Printed on acid-free paper

Contents

Preface *xi*

1 Introduction into Nano- and Biomaterials *1*
1.1 Definition of Nano- and Biomaterials *1*
1.2 History of Nano- and Biomaterials Application *1*
1.3 Methods for Preparing of Nanomaterials *2*
1.3.1 Mechanical Dispersion Methods for Nanomaterial Synthesis *2*
1.3.2 Intensive Plastic Deformation Methods for Nanomaterial Synthesis *5*
1.3.3 Obtaining of Nanomaterials by Mechanical Interaction of Various Mediums *8*
1.3.4 Physical Dispersion Methods for Nanomaterials Preparation *9*
1.3.5 Preparation of Nanomaterials by Evaporation–Condensation Method *10*
1.3.6 Obtaining of Nanomaterials by Vacuum-Sublimation Technology *13*
1.3.7 Obtaining of Nanomaterials by Using Solid Phase Transformations *14*
1.3.8 Chemical Dispersion Methods for Nanomaterial Preparation *14*
1.3.9 Obtaining of Nanomaterials by Using Chemical Reactions *15*
1.3.10 Preparation of Nanomaterials by Electrochemical Methods *20*
1.3.11 Preparation of Nanomaterials by Combinations of Physical and Chemical Transformations *21*
1.4 Main Achievements in Nanotechnology *22*
Case Study 1: Synthesis of Nanoparticles and Environmental Safety Considerations *22*
Case Study 2: Property Control of Nanomaterials by Setting Experimental Conditions during Synthesis *23*
Control Questions: *23*
References *24*
Further Reading *25*

2 Classification of Nanomaterials *27*
2.1 Dispersive Systems and Their Classifications *27*
2.1.1 Classification of Dispersive Systems According to their Aggregation States *27*
2.1.2 Classification of Dispersive Systems According to Size *28*
2.1.3 Classification of Dispersive Systems According to Dimension *31*

2.2 Fullerenes 32
2.2.1 History of Fullerenes 34
2.2.2 Tetrahedral Fullerenes 34
2.2.3 Icosahedral Fullerenes 42
2.2.4 Physical Properties of Fullerenes 47
2.3 Carbon Nanotubes 49
2.3.1 Types and Classification of Carbon Nanotubes 49
2.3.2 Mechanical Properties and Physical Parameters of Carbon Nanotubes 52
Case Study 1: Comparison of Structural Characteristics between Carbon Nanotubes and Fullerenes 54
Control Questions 54
References 55
Further Reading 56
Online Sources 56

3 Nanocomposite Materials and Their Physical Property Features 57
3.1 Nanocomposite Materials 57
3.2 Size Dependence as Nanomaterial Property 57
3.3 Thermodynamical Features of Nanomaterials 58
3.4 Phase Equilibrium Changes in Nano-sized Systems 60
3.5 Melting Temperature Changes in Nanomaterials 61
3.5.1 Polymorphic Characteristic Changes in Nanosystems 61
3.6 Structure of Nano-sized Materials 62
3.7 Crystal Lattice Defects in Nanomaterials 65
3.8 Microdistorsions of Crystal Lattice in Nanomaterials 66
3.9 Consolidation of Nano-sized Powders 68
Case Study 1: Applications of Composite Nanomaterials Due to Their Improved Mechanical Properties 74
Control Questions 75
References 76
Further Reading 76
Online Source 77

4 Mechanical Characteristics of Dispersive Systems 79
4.1 Dispersion Characteristics of Nanomaterials 79
4.1.1 Specific Surface Area 79
4.1.2 Size Distribution in Nanomaterials 80
4.1.3 Surface, Boundaries, and Morphology of Nanomaterials 89
4.1.4 Grain Boundaries in Nanomaterials 91
4.1.5 Morphology of Nanodisperse Particles 92
4.2 Electrical Properties of Nanomaterials 95
4.2.1 Change in Length of Electron Free Path in Nanomaterials 95
4.3 Electrical Conductivity in Nanomaterials 97
4.4 Electron Work Function in Nanomediums 99
4.5 Superconductivity Phenomenon in Nanomaterials 101

Case Study 1: Surfactant Effects on Dispersion Characteristics of Copper-Based Nanomaterials *105*
Case Study 2: Applications of Superconducting Nanomaterials *105*
Control Questions *106*
References *106*
Further Reading *106*

5 Physical Properties of Nanomaterials: Graphene *109*
5.1 Ferromagnetic Characteristics of Nanomaterials *109*
5.1.1 Substance in Single-Domain Condition *109*
5.1.2 Superparamagnetism in Nanoparticles *111*
5.1.3 Size Dependence on Coercive Force *112*
5.1.4 Size Dependence on Saturation Magnetization *114*
5.1.5 Size Dependence on Curie Temperature *115*
5.2 Thermal Property Features in Nanomaterials *115*
5.2.1 Size Dependence on Heat Conductivity *116*
5.2.2 Heat Conductivity of Crystal Lattice in Nanomaterials *120*
5.2.3 Debye Temperature in Nanomaterials *121*
5.3 Optical Characteristics of Nanomediums *122*
5.3.1 Light Scattering Features of Tiny Particles *123*
5.3.2 Extinction by Dielectric Nanoparticles *125*
5.3.3 Extinction in Metallic Nanoparticles *128*
5.3.4 Influence of Morphology and Polydispersity on Optical Properties of Nanomaterials *131*
5.4 Diffusion in Nanomaterials *133*
5.4.1 Diffusion in Nanopowders *133*
5.5 Graphene *136*
5.5.1 Structure of Graphene *137*
5.5.2 Electronic Properties of Graphene *138*
5.5.3 Topology of Hexagonal Lattice *138*
5.5.4 Physical Properties and Ionization Potential of Graphene *139*
5.5.5 Approaches in Graphene Synthesis *141*
5.5.6 Characterizations of Graphene *142*
5.5.7 Applications of Graphene *145*
Case Study 1: Structural Features of Graphene, Lattice Directions, Edge Location, Crystal Structure, and Energy in Reciprocal Space *145*
Control Questions *147*
References *148*
Further Reading *149*

6 Chemical Properties and Mechanical Characteristics of Nanomaterial Characterization Tools in Nanotechnology *151*
6.1 Chemical Properties of Nanomaterials *151*
6.1.1 Size Effects in Chemical Processes *151*
6.1.2 Oxidation Processes in Nanomediums *153*
6.1.3 Spontaneous Combustion and Pyrophoricity of Nanomediums *157*
6.1.4 Catalysis Involving Nanomaterials *160*

6.2 Mechanical Characteristics of Nanomaterials *163*
6.2.1 Hardness, Strength, and Plasticity in Nanomaterials *163*
6.2.2 Superplasticity Phenomenon in Nanomaterials *170*
6.3 Concept Map of Characterization Tools in Nanotechnology *172*
6.4 Diffraction Methods for Nanomaterial Characterization *173*
6.5 Microscopical Characterization of Nanomaterials *174*
6.5.1 TEM Characterization of Nanomaterials *174*
6.5.2 HRTEM Characterization of Nanomaterials *177*
6.5.3 AFM Characterization of Nanomaterials *177*
6.5.4 SEM Characterization of Nanomaterials *178*
6.6 Spectroscopical Characterization of Nanomaterials *181*
6.6.1 FT-IR Spectroscopy of Nanomaterials *181*
6.6.2 X-ray Photoelectron Spectroscopy of Nanomaterials *182*
Case Study 1: Oxidation of Fe Nanoparticles *182*
Case Study 2: Microscopical Characterization of Nanomaterials and Sample Preparation *183*
Case Study 3: Nanomaterials Strength *184*
Control Questions *185*
References *185*
Further Reading *187*
Online Sources *187*

7 Introduction to Biomaterials *189*
7.1 Biomaterials: Subject, Purpose, and Problems *189*
7.1.1 Current Goals of Biomaterials Field *189*
7.2 General Requirements for Biomaterials *190*
7.3 Biomaterials in Body Systems *191*
7.4 Types and Classification of Biomaterials *192*
7.4.1 Metallic Biomaterials *193*
7.4.2 Composite Biomaterials *199*
7.4.3 Nanostructured CaP Composites *200*
Case Study 1: Mechanical Properties of Bone Cements and Tissue Interface Formation after Implantation *203*
Control Questions *204*
References *205*
Further Reading *207*

8 Properties of Biomaterials *209*
8.1 Mechanical Properties of Biomaterials *209*
8.1.1 Mechanical Properties of Biomaterials *209*
8.1.2 Titanium Alloy with Self-Adjustable Young's Modulus *211*
8.1.3 Wear Resistance of Biomaterials Used in the Living Body *212*
8.2 Biological Properties of Biomaterials *215*
8.2.1 *In Vivo* Tissue Biocompatibility *215*
8.3 Chemical Properties of Biomaterials *220*
8.3.1 Ceramic Biomaterials *222*
8.3.2 Polymer Biomaterials *230*

Case Study 1: Polymeric Biomaterials Used in Load-Bearing Medical Devices *235*
Control Questions *236*
References *237*
Further Reading *238*

9 Implants and Artificial Organs *239*
9.1 Implants *239*
9.2 Types of Implants *239*
9.2.1 Intraocular Lenses *239*
9.2.2 Cochlear Implants *241*
9.2.3 Brain Implants *242*
9.2.4 Heart Implants *243*
9.2.5 Joint Implants *246*
9.2.6 Other Organ Replacement Implants *247*
9.3 Processes between Living Tissue and Implant Interface *249*
Case Study 1: Iris-Fixated Phakic Intraocular Lens Implantation after Retinal Detachment Surgery: Long-Term Clinical Results *252*
Case Study 2: Cardiac Pacing Systems and Implantable Cardiac Defibrillators (ICDs): A Radiological Perspective of Equipment, Anatomy, and Complications *254*
Control Questions *255*
References *256*
Further Reading *258*

10 Tissue Engineering, Scaffolds, and 3D Bioprinting *259*
10.1 Definition of Tissue Engineering *259*
10.1.1 Biomaterials Used for Tissue Engineering *259*
10.1.2 Principles of Tissue Engineering *260*
10.1.3 Components of Tissue Engineered Constructs *260*
10.2 Scaffolds and Scaffolding *262*
10.2.1 Scaffolds for Bone Tissue Engineering *262*
10.2.2 Tissue Engineering of Heart Valves *264*
10.3 3D Bioprinting *266*
10.4 Foreign Body Reaction *271*
10.4.1 Inflammatory Response Following Material Implantation *273*
10.4.2 Monocytes, Macrophages, and Foreign Body Giant Cells *274*
10.5 Wound Healing *275*
Case Study 1: Bioactive Glass and Glass-Ceramic Scaffolds for Bone Tissue Engineering *275*
Case Study 2: Regulatory Considerations in the Design and Manufacturing of Implantable 3D Printed Medical Devices *276*
Control Questions *279*
References *279*
Further Reading *282*

Index *283*

Preface

If you are the person who is trying to bend the hills of Nano- and Biomaterials science, here is the textbook, carefully designed and addressed to you, students, as well as instructors and to all, who need to master the basic phenomena, terms, determinations and examples of Nano- and Biomaterials course. The main goal of this book is to foster an easy perception and conceptualizing ability in readers. Systematical representation and logical sequence are one of specific aspects, helping in assimilation of obtained knowledge.

Chapter 1 of this textbook starts with introduction into Nano- and Biomaterials, describing definition, history and application of Nano-and Biomaterials. Body of the chapter 1 covers various methods for nanomaterials preparation, and end with the main achievements in Nanotechnology. Chapter 2 is focuses on classification of nanomaterials, including classification of dispersive systems, fullerenes and nanotubes. Chapter 3 presents nanocomposite materials and their physical property features, mainly of size dependence, thermodynamic, phase equilibrium and melting temperature changes, structure of nanomaterials, crystal lattice defects, microdistorsions of crystal lattice and consolidation of nano-sized powders. Chapter 4 covers mechanical characteristics of dispersive systems, electrical properties, electrical conductivity, electrical work function and superconductivity phenomena in nanomaterials. Chapter 5 gives the theory of physical properties for nanomaterials and Graphene, particularly, ferromagnetic characteristics, thermal and optical property features, diffusion in nanomaterials, graphene and its structure, synthesis approaches and characterization of graphene. Chapter 6 presents chemical property and mechanical characteristics of nanomaterials, as well as characterization tools in nanotechnology, diffraction methods, microscopical and spectroscopical characterization tools for nanomaterials. Chapter 7 reviews introduction into biomaterials, subject, purpose and problems of biomaterials science, general requirements for biomaterials, biomaterials in body systems, types and classification of biomaterials, metallic and composite biomaterials. Chapter 8 gives theory of biomaterials properties, such as mechanical, chemical and biological, also describing ceramic and polymeric types of biomaterials. Chapter 9 covers implants and artificial organs, clarifying their definitions, types, explaining the processes between living tissue and implant interface. Chapter 10 focuses on tissue engineering, scaffolds and 3D bioprinting, provides conclusion by foreign body reaction and wound healing.

Each chapter ends with answer-required questions for control of obtained knowledge. Case studies given after control questions are providing additional explanatory support related to the key concepts along the chapter, which are helpful for readers in building of basic knowledge and learning skills.

1

Introduction into Nano- and Biomaterials

Translated materials from the original work of Ryzhonkov, D.I., Levina, V.V., Dzidziguri, E.L. were used in this chapter.

There is no substitute to hard work....

Thomas Edison, inventor (1847–1931)

1.1 Definition of Nano- and Biomaterials

Nano (from Greek, *nannos*), meaning dwarf, is one billionth of or 10^{-9} part of a thing, for example, $1\,nm = 10^{-9}\,m$. *Nanomaterials* consist of nanostructured materials and *nanoparticles,* which can be defined as nano-sized complexes of interrelated atoms and/or molecules. *Nanotechnology* is defined as the knowledge and management of processes on a scale from 1 to 100 nm and application of object properties on a nanometer scale. Significant works in nanotechnology started in 1980. Definition for the term *nanotechnology* was given for the first time by Norio Taniguchi, a professor of Tokyo University, in 1974 in his paper *Basic concepts of Nanotechnology,* which mentioned "Nanotechnology mainly consists of the processing of separation, consolidation, and deformation of materials by one atom or one molecule."

Biomaterials can be defined as "materials intended to interface with biological systems to evaluate, treat, or replace any tissue, organ or function of the body" [1] or "any synthetic material which is used to replace part of a living system or to function in intimate contact with the living tissue [2]."

1.2 History of Nano- and Biomaterials Application

Nanomaterials and biomaterials are important because of their primal and initial applications, which date back to ancient times and the Middle Ages, when glassblowers insensibly used nanotechnology. They added gold chloride ($AuCl_3$) to melted glass to change its color to ruby. Thousands of years BC, people knew and used natural fabrics such as cotton, silk and flax, and wool [3]. The Romans had the Lycurgus Cup during the fourth century AD (Anno Domino), which comprises silver and gold nanoparticles at a ratio of roughly 7 : 3, with a diameter

Nano- and Biomaterials: Compounds, Properties, Characterization, and Applications,
First Edition. Zhypargul Abdullaeva.

size of 70 nm, as disclosed by modern analytic methods. The cup demonstrates a unique color display because of the presence of these metal nanoparticles. It appears green when observed in reflected light, for instance, in daylight, but turns red when light is propagated through it, which is now in the British museum. Historical applications of biomaterials include the use of linen threads by ancient Egyptians to close wounds. Europeans used a fiber made from catgut to close the wounds during the Middle Ages 4000 years ago. Inca surgeons repaired cranial fractures with gold plates in neurosurgery. Mayans used sea shells to create an artificial teeth. In the nineteenth and early twentieth centuries, a number of physicians began to explore the way in which the body reacted to implanted materials. After World War II, observations began to demonstrate the tolerance of the human body to some metals *in vivo*. Physician Harold Ridley who worked with World War II aviators had noticed that pieces of shattered cockpit canopies inadvertently embedded in the eyes of pilots were well tolerated; thus, he made the 1st formal assessment of "biocompatibility." Later he created implantable intraocular lenses from polymethylmetacrylate [1].

1.3 Methods for Preparing of Nanomaterials

Recently, a huge number of methods for nanomaterial preparation were developed, which led to a variety of nanomaterial properties and expanded the ranges of nanomaterial classes with the creation of a new and unique materials. The formation of high-dispersive structures might happen during phase changes, chemical interactions, recrystallization, amorphization, high mechanical stress, and biological synthesis. Improvement of primary methods for nanomaterials syntheses defined the main requirements such as:

- Method should provide control of composition and properties for obtaining of nanomaterials.
- Method should provide permanent stability of nanomaterials, principal protection of particle surfaces against oxidation and sintering during synthesis.
- Method should be highly productive and economical.
- Method should allow acquisition of nanomaterials with definite sizes or grains.

Basically, preparation of nanomaterials can be divided into *up-bottom* and *bottom-up* processes, which are based on crushing and integration, respectively. These processes are essential for nanomaterials syntheses, especially of mechanical, physical, chemical, and biological methods. Mechanical dispersion methods are based on the interaction between pressure, curve, vibration, friction, and cavitation processes. *Physical methods* for nanomaterial syntheses are based on physical transformations: evaporation, condensation, sublimation, hardening, thermocycling, and so on. *Chemical methods* are based on chemical dispersion process, chemical reaction, electrolysis, reduction, and thermal decomposition. *Biological methods* for nanomaterials syntheses are based on the use of biochemical processes in the protein-containing body.

1.3.1 Mechanical Dispersion Methods for Nanomaterial Synthesis

Most mechanical dispersion methods involve mechanical milling, intensive plastic deformation, and mechanical interactions between various mediums.

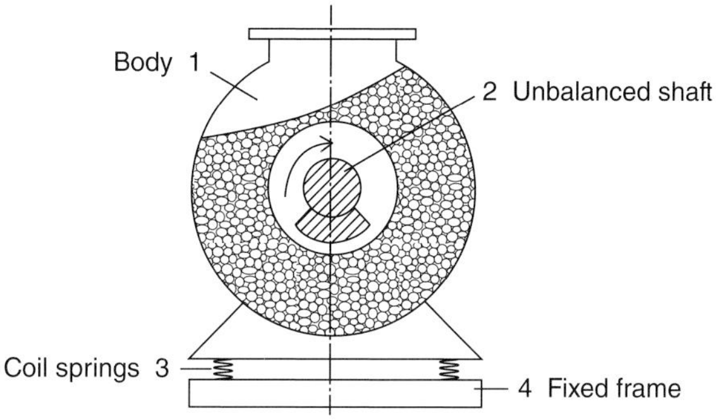

Figure 1.1 Scheme of vibration mill for nanomaterial preparation (reproduced with permission of BKL Publishers).

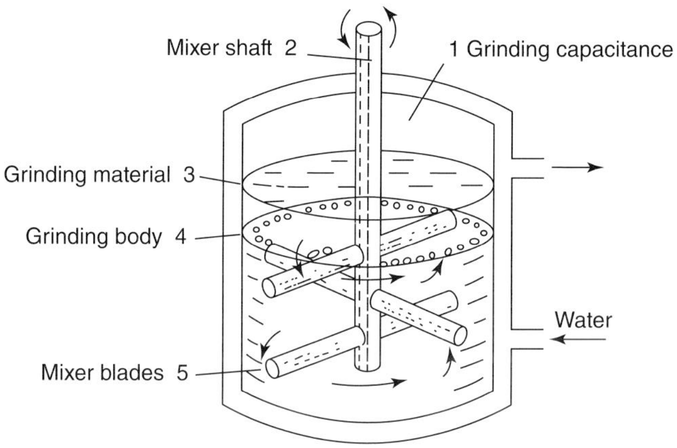

Figure 1.2 Scheme of attrition milling device for nanomaterial preparation (reproduced with permission of BKL Publishers).

Mechanical milling is determined by local mechanical interactions appearing in the strain field of the given material. Due to locality and impulsivity in the area of dispersing material, loads can be focused for a short time and cause formation of particle defects, stacking faults, deformations, and cracks. Finally, milling of materials will occur, as well as acceleration of mass transfer, mixing of components in material, and activation of chemical interactions between solid reagent compounds. Mechanical milling or grinding is conducted by using of various equipment such as vibration mills (Figure 1.1), ball mills, hygroscopic mills, attrition mills (Figure 1.2), vortex mills (Figure 1.3), and jet mills.

Grinding in vortex mills is primarily intended for ductile metal conversion into nanopowders. In these devices, collisions between the abrasive particles of grinding material will occur. Inside the working chamber of a jet, mill propellers rotate in opposite directions with a speed of 3000 rotations per minute (Figure 1.3). Depending on the nature of the grinding material, particles might be obtained in splintered, flaky, and rounded forms.

Another type of mill for nanomaterial preparation is the planetary *centrifugal mill*, which allows fast and fine crushing of hard milling materials. In hygroscopic mills, the grinding drum rotates horizontally and vertically at the same time.

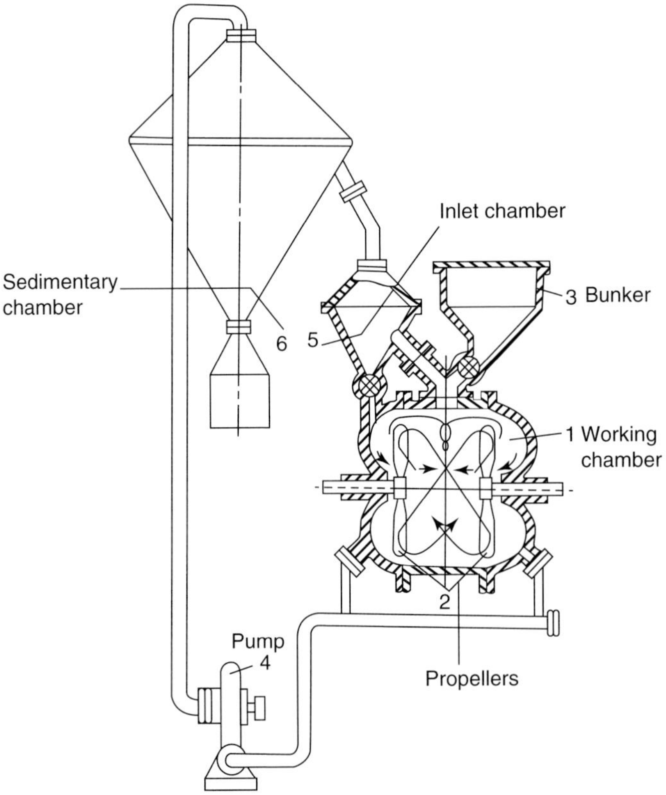

Figure 1.3 Scheme of vortex mill device for nanomaterial preparation (reproduced with permission of BKL Publishers).

Jet mills are designed for the effective production of nanopowders. They provide fine crushing of material by inserting compressed gas jet (air, nitrogen, etc.) or hot steam into working chamber from the nozzles, with sonic or ultrasonic velocity. Inside the working chamber, grinding materials undergo vortex motion and multiple collisions, resulting in their intensive abrasion. Jet mills are used for grinding of metals, ceramics, polymers, and their different combinations.

Also, the grinding of fragile and specially embrittled materials, for example, electrolytic sediments and spongy metals, can be conducted inside jet mills. An inert atmosphere can prevent the oxidation inside the working chamber of jet mills.

Moreover, for effective grinding, it is recommended that the grinding process be conducted in liquid organic mediums, such as hydrocarbons and oleic acid. Nanoparticles obtained by mechanical milling methods usually have various shapes, ranging from uniaxial to flaky or lamellar. As-obtained powder size depends on synthesis conditions and ranges from 1 to 100 nm.

Mechanochemical method is one of the means to grind materials and involves increase in the physical interaction between mixtures of various components, as well as *mechanochemical reactions* likely initiated or accelerated by mechanical interactions due to the deformation and destruction of the grinding material. Thus, in the solid phase, chemical reactions might occur in solutions and melts at high temperatures. The flow of mechanochemical reaction depends on the dispersity of initial substances, their characteristics, and conditions of grinding. The effect of deformation on material properties can be characterized by *mechanical activation*, referred to mechanical processes, during which reaction ability of solid material will increase.

1.3.2 Intensive Plastic Deformation Methods for Nanomaterial Synthesis

In order to form nanostructures in bulk materials, special mechanical schemes for deformation are applied. They allow significant distortions in samples at relatively low temperatures. Intensive plastic deformation methods include the following:

a) Torsion under high pressure
b) Equal-channel angular pressing
c) Comprehensive forging method
d) Equal-channel angular extraction
e) Hourglass method
f) Intensive sliding friction method.

Among these, torsion under high pressure and equal-channel angular pressing are mostly applied. There are several requirements to form nanostructures in bulk materials by using of plastic deformation:

- The final result of the aforementioned methods is the formation of nanostructures with large angular borders of grains.
- These methods should form homogenous nanostructures within the whole volume of material.
- The material obtained should not have any mechanical damages and destructions.

For the implementation of deformation by *torsion under high pressure*, initial substances should have disk-like shapes. The initial material is inserted between punches and pressed under pressure of several gigapascal (Figure 1.4).

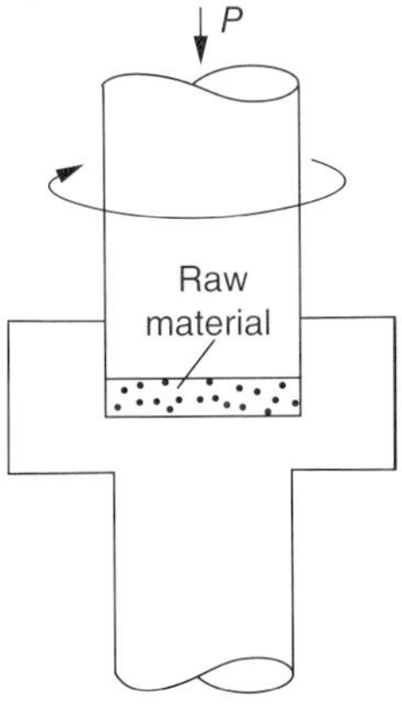

Figure 1.4 Schematic illustration of deformation by torsion method under high pressure (reproduced with permission of BKL Publishers).

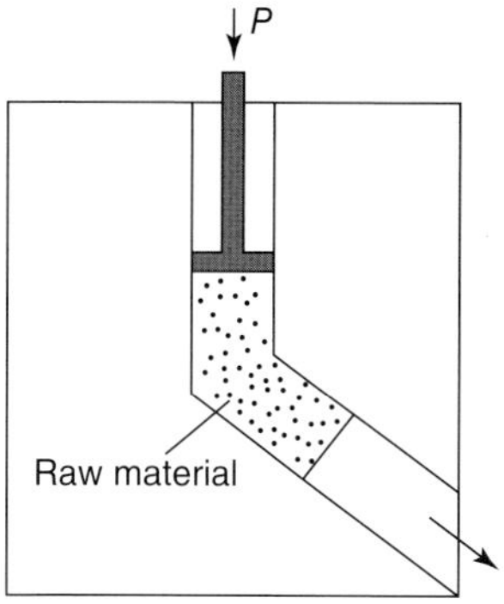

Figure 1.5 Principle of equal-channel angular pressing method for nanomaterial preparation (reproduced with permission of BKL Publishers).

Only the upper punch will be rotated, deforming the main volume of material by friction force. Hydrostatical compression and applied pressure lead to nondestruction of the sample by deformation. The process occurs at room temperature, as well as at temperatures up to $0.4T_{melt}$. The obtained samples by intensive plastic deformation have disk-like shapes, with sizes of 10–20 mm and thickness of 0.2–0.5 mm; significant grindings of sample structure can be observed right after the deformation at half turnover, but for the preparation of homogenous nanostructure, deformation at multiple turnovers is required.

Raw materials for *equal-channel angular pressing* are samples with round or square transverse section and a diameter of 20 mm; for example, the maximum diameters of raw materials treated through this method are 40 mm for Ti, 90 mm for Al, and 150 mm for Mo. The length of raw materials was 70–100 mm. To obtain the necessary level of deformation, the sample was repeatedly pressed inside a special equipment through two channels with similar transverse section, crossing at an angle of 90° (although this angle might be larger (Figure 1.5)). The quantity of passages depend on the nature of deformation material. For example, Cu tolerates sixteen passages, while the Al–Cu–Mg alloy is destroyed after three passages.

The transformation speed of the sample during pressing depends on temperature, with the average being 60 mm min^{-1}, that is, one passage being finished in 10 seconds.

There are several routes for deformation such as (Figure 1.6):

- Orientation of raw material does not change (route A).
- After each passage, the raw material turns around its cross-sectional axis to 90° direction (route B).
- After each passage, the raw material turns around its cross-sectional axis to 180° direction (route C).

The direction of shift during repeatable passages through the crossing channels for the raw material changes according to the aforementioned routes, leading to the formation of various structures in the raw material.

Comprehensive forging is another way of nanostructure formation in bulk samples and is based on the use of multiple (up to 20 times) repetitions of free forging (Figure 1.7). By starting the treatment at high temperatures $(0.3–0.6)T_{melt}$ through this technique, it is possible to obtain a nanostructured condition for

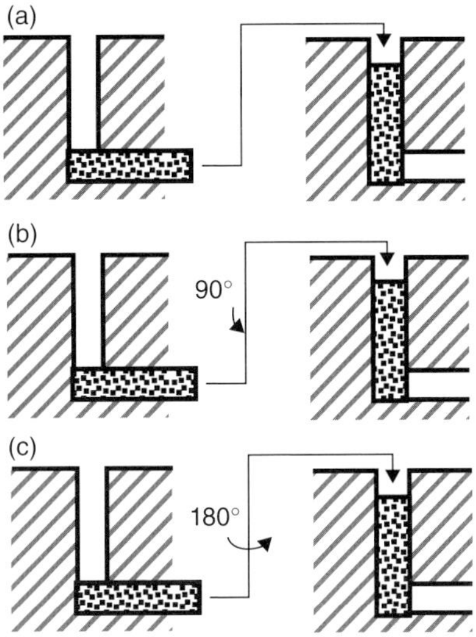

Figure 1.6 Routes for raw material orientation during equal-channel angular pressing: (a) orientation of raw material does not change during all passages; (b) the raw material turns to 90° after each passage; (c) the raw material turns to 180° after each passage (reproduced with permission of BKL Publishers).

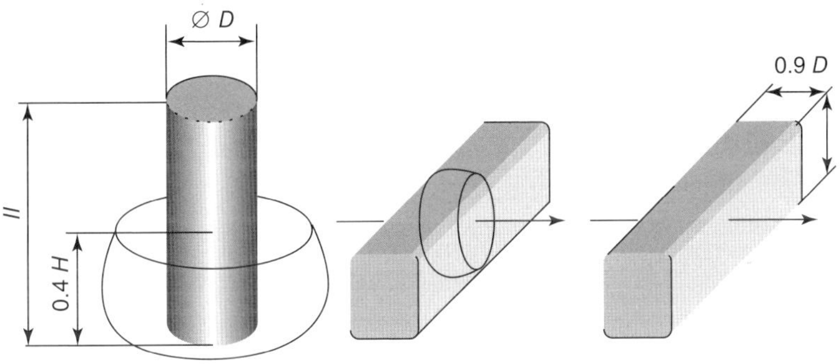

Figure 1.7 Scheme for comprehensive forging method (reproduced with permission of BKL Publishers).

fragile materials. By increasing the deformation percentage, the temperature can possibly decrease.

Intensive plastic deformation methods exhibit a number of certain advantages:

- The possibility for obtaining of bulk materials, and also nanostructures with complex profiles, at a single stage
- The possibility for the formation of continuous process based on equal-channel angular pressing.

Below are some goals, which can be achieved by the improvement of technology:

- Small size of product
- Nonhomogenous microstructure of the final product
- Complicated and expensive technical equipment.

1.3.3 Obtaining of Nanomaterials by Mechanical Interaction of Various Mediums

Recently developed methods are hydrodynamic cavitation, vibration, shock wave, grinding by ultrasound, and detonation synthesis.

Hydrodynamic cavitation aims to synthesize suspensions of nanopowders in various dispersion mediums. *Cavitation* comes from the word *cavitas,* which means hollow, and hence is defined as the formation of hollows (cavitation bubbles or caverns) in liquids filled with gas, steam, or gas–steam mixture. Cavitation results from a decrease in the local pressure of liquid, which might happen due to the increase of its velocity (hydrodynamic cavitation) or due to the passing of most intensive acoustic waves during the intensity subperiod (acoustical cavitation). During the transfer to the large flow region with high pressure or during subperiodical pressing, cavitation bubble slams, thus emitting a shock wave. The destruction caused by cavitation impact is also used in the grinding of nanomaterials by ultrasound.

Vibrational method is based on the synthesis of nanomaterials by resonance. This allows minimal energy use and high level of homogenization in multiphase mediums. The procedure is based on definite vibrational interaction of the dispersing reagent vessel. *Shock wave* in mechanical interaction can be used to obtain nanomediums. Nanodiamond powders with an average particle size of 4 nm are synthesized by shock wave treatment of graphite and metal mixture under a pressure several tenths of gigapascal and for an interaction period of 10–20 μs. Also, the shock wave treatment is used for grinding of porous structures. Investigations done on the ZrO_2–Y_2O_3 system showed that shock wave completely grinds initial dimensional compounds into fragments with size not less than 100 nm and with a particle size of 10 nm. Diamond particles are also obtained by using the *detonation synthesis* method. In this method, explosion energy is used to reach pressures up to hundreds of atmosphere and temperatures up to several thousands of degrees. These conditions are suitable in the thermodynamical stability region for diamond phase. In order to achieve a significant production of diamond powder, a mixture of trinitrotoluol and hexane (with mass ratio of 50 : 50 or 60 : 40) is used under a pressure of 15 GPa in detonation wave and a temperature of 3000 K. The detonation synthesis is carried out inside a special chamber, with a capacity of 10 g to several kilograms of initial reaction mixture. To prevent the reduction of diamond powder and its transformation into graphite, reaction chambers are filled with inert carbon dioxide gas. Synthesis lasts for 0.2–0.5 μs. In order to remove the carbon soot and other contaminants after synthesis, condensed product is treated with hot acids and then dried after multiple washings. The productivity of diamond powder is 8–9% of the total initial reaction mixture mass. The amount of main synthesizing product has a particle size of 4–5 nm. Explosive compounds containing carbon have an important role during the synthesis procedure. Carbon exists in the form of several complex morphologies: nanotubes, funnels, hollow spherical particles, and plates. Also, synthesis products plaques by carbon layer with a thickness of 10–20 nm. Mechanical interaction methods have the following advantages:

- High productivity
- Possibility for waste utilization
- Possibility for formation of protective layers during dispersion.

However, the following disadvantages are present:

- Contamination of product by material of reaction medium
- Necessity of a special complex equipment.

1.3.4 Physical Dispersion Methods for Nanomaterials Preparation

This group of methods includes spraying, evaporation–condensation processes, vacuum-sublimation technology, and solid state transformation methods.

Solid spraying method is one of the common methods for spraying of melt flow by liquid or gas (Figure 1.8). In this complex physical process, aerodynamical forces play a main role, determined by the relative speed of transferring dispersive material and its density. The mechanism of liquid stream dispersion is determined by a step-by-step splitting of more disperse particles into primary drops and then into secondary drops.

In contrast to gas dispersion, *liquid spraying* method is characterized by a high-density medium, which influences the kinetic energy of the liquid stream. The high density of the separating liquid provides high-speed preservation at significantly large distances from the nozzle section, which allows relative position of stream and makes construction of streaming equipment easier. One of the possible schemes for the dispersion of metal alloy melt is presented in Figure 1.9.

Taking out of the working liquid happens through holes in the circular disk, which rotates at a high speed. For example, to obtain nanomaterials with a particle size less than 100 nm, the jet undergoes cold gas spraying to cool the sedimentation surface. The particle size can be influenced by the working pressure of the separating jet: the larger the pressure, the smaller the particle size of the dispersing material. Also, particle size distribution and powder particle morphology can be affected by melt temperature during spraying and the square jet cross section. It is possible to obtain powder with a particle size of 50–100 nm. The shape of

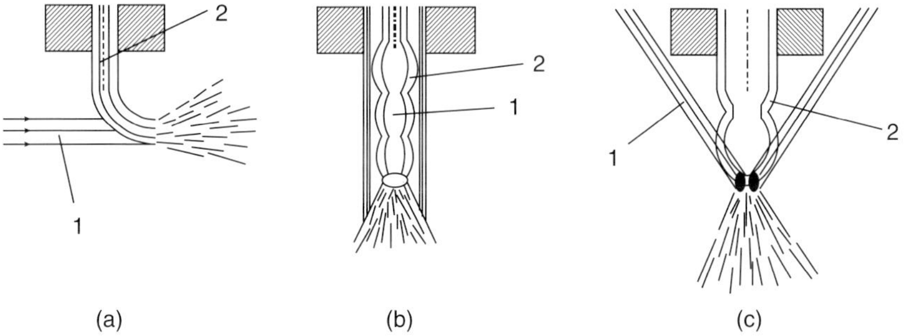

Figure 1.8 Scheme of jet melt spraying method: (a) gas flow, directed perpendicular to the melt jet; (b) spraying by subaxial gas flow; (c) gas flow, directed under the angle to melt jet. 1 – breaking gas flow; 2 – dispersing melt flow (reproduced with permission of BKL Publishers).

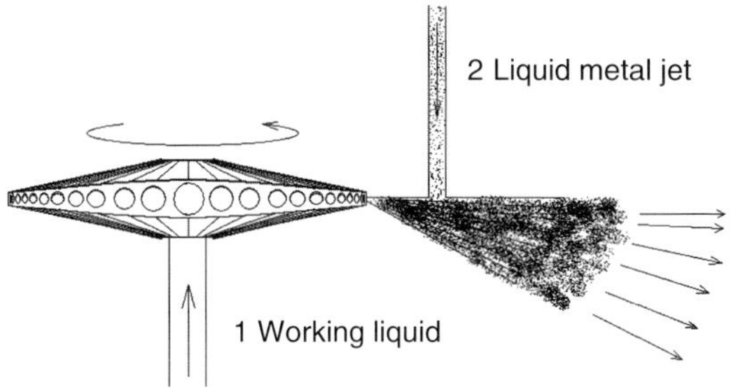

Figure 1.9 Spraying method of metal melt by liquid jet.

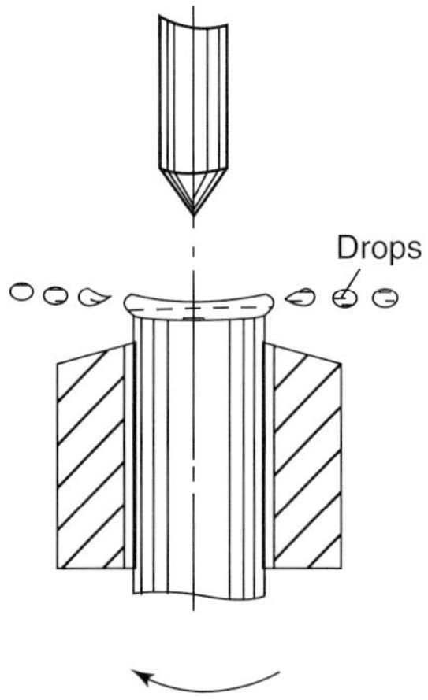

Figure 1.10 Scheme of centrifugal spraying method under centrifugal force or rotating method (reproduced with permission of BKL Publishers).

spraying material is usually drop-like or spherical. However, during high-speed cooling, the formation of particles with an inappropriate shape is possible.

During *centrifugal spraying* method, nanopowder is obtained through melt material spraying in nonoxidative atmosphere by centrifugal force. During melting in the electric arc furnace or in the low-temperature plasma, the electrode (Figure 1.10) rotates at high speed.

From the surface of being melted and fast rotating electrode end, liquid drops are separated and converted into dispersive powder during solidification. The main advantage of this process under centrifugal force is the possibility for dispersion in inert gas or vacuum. By regulating the atmosphere inside the furnace, it is possible to disperse refractory metals and metals with affinity to oxygen. The particle size obtained by using this method is about 100 nm.

Spinning is a method for nanomaterial formation by hardening the liquid phase. This method is based on obtaining thin tapes at fast cooling stage, with a speed not less than 10^6 K s^{-1}, and cooling the melt on the surface of a rotating cylinder.

1.3.5 Preparation of Nanomaterials by Evaporation–Condensation Method

All *evaporation–condensation* methods are based on the synthesis of nanomaterials by fast change in aggregate condition and by phase transformations: steam–solid matter or steam–liquid–solid substance. The final material evaporates by intensive heating and then is sharply cooled. Evaporation–condensation methods are classified according to the heating type of evaporating material,

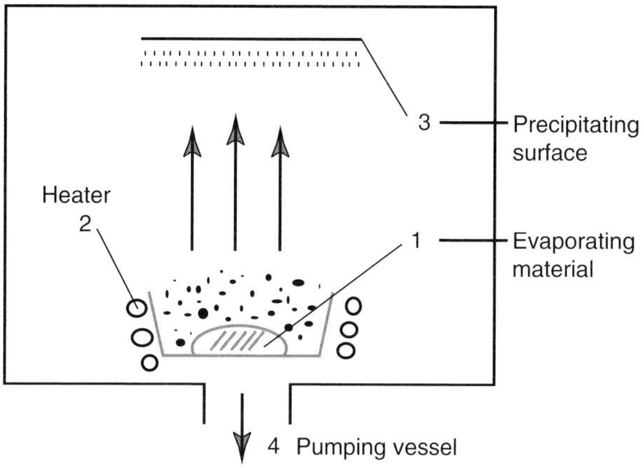

Figure 1.11 Scheme of equipment for obtaining nanopowder by evaporation–condensation method (reproduced with permission of BKL Publishers).

such as resistive, laser, plasma, electric arc, induction, ionic, and so on. In addition, evaporation–condensation process can be conducted in vacuum or neutral gas medium and can also be applied in various cooling ways. The evaporating material is usually inserted inside the crucible or vessel made from refractory, chemically inert materials, such as wolfram, tantalum, graphite, and glass carbon (Figure 1.11).

Plasma technology is widely used for metal nanoparticle preparation. Plasma can be defined in terms of partially or fully ionized gas, forming as a result of thermal ionization of atoms and molecules at high temperature. There are several types of plasma: weakly ionized or low-temperature plasma, moderately or fully ionized plasma, and high-temperature plasma. In technological processes, low-temperature plasma is usually used, obtained at a temperature of 2000–20 000 K and pressure at diapason of 10^{-5}–10^{3} MPa. For the generation of plasma, electric arc, high-frequency, and super-high-frequency high-power plasma torches, which are able to heat gas up to high temperatures, are applied. Stable and low-pressure plasma can be achieved by using an inert gas and hydrogen. Figure 1.12 shows the scheme of equipment for obtaining of nanopowders by plasma jet. Heating and evaporation of dispersing material is achieved by low-temperature plasma jet energy, followed by discharging from the plasma torch. The evaporating material is inserted into the plasma zone in the form of powder or consumable electrode (or anode). The cooling speed of the formed strongly heated gas bears importance for the dispersity, powder structure, and production process. Condensation of the dispersing material in the plasma processes is achieved using the cooling gas stream and cooling surfaces, which permits the temperature gradient to be more than 10^5 °C min^{-1}, which is suitable for refractory metal powders with a particle size of 5–100 nm. At a cooling speed of 10^5–10^8 °C s^{-1}, it is possible to obtain Al powder with a particle size of 0.5–50 nm.

Combined plasma allows an effective evaporation of the dispersing material. In this method, two kinds of plasma are used: plasma by constant electricity to heat

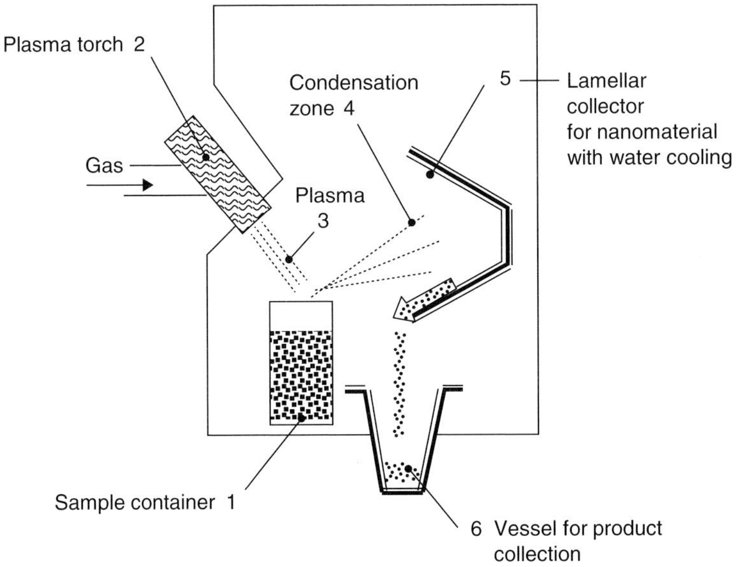

Figure 1.12 Scheme of equipment for the synthesis of nanopowders by plasma jet (reproduced with permission of BKL Publishers).

the material and high-frequency plasma, which permits melting and evaporation of final large-size powder or flakes. This method enables the acquisition of powders of most metals and metallic compounds with spherical shape and size of more than 50 nm.

Laser heating is used to avoid disadvantages associated with plasma method by keeping the working temperatures stable. Using this evaporating technology, nanopowders of Ti, Ni, Mo, Fe, and Al with an average particle size of several nanometers can be obtained. *Laser,* determined as an optical quantum generator, is a source of optical coherent radiation, characterized by high focus and large energy thickness. Laser types include gas, liquid, and solid.

Electric arc melting is one of the effective ways for metal nanopowder synthesis. Figure 1.13 shows the scheme of reactor with electric arc plasma torch and direct current.

Electric detonation of semiconductors is considered as an evaporation–condensation method wherein thin metal wires with diameters of 0.1–1 mm are inserted into the camera, where high electricity is applied (Figure 1.14).

As mentioned previously, evaporation–condensation methods depend on the working medium and cooling.

Conducting the synthesis process in vacuum is effective for obtaining powders with special properties and a large number of heavy and refractory materials. Through this method, Ni, Al, Zn, Pb, Mn, Fe, and Co with a particle size of 50–100 nm can be obtained.

Condensation of steam in the inert gas is usually maintained at $10–10^2$ Pa. Inert gases such as He, Ar, Xe, or N_2 are used. The size of as-obtained particles is 10–100 nm.

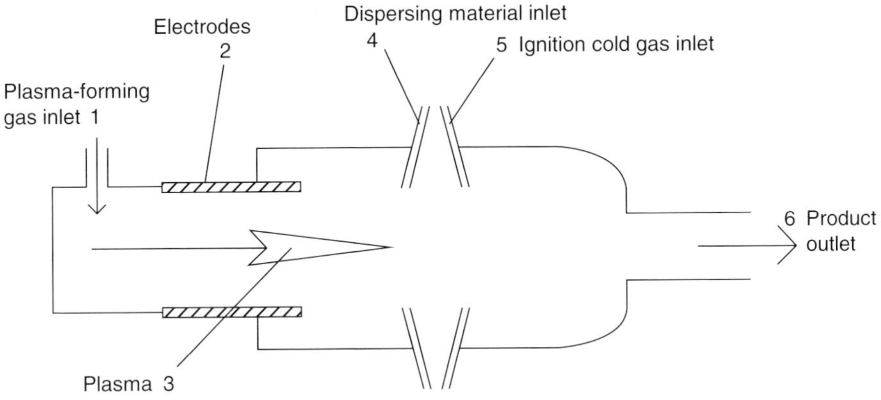

Figure 1.13 Scheme of reactor with direct current electric arc plasma torch (reproduced with permission of BKL Publishers).

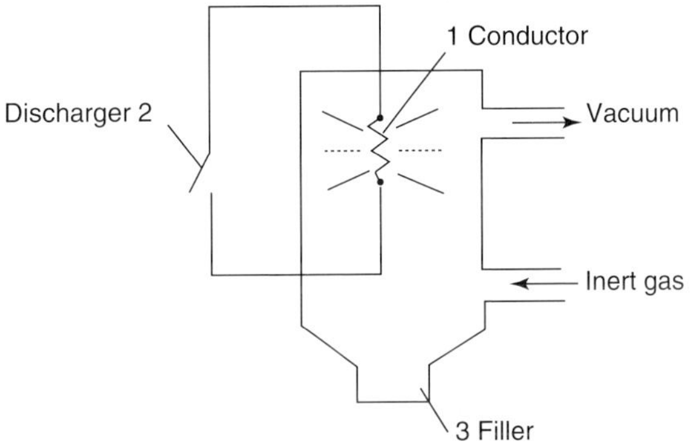

Figure 1.14 Principal scheme of equipment for obtaining nanopowder by semiconductor detonation method (reproduced with permission of BKL Publishers).

1.3.6 Obtaining of Nanomaterials by Vacuum-Sublimation Technology

The change in the aggregate state of material sublimation underlies the physical methods for obtaining of nanomaterials.

Vacuum-sublimation technology is a process of obtaining nanomaterials that involve three basic stages. In the first stage, an initial mixture of processed materials is prepared. The second stage is called solution freezing, aims to fix the uniform dimensional distribution of components in the liquid to achieve crystallite sizes as small as possible in the solid phase. During the third stage, crystallites are removed from the freeze solution by sublimation. After completion of these three stages, a porous material is obtained, which consists of crystallites of solvent particles. *Evaporative freezing* (or self-freezing) of solution is realized by intensive evaporation of solvent in vacuum. Figure 1.15 shows the principal scheme for obtaining of nanomaterials using this method. The working pressure is 0.05 mmHg and the temperature is not higher than 40 °C. In this case, liquid jet disperses into drops, which undergoes freezing during flight. The formed cryogranules fill the volume of the entire heater, in which sublimation from solvent will take place. As a result, a spherical mass-like product consisting of dissolved substances will form.

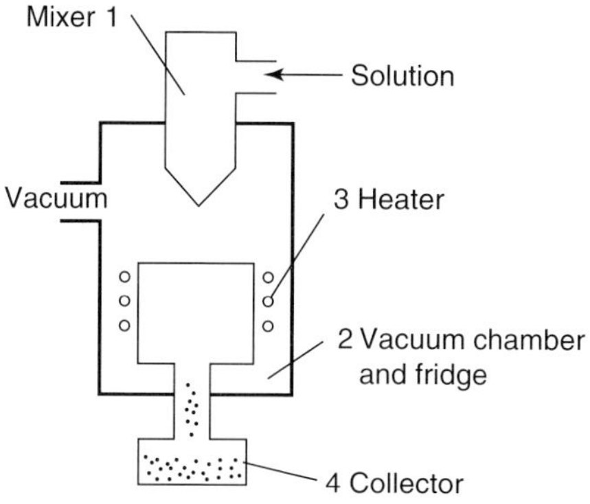

Figure 1.15 Scheme of equipment for obtaining nanopowders by vacuum-sublimation technology (reproduced with permission of BKL Publishers).

Using the vacuum-sublimation technology, a wide range of nanomaterials can be produced, including ferrites, oxides, nitrides, carbides, and high-temperature and high-superconductivity compounds. Advantages of vacuum-sublimation technology are:

- Granularity of product, which allows its transportation with minimal dusting and ability to be kept for a long time without significant property changes
- Low dusting, which increases safe synthesis of nanomaterials
- Good background for organization of continuous production.

However, the following disadvantages still exist:

- Limitation on solubility, which narrows the number of obtained products
- Necessity of special equipment for conducting the sublimation process.

1.3.7 Obtaining of Nanomaterials by Using Solid Phase Transformations

There are a number of methods for nanomaterial acquisition, in which the dispersing process is carried out in the solid material without a change in its aggregate state. *Controlled crystallization from amorphous state* is one of the ways for obtaining the bulk material. The method is based on obtaining amorphous material, with hardening from liquid state and then crystallization in controlled heating conditions. Through this method, it is possible to obtain the following nanomaterials (various transition metal and nonmetal alloys) prone to amorphization: Fe–B, Fe–Si, Fe–Si–B, Fe–Cr–B, Fe–Mo–Si–B, Fe–Mo–Si–B, Ti–Ni–Si, Ni–P, Fe–Cu–Nb–B, Se–Fe–Zr, and Al–Cr–Ce–Co. The sizes of the obtained crystallites depend on the nature of materials and the type of thermal treatment. In thermal annealing, the grain size of Se crystallites with hexagonal modification varies from 13 to 70 nm, and the size of Fe–Mo–Si–B alloy is from 15 to 200 nm.

1.3.8 Chemical Dispersion Methods for Nanomaterial Preparation

Methods for the synthesis of nanomediums by chemical reactions are very diverse but can be grouped into three: the first group includes methods in which dispersing occurs during the chemical reaction. The second group includes methods based on the different variants of electrochemical reactions. The third group includes methods that combine chemical and physical transformations.

1.3.9 Obtaining of Nanomaterials by Using Chemical Reactions

Precipitation method is widely used and is based on the sedimentation of metals from their salt solutions using precipitators. Base solutions such as NH_4OH, NaOH, KOH, and so on are used. In general, the process is as follows:

$$Me_x(A)_y + K(OH) \rightarrow Me_x(OH)_y + KA$$

where A denotes anions: NO^{3-}, Cl^-, $SO_4{}^{2-}$; *K* is for cations: and Na^+, $NH_4{}^+$, K^+; *x*, and *y* are coefficients.

By regulating the pH and temperature of the solution, it is possible to produce optimal sedimentation conditions to obtain nanomaterials. Under these conditions, high-speed crystallization and highly dispersive hydroxide can be achieved. The produced precipitate goes through washing, drying, annealing, and, when needed, reduction. Metal nanoparticles obtained through this method have a particle size range from 10 to 150 nm. By varying the process parameters, it is possible to alter the shapes of particles, including spherical, needle-like, lamellar, and other shapes.

Coprecipitating is used for the synthesis of complex metal hydroxide compounds. In this case, in a reaction vessel, precipitant–metal–salt mixture is supplied. Under constant mixing and heating conditions, the following reaction occurs:

$$Me'_a(A)_b + Me''_c(A)_d + K(OH) \rightarrow (Me', Me'')_x(OH)_y + KA$$

where A are anions; Me′ and Me″ are various metal cations and bases, respectively; and *a, b, c,* and *d* are coefficients. Then, analogous to the precipitation method, the obtained powder is thoroughly washed to separate dissolved anions, is dried, and then undergoes thermal decomposition or reduction. The given method allows to obtain complex oxygen-containing compounds with specified ratio of cations, which leads to an increased solubility of metals in each other. Emulsion precipitation is an example of this method, occurring in non-mixing solvents. Through this way, it is possible to obtain nanoparticles covered with shell or layer of organic molecules. For example, for the synthesis of α-Fe_2O_3 with shell, a water solution of $FeCl_2$ at a concentration of 0.01 mol l^{-1} and sodium dodecylbenzol sulfonate and benzene are used. Emulsion is obtained after intensive mixing of liquids. For the precipitation of Fe compounds in organic mediums, NaOH is added. The average particle size of α-Fe_2O_3 covered with shell from organic molecules is 2.1 nm, as observed using transmission electron microscope (TEM). Through precipitation and coprecipitation, oxide, metal, and metalloxide powders and composites and ferrites and salts (e.g., $BaTiO_3$) with various particle shapes, chemical and physical compositions, dispersities, and size distributions in nanostate can be obtained. Additionally, materials synthesized using this method are characterized by chemical homogeneity and reaction ability.

Obtaining of nanomaterials through *heterophase interaction method* is based on the replacement of solid phase cations or anions by ions of the surrounding medium. This method is used to obtain composite particles, in particular, nanoparticles comprising one material and covered by a layer of another material. For example, CdS nanoparticles covered by PbS layer can be obtained by replacing the Cd ions with Pb ions. For this purpose, CdS nanoparticles stabilized by polyvinylpyrrolidone are placed in a solution containing Pb^{2+} cations. Depending on the concentration of Pb^{2+} and the length of time of interaction, it is possible to replace one part or all Cd with Pb. For CdS nanoparticles with a size of 6 nm, the time of full transformation to PbS can be over 2 h. This method also allows to obtain a variety of metallic powders with a particle size of 10–100 nm when solid salt interacts with base solution. For example, the particle size of as-obtained Ni nanopowder is 20 nm. The shape of final metal nanoparticles is determined by crystal morphology of initial solid salts.

Initially, *sol–gel method* was developed for obtaining of Fe powder. The method is based on the precipitation of metallic compounds from water solutions in the form of gel and their further reduction. As practically shown, chemical purification of product will occur in the process. For example, the composition of Fe in the final powder is 98.5–99.5%. As initial substances, Fe salts are used, as well as metallurgical industry waste: metal scrap or waste pickle liquor. The use of secondary raw materials provides the opportunity for pure and relatively cheap Fe nanopowder. Other materials in nanostate, such as oxide ceramics, alloys, and metal salts, can be obtained also. In the sol–gel method, sol is obtained first, followed by gel after drying, which can be used in obtaining of films and monolithic materials.

Solvent evaporation is important in the precipitation process, which is complicated by long-term stages. *Cryogenic technology* is one of the ways for solvent evaporation, in which a solvent with necessary composition is prepared and sprayed inside a camera under cryogenic conditions and fast freezing, for example, liquid nitrogen. On the next stage, the pressure of gaseous medium will decrease below the triple point value of dispersion system equilibrium, and the temperature will increase for solvent sublimation. As a result, product consisting of thin porous granules will be obtained. By annealing of granules in the air, it is possible to obtain oxides; by reduction, it is possible to achieve metal powders, for example, Cu, W, and their salts; by selective reduction, oxide mixtures and metals, such as $Cu–ThO_2$.

Sublimated drying is based on spraying a metal saltwater solution in organic liquid at low temperature. In this process, immediate freezing will occur and then water from the precipitate under low-temperature and low-pressure conditions will evaporate. The final product will be obtained after thermal decomposition. For example, Li-doped Ni nanooxide used in the fuel cells can be obtained through this method.

In *evaporative thermal decomposition* method, a metal solution is sprayed into the surrounding atmosphere heated at high temperature. Evaporation of solution and thermal decomposition of metal salts occur as a result. Using heat generated during burning, alcohols are used as solvents. This method allows one-stage acquisition of ferrite nanopowders, which is further used for the production of high-quality ceramics.

In *reduction methods,* nanomaterials, particularly, metals, are obtained by reducing them from initial oxygen-containing compounds. The reduction process can also be the final step in obtaining metal nanopowders by other methods.

Reduction of metal oxides and other solid compounds is a cheap and popular method for obtaining of nanomaterials by using of hydrogen, carbon monoxide, natural gas, solid reductants – carbon, (coke, soot), metals (sodium, potassium), and metal hydroxides. The final products include oxides, hydroxides, other chemical metal compounds, mine, and concentrates after preparation (enrichment, removal of impurities), waste and impurity materials after metallurgy manufacturing. The size and shape of synthesizing powder depends on the composition and properties of the initial and reductant materials, as well as on the reaction temperature and reaction time.

Upon the *interaction between metal oxides and gases* (H_2, CO) and carbon, the following metals can be obtained: Fe, W, Ni, Re, Mo, Cu, and Co. This process is expressed by the following chemical equations:

$$MeO + H_2 \rightarrow Me + H_2O$$

$$MeO + CO \rightarrow Me + CO_2$$

$$MeO + C \rightarrow Me + CO$$

By using of hydrides as reductants, it is possible to obtain Zr, Ta, Hf, Cr, Nb, and B nanopowders. In this case, chemical reaction will flow as follows:

$$MeO + CaH_2 = Me + CaO + H_2$$

where MeO is a metal oxide. To obtain high-purity nanomaterials, the use of reagents containing fewer impurities is a necessity, since the purity of the final products depend on the purity of the initial substance and the reductant.

Metallothermic method is used for Pt, Ag, Cu, Zn, Co, Ni, Fe, Mo, and Cr nanopowders. Reduction process is conducted in the presence of naphthalene in anhydrous medium:

$$Me'_a(A)_b + Me'' = Me''_c(A)_d + Me'$$

The average particle size of as-obtained particles in Au, Ag, and Pt is 10 nm, and for other metals, it is about 30 nm. Particle size distribution is narrow. Obtained powders are pyrophoric and thus require specific conditions to keep them. Metal ions are reduced in water solutions and salts by reductants such as H_2, CO, hydrazine, hypophosphate, and formaldehyde. In the case of gaseous hydrogen or carbon monoxide used as reductants, the process is conducted at high temperatures (about 200 °C) and high pressures (more than 5 MPa) in autoclaves. In this case, the initial raw materials are sulfuric acid and ammonia solutions of metal salts. Using this method, Cu, Ni, Co, Ag, and their composites were obtained. Synthesis of metal nanopowders from their salt solutions is possible using strong reductants such as hydrazine, hypophosphite, formaldehyde, and so on. In this method, nanopowders of Fe, Ni, Co, Cu, and their composites with spherical particles and size not less than 5 nm were obtained.

Obtaining of nanoparticles on carriers is one of the important ways aimed for decreasing the reaction ability of material. As for carriers, activated carbon is fed into metal salt solutions. Advantages of reduction method for the synthesis of nanomaterials depend on the following:

- Obtaining of alloy powders with component composition from 0% to 100%,
- Obtaining of homogeneous product (solid solution and chemical compound) as well as heterogonous system,
- Using cheap raw material for economy purpose.

However, disadvantages of this method are existing, such as:

- Limitations based on metal activity against various reductants,
- Pollution of nanomaterials by reductants.

Gas phase chemical reaction method is based on the synthesis of nanomaterials during chemical interaction, taking place in the atmospheric steam of volatile compounds. It is possible to divide all gas phase chemical reactions into decomposition reaction, occurring by participation of one of the initial chemical compounds ($A = B + C$), and the reaction between two or more chemical compounds ($A + B = C + D$). A mandatory condition for the use of the first type of gas phase chemical reaction is the existence of suitable chemical compound containing all the elements of final product, which is a rare case. The second type of gas phase chemical reaction is a common case. For conducting the gas phase reaction, initial substances should be volatile. As initial compounds, halogenides are used, especially metal chlorides, MO_nCl_m, metal steams, and so on. Equipment used for conducting the gas phase reaction is shown in Figure 1.16.

Pipes I and II are used for inserting of gas into the reaction vessel. Furnace 1 allows the heating of the reaction zone. An additional furnace 2 is used for heating of an substance 3; when needed, the evaporation occurs directly inside the reaction vessel (Figure 1.16). Reaction products in gas phase will enter vessel 4, where they undergo cooling and condensation. As a rule, reaction vessel is made of quartz, ceramic material, or clay. The main problem with this method is the

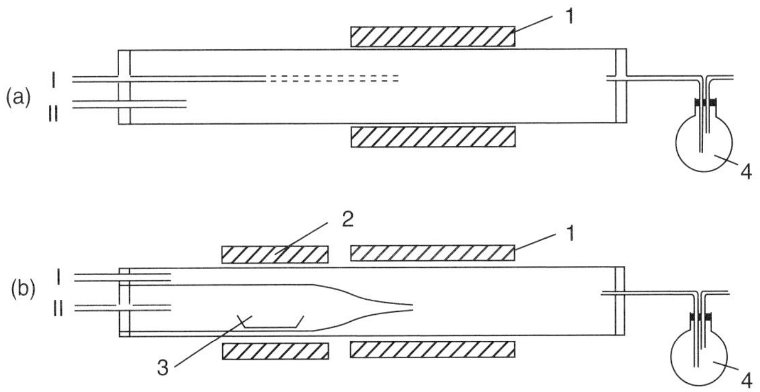

Figure 1.16 Scheme for obtaining nanopowders by outer heating of reaction zone: (a) inlet of initial gaseous substances; (b) use of initial solid substances. Number labels are explained in the text (reproduced with permission of BKL Publishers).

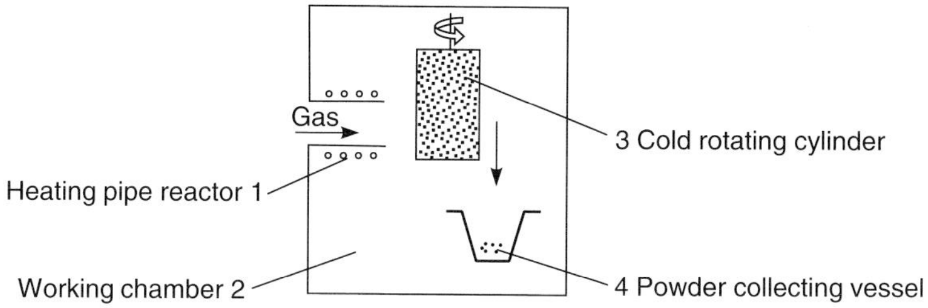

Figure 1.17 Scheme for obtaining nanopowders by gas phase chemical reactions (reproduced with permission of BKL Publishers).

separation of nanoparticles from the gas phase. For particles with nanosize and low gas flow concentration, the gas temperature is significantly high.

For trapping of nanoparticles, special filters, such as ceramic filters and electrofilters, as well as cyclones with liquid films, special gas centrifuges, and cold rotating barrel for gravitational precipitation, are used (Figure 1.17).

Advantages of gas phase reactions are:

- Possibility for synthesis of unique compounds
- Narrow size distribution of particles
- High purity of product

This method requires a special equipment, which is a disadvantage.

Thermal dissociation or pyrolysis is used for preparation of nanopowders of various compounds, as well as individual materials. As for initial substances, salts of low-molecular-weight organic acids, including metal formates, metal oxalates, metal acetates, metal carbonates, and carbonyls, are used. Dissociation is carried out at temperature intervals of 200–400 °C. Decomposition can be initiated by several methods. Heat energy is often used, as well as high-quality radiation, laser radiation, ionizing radiation, plasma flow, electron flow, and heat generation during friction.

Formiate pyrolysis can be expressed by the following equations:

$$(HCOO)_2Me \rightarrow MeO + H_2 + CO + CO_2 + H_2O + Me$$

Metal oxide reduction by CO and H_2 gases, generated during pyrolysis, is considered as secondary reduction reaction in this case. According to the above equation, decomposition of Cu and Zn formiates will occur. In the case of Mn, Fe, Co, Ni, Zn, and Ca preparations, in the first stage, decomposition of formiates will occur as:

$$(HCOO)_2Me \rightarrow Me + H_2 + 2CO_2$$

Decomposition of Mn, Fe, and Cu metal oxalates is expressed as:

$$MeC_2O_4 \rightarrow MeO + CO + CO_2$$

Co, Ni, Cu, and Zn oxalates are dissociated, as in the following equation:

$$MeC_2O_4 \rightarrow MeO + 2CO_2$$

Through pyrolysis of metal formates, oxalates, and other metal salts, powders with a particle size of 100 nm can be obtained. Thermal decomposition of carbonyls occurs as follows:

$$Me_x(CO)_y \xrightarrow{t} xMe + yCO$$

There is a possibility for obtaining Ni, Mo, Fe, Cr, and W nanopowders by this reaction. Also, carbonyl dissociation method is used to obtain polymetallic films with nanostructures. Reaction is conducted at a temperature of 500 °C; crystallite size in films is 20 nm.

Methods for obtaining of nanomaterials based on the oxidation of initial substances have been developed recently. To obtain the carbon soot–amorphous carbon, low-temperature burning method of hydrocarbons was developed. The process is carried out inside the double section reactor. Inside the first section, where the temperature is 423–773 K, preliminary heating occurs. In the second section, at a temperature of 1073–1173 K, flaming and controlled heating occurs, with the formation of soot, which has a particle size of 100 nm.

Precipitation from the metal alloy is based on the oxidation of metals or alloys by gases. For example, during the passage of an air after the completion of the precipitation process, material with metal and metal oxide particles.

Metal salt hydrolysis is used to obtain colloidal particles, in particular, nanooxides of Ti, Zr, Ir, and Al, by hydrolysis of appropriate chlorides, hypochlorites, and sulfates. In order to avoid nanoparticle coagulation, for stabilization of colloidal solutions, polyphosphates, amines, and hydroxyl ions are used. For example, Si alcooxide hydrolysis gives an opportunity for SiO_2 synthesis, which has less number of soluble salts and does not contain cations of alkali metals. Also, alcooxides are well dissolved in alcohols (ethanol); they are easily obtained by mixing of metals with alcohols.

1.3.10 Preparation of Nanomaterials by Electrochemical Methods

The use of electricity allows conducting processes that are not possible under usual conditions.

Electric precipitation method is based on the passage of direct current electricity through saltwater solutions during the precipitation process. Procedure of electric precipitation can be expressed as follows: cathode and anode as a rule have a film shape and are submerged into specially chosen electrolyte solution. To provide a product with purity, as anode, the same metal as precipitating metal should be used. But this condition is not always possible. For this reason, during the production of Cu powder, alumina anode is used, and for the production of Fe powder, Mo or Cr–Ni alloy anode is used. By this method, it is possible to obtain about 30 metals. Refining occurs in this process, which allows achieving materials with high purity. Metals precipitating on cathode, depending on the process conditions, can be obtained in the form of easily crushable powders, pores, or dendrites.

Electroflotation is a method for obtaining disperse powder based on crystallization of metals in double-layer bath with the presence of surfactants in the organic medium. Obtained dispersive powder has needle- and rod-like shapes (Fe, Co) and is applied in the production of magnets and magnetic varnishes.

Salt melt electrolysis is a process carried out at high temperatures. As for electrolytes, metal salts are used. By this method, it is possible to obtain metal powders of Fe, Ni, Cr, Ag, Th, Nb, Ti, Zr, and Be.

Obtaining nanopowders is also possible by using the *liquid metal cathode*. In this case, liquid metal such as mercury is used as a cathode, in which metal powder is precipitating. The process is carried out in inorganic acid solution. By this method, Fe, Co, Zr, or Fe–Co alloys can be obtained. Particle shape is usually dendritic (10–20 nm). Obtained powders are mainly used for magnets.

Electrochemical synthesis method is based on obtaining chemical compounds inside liquid baths by passage of electric current. Reaction occurs at high temperatures, which allows the synthesis of high-temperature phase materials. By changing the electric parameters in this process, it is possible to control the sizes of obtained materials.

1.3.11 Preparation of Nanomaterials by Combinations of Physical and Chemical Transformations

Dispersion in this method on one hand is directly related to physical interactions and chemical reactions. In particular, physical interactions are caused by the decomposition of metal steams by various radiations during chemical reactions.

If the *laser* is used for the reaction, the reactor should have transparent windows for the passage of beams. In the simplest way, one of the laser beams that are directed to each other will pass through the first and second reactor windows. Reaction mixture flow will cross the laser beam perpendicularly. Particle size depends on the pressure inside the reaction chamber (reactor) and on the intensity of laser beam radiation. By this method, silicon nitride is obtained, with a particle size of 10–20 nm, from the SiH_4 and NH_3 mixtures.

γ-Radiation was used for obtaining Cu and Ag powders by decomposition of heavy metal azides (MeN_n). The main advantage of this method is the acquisition of non-defect metal particles.

In the *arc-discharge method*, the anode is made of Ni, Fe, or W metal or metal compounds. Arc discharge is produced in the atmosphere of reaction gas. As an example, high-density magnetic recording carriers are synthesized by metal halogenides with hydrogen at an atmospheric pressure of 50–600. Size of obtained particles is 17–39 nm.

Chemical flame in gas mixtures is used for nanomaterial synthesis. As initial substances, fluorides, chlorides, and metal oxides are used, and the chemical flame is produced by hydrogen and fluorine, hydrocarbon, and oxygen gas mixtures. By this method, Mo, Cu, and Ni alloys and oxides are obtained. Spherical nanopowders have particle sizes of less than 100 nm.

In the *plasma method* the metal source undergoes evaporation and the steam interacts with the reaction gas that contains metal compounds, and directed to the plasma burn. Figure 1.18 presents the scheme of equipment for obtaining nanopowders in impulse plasma with condenser-type discharge.

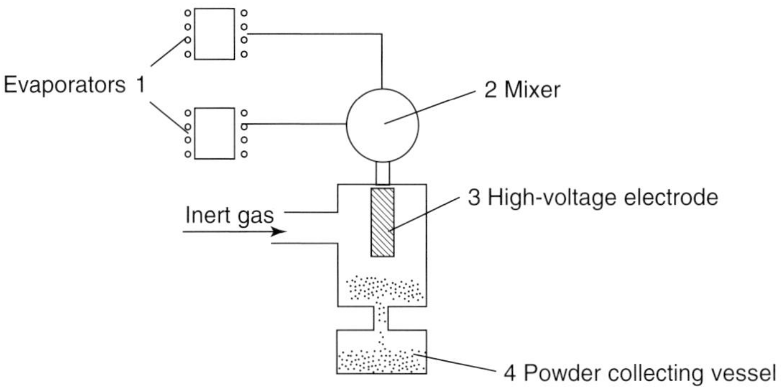

Figure 1.18 Scheme of equipment for obtaining nanopowders in impulse plasma with condenser-type discharge (reproduced with permission of BKL Publishers).

Obtaining nanopowders is also possible by *shock wave loading* of porous metals. In this method, a layer of initial powder undergoes physical loading by contact charge of detonating material. As a result, nanooxides with a particle size of 50–100 nm were produced [4].

1.4 Main Achievements in Nanotechnology

Table 1.1 shows the significant achievements in nanotechnology and Nobel Prize awards in the field of chemistry and physics.

Table 1.1 Significant achievements in the nanotechnology.

Nobel Prize in chemistry	Nobel Prize in physics
1996 Discovery of fullerenes	1986 Creation of HRTEM and TEM
1998 Development of quantum chemistry	1998 Discovery of quantum Hall effect
2000 Discovery of conductive polymers	2000 Creation of semiconductor
2008 Development of fluorescent protein	2010 Graphene research

Case Study 1: Synthesis of Nanoparticles and Environmental Safety Considerations

- Several methods exist for nanomaterial synthesis, such as physical, chemical, and biological methods. Nanomaterial synthesis requires a number of chemicals, conditions, and techniques. Each synthesis method is characterized by definite equipment, necessary laboratory glassware, and utensils for the synthesis process.
- Also, nanomaterial synthesis process is followed by structural, phase composition, and morphological characterizations and analyses of obtained nanomaterials. The person conducting X-ray diffraction analysis of synthesized nanomaterials should obey safety rules in order to not suffer from radiation.

- Synthesis and characterization analyses require knowledge and technical skills. Being informed about chemical hazards and laboratory safety rules is mandatory. Also, the conducting person should know and follow environmental safety rules without polluting or harming nature. Laboratory waste subproducts and end products should be collected and kept in preferred and appropriate places and their disposal should also be arranged.
- Working in the laboratory requires responsibility, good communication, and comprehensive skills. Working in agreement with other members of the research team is preferred, which helps eliminates undesirable conditions. Every person conducting synthesis must be responsible to keep the working space clean and well organized.
- The above problem is related to that in the article of Groso *et al.* [5] in which management of nanomaterials safety in research environment was described.

Case Study 2: Property Control of Nanomaterials by Setting Experimental Conditions during Synthesis

- A set of experimental conditions such as equipment settings (temperature, pressure, reaction time, etc.), initial chemical types, concentration, and pH allows the synthesis of nanomaterials with definite properties (shape, size distribution, phase composition, etc.).
- Subnanometer control of mean core size during mesofluidic synthesis of small ($D_{core} < 10$ nm), water-soluble, ligand-stabilized gold nanoparticles was reported by Elliott *et al.* [6] in *Langmuir*. A key advantage of this synthesis is that simply adjusting the pH of the gold salt solution led to control over the Au NP core size. The synthesis involved the reduction of an Au(III) species with sodium borohydride in the presence of a functionalized alkyl thiosulfate (Bunte salt) to yield thiolate-protected Au NPs. The average core size increased as the pH was raised for each ligand studied.
- Another study focused on the controlled synthesis and electric conduction properties of anatase TiO_2 nanoparticles via the polyol method [7]. In this work, the preparation state and particle size were controlled by varying the synthesis parameters such as the precursor concentration, hydrolysis rate, and synthesis time.

Control Questions:

1) Define the term of nano- and biomaterials.
2) List the main achievements in nanomaterial and biomaterial application history.
3) Describe the basic methods and requirements for nanomaterial preparation.
4) Discuss the mechanical dispersion method and its features in nanomaterial preparation process.

5) Define and describe the intensive plastic deformation method for nanomaterial synthesis.
6) Describe the process of obtaining nanomaterials by mechanical interaction of various mediums.
7) Which kinds of methods are included in physical dispersion methods for nanomaterial preparation?
8) Discuss evaporation–condensation method and its difference to other preparation methods of nanomaterials.
9) Describe vacuum-sublimation technology and its features for the synthesis of nanomaterials.
10) What kind of methods are available for obtaining of nanomaterials by using the chemical reactions?
11) Describe the preparation of nanomaterials by electrochemical methods and its specific difference to other methods.
12) Define electric precipitation method for the synthesis of nanomaterials and its main requirements.
13) List chemical reaction synthesis methods suitable for the preparation of metal nanomaterials.
14) Describe laser-based method for the preparation of nanomaterials.

References

1 Gentleman, E., Ball, M.D., and Stevens, M.M. *Encyclopedia of Life Support Systems*, Vol. 2: Biomaterials. Medical Sciences, p. 3, http://www.eolss.net/Sample-Chapters/C03/E6-59-13-07.pdf (accessed 30 December 2016).

2 Wong, J.Y., Bronzino, J.D., and Peterson, D.R. (2012) *Biomaterials: Principles and Practices*, CRC Press.

3 Tolochko, N.K. History of Nanotechnology, http://www.eolss.net/sample-chapters/c05/e6-152-01.pdf (2009).

4 Ryzhonkov, D.I., Levina, V.V., and Dzidziguri, E.L. (2008) *Nanomaterials, BINOM*, BKL Publishers, Moscow.

5 Groso, A. *et al* (2010) Management of nanomaterials safety in research environment. *Part. Fibre Toxicol.*, 7 (1), 40.

6 Elliott, E.W. *et al.* (2015) Subnanometer control of mean core size during mesofluidic synthesis of small (D_{core} < 10 nm) water-soluble, ligand-stabilized gold nanoparticles. *Langmuir*, **31** (43), 11886–11894.

7 Bargougui, R. *et al.* (2016) Controlled synthesis and electrical conduction properties of anatase TiO_2 nanoparticles via the polyol method. *Appl. Phys. A*, **122**, 309.

Further Reading

Huczko, A. (2000) Template-based synthesis of nanomaterials. *Appl. Phys. A*, **70** (4), 365–376.

Huebsch, N. and Mooney, D.J. (2009) Inspiration and application in the evolution of biomaterials. *Nature*, **462** (7272), 426–432.

Mackenzie, J.D. and Bescher, E.P. (2007) Chemical routes in the synthesis of nanomaterials using the Sol–Gel process. *Acc. Chem. Res.*, **40** (9), 810–818.

Song, J.Y. and Kim, B.S. (2009) Rapid biological synthesis of silver nanoparticles using plant leaf extracts. *Bioprocess. Biosyst. Eng.*, **32** (1), 79–84.

Virender, K., Sharma, R.A., and Yngard, Y.L. (2009) Silver nanoparticles: green synthesis and their antimicrobial activities. *Adv. Colloid Interface Sci.*, **145** (1–2), 83–96.

Vollath, D. (2013) *Nanomaterials: An Introduction to Synthesis, Properties and Applications*, 2nd edn, Wiley-VCH Verlag GmbH.

Williams, D. (2014) *Essential Biomaterials Science*, Part of Cambridge Texts in Biomedical Engineering, Cambridge University Press.

Yu, C.H., Tam, K., and Tsang, E.S.C. (2008) *Metallic Nanoparticles*, Handbook of Metal Physics, Elsevier, vol. **5**, pp. 113–141.

2

Classification of Nanomaterials

Translated materials from the original works of Ryzhonkov, D.I., Levina, V.V., Dzidziguri, E.L. and Glukhova, O.E. were used in this chapter.

The early bird catches the worm.

Proverb

2.1 Dispersive Systems and Their Classifications

Understanding nanomaterials classification allows us to also comprehend *dispersive systems.* Recent studies on technology of nanomaterials as dispersive systems have generated a large number of terms and definitions. Structural and morphological elements of materials having sizes ranging from 10^{-8} to 10^{-9} m are associated with terms such as nanomaterials, nanocrystals, nanoparticles, nanocomposites, nanophases, and nanosized mediums; clusters and micro clusters; small, ultrasmall, colloidal, and sub-colloidal particles; and ultra-dispersive, high dispersive, sub-microcrystal and ultrathin powders, as well as molecular aggregations, crystal clusters, metal fluids, and molecular dispersive, colloidal dispersive, and microheterogeneous systems. Furthermore, terms such as sol, gel, aerosol, and aerogel are used in colloidal chemistry. *Dispersive systems* are those systems that consist of two or more phases with high surface area interface between them. One phase of the dispersive system is distributed in another solid phase of this system in the form of small fine particles. The granulated part of this system is called dispersive phase, and the non-granulated part as dispersive medium [1].

2.1.1 Classification of Dispersive Systems According to their Aggregation States

The first classification of dispersive systems was suggested by *V. Ostwald* in 1891. According to this classification, there are nine combinations of dispersive systems and dispersive phases, whether in gaseous, liquid, and solid matter. Practically, eight of these combinations are possible, because gases in normal state are soluble in each other in non-limited amounts, thus forming the homogenous system. Table 2.1 shows classification of dispersive systems according to their

Nano- and Biomaterials: Compounds, Properties, Characterization, and Applications,
First Edition. Zhypargul Abdullaeva.

Table 2.1 Classification of dispersive systems according to their aggregation state.

	Dispersive phase		
Dispersive medium	**Gaseous**	**Liquid**	**Solid**
Gaseous	—	Aerosols, fogs, drops	Aerogels, aerosols, powders, smokes, dust
Liquid	Foams, gaseous emulsions	Emulsions, creams	Sols, gels, emulsions, pastes
Solid	Solid foams, filters, sorbents, membranes	Solid emulsions	Solid sols, alloys, composites, coatings, sheets

Source: Ryzhonkov *et al.* 2008 [1]. Reproduced with permission of BKL Publishers.

aggregation states and gives definition for some terms. Sedimentary stable sol is highly dispersed system consisting of solid dispersive phase and liquid dispersive medium. Traditionally, sols are called as *colloidal solutions*. *Colloidal systems* are high dispersive, microheterogeneous systems. Dispersive phase particles in the colloidal system usually have sizes ranging from 1 to 100 nm. In gas and liquid phases, they are freely and independently involved in the Brownian motion, filling uniformly the entire volume of the dispersive system.

Aerosols are gaseous dispersive systems containing suspensions of solid or liquid dispersive phase. *Gels* are high dispersive systems with liquid dispersive medium, containing structural framework formed by particles of the dispersive phase. Typical gels in the form of jelly precipitates are formed upon coagulation of sols during allocation of new phase from supersaturated solutions. In the case of gaseous dispersive medium, aerosols can form. *Powders* are double-phase systems containing solid particles of dispersive phase, which are distributed in air or another gaseous phase. Or, in other words, powders constitute complex of individually contacting solid substances or their agglomerates (*aggregates*), for example, friable materials with particle sizes from 0.001 to 1000 μm. Dispersive systems with particle sizes not exceeding 0.001 μm are called clusters, and those with particle sizes of 1000 μm and over called *granules*. Powders consisted of particles with sizes not larger than 1 μm, suspended in a gaseous phase, and involved in the Brownian motion form aerosols, dusts, and smokes. *Particle* is the basic unit of powder, which is impossible to separate through conventional separation methods. Particle can be consisted of several grains (Figure 2.1); therefore, the term *grain* is not synonymous with the term particle. *Agglomerate* (or aggregate) will be formed when several particles combine together. Aggregates and agglomerates are different from each other by the existence of inner porosity. In agglomerates interparticle holes are present, while in agglomerates they are absent (Figure 2.2).

2.1.2 Classification of Dispersive Systems According to Size

Initially, dispersive systems can be classified into (i) coarsely dispersed and (ii) thinly (or highly) dispersed groups (also called colloidal dispersive or colloid systems). In coarsely dispersed systems, particles have sizes from 1 μm and

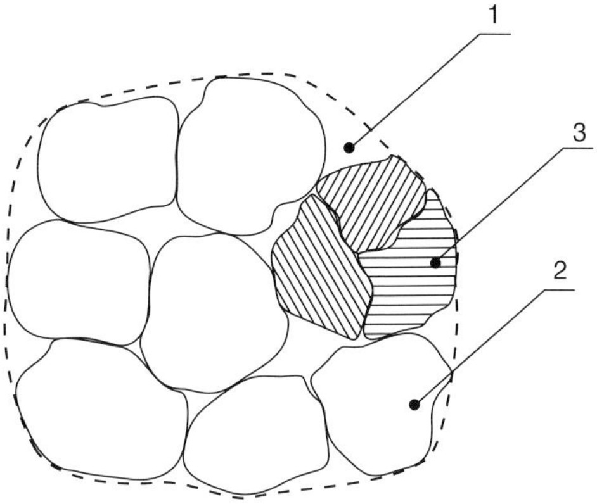

Figure 2.1 Ratio of aggregates, particles, and coherent scattering regions (CSR): 1 – aggregate; 2 – particle; 3 – coherent scattering region. (Ryzhonkov *et al.* 2008 [1]. Reproduced by permission of BKL Publishers.)

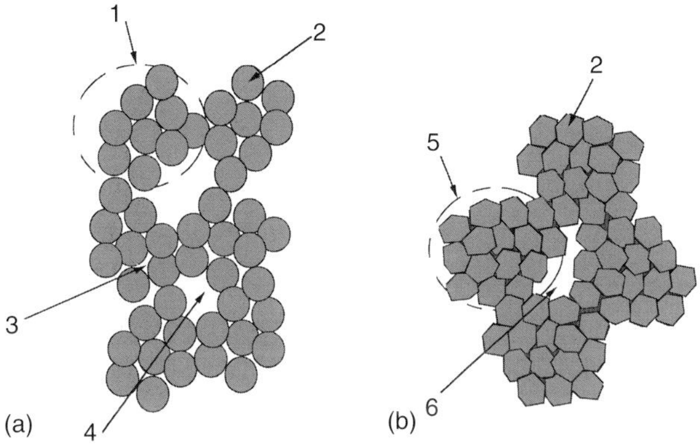

Figure 2.2 Schematic representation of (a) agglomerated and (b) aggregated powder; 1 – agglomerate, 2 – primary particle, 3 – within the agglomerate pore, 4 – between agglomerate pore, 5 – aggregate, 6 – between aggregate pore. (Ryzhonkov *et al.* 2008 [1]. Reproduced by permission of BKL Publishers.)

over and a specific surface area of 1 $m^2\ g^{-1}$, while in colloidal systems particles have sizes from 1 nm to 1 μm and a specific surface area of 100 $m^2\ g^{-1}$. At the beginning of the last century, dispersive systems were classified based on the possibility of microscopical characterizations. For this purpose, particles were of sizes less than 0.2 μm, suitable for observation by optical microscope; sizes between 0.2 and 0.02 μm, suitable for ultramicroscopic observations; and sizes from 0.02 to 0.05 μm, also called zero-dimensional, which cannot be detected by ultramicroscopy. In colloidal chemistry, dispersive systems are classified as molecular dispersive (with dispersive phase size no more than 1 nm), high dispersive (1–100 nm), middle dispersive (100 nm–10 μm), and coarse dispersive (more than 10 μm). According to this classification, middle dispersive systems are microheterogeneous, and high dispersive systems ultramicroheterogeneous. Powders used in metallurgy can be classified into ultrathin powders (particle size no more than 500 nm), very thin powders (500 nm–10 μm), thin powders (10–40 μm), medium-sized powders (40–150 μm), and coarse (or large) powders (150–500 μm). Powders produced in huge tons of mass are classified separately. For example, iron powders are divided into four groups: large (particle size is more than 450 μm), middle (160–450 μm), small (less than 160 μm), and very small (less than 56 μm). Powders synthesized by plasma are divided into following types:

- Nanosized (nanocrystal, ultra-dispersive) – 1/30 to 50 nm
- High dispersive (sub-microcrystal) – 30–50 to 100–500 nm
- Micron or large crystal – 100–500 nm to 10 μm

Up until now, there is no development of a definite physically grounded classification for dispersive systems. This class of dispersive systems is called nanopowders, nanosized mediums, and nanocrystal materials. In other words, if the particle value for morphological elements agrees with their physical parameters, changing in appropriate properties is related to nanosystems. Often, these effects appear in the dispersive system with particle size less than 10 nm (Figure 2.3). Figure 2.3 shows schematically that the properties of nanomaterials might increase by reducing their sizes and have extremal or oscillating dependence.

It is important to note that the size from which changes will start varies for each property. Objects with a size of 1–10 nm are recently called *nanoparticles.* The lowest limit for the existence of nanoparticle is quite blurred. It can be determined through transition from crystal phase to quasi-molecular or icosahedral structure, which has a fifth-order symmetry. Such tiny formations are called *clusters.* Clusters (bundle or collection) are determined by a group of closely located atoms, molecules, or ions tightly bound with each other. Upper size limit for nanoparticle could be determined by means of the ratio of inner and outer atoms. Particularly in chemistry, classification criteria of objects as nanoparticles (not as ultra-dispersed media) are considered by equal quantities of surface and inner atoms. Depending on the shape of nanoparticles, 10^3–10^5 atoms are included in this criterion. By summarizing the above interpretation, it can be concluded that during the motion through size axis of unit atom to massive

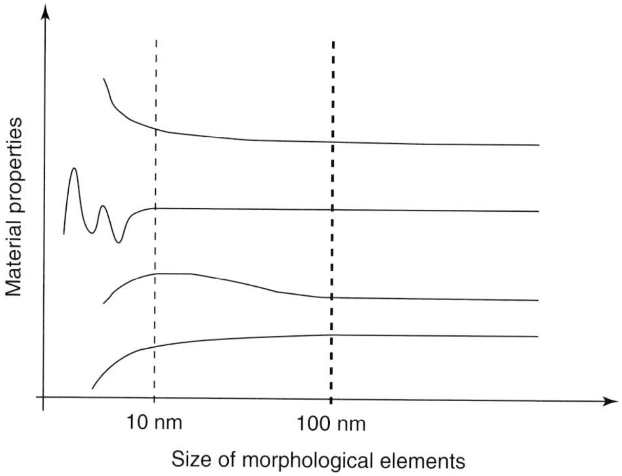

Figure 2.3 Schematic illustration of variations in physical properties of materials upon the decrease of their morphological size. (Ryzhonkov *et al.* 2008 [1]. Reproduced with permission of BKL Publishers.)

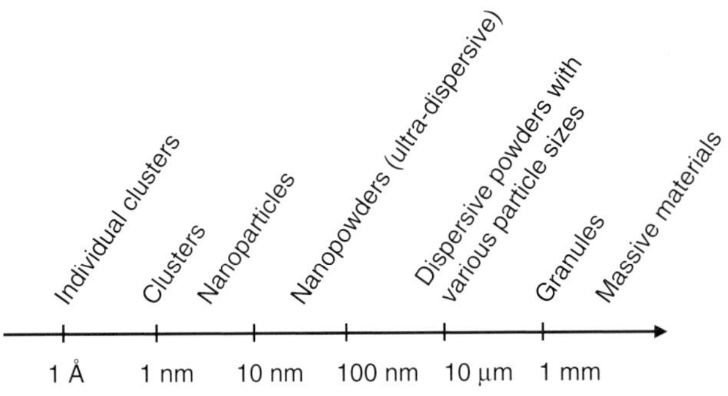

Figure 2.4 Classification of dispersive materials according to the size of dispersive phase. (Ryzhonkov *et al.* 2008 [1]. Reproduced with permission of BKL Publishers.)

condition, the dispersive system will have steps under intermediate conditions, including formation of clusters, nanoparticles, nano-, and ultra-dispersive systems (Figure 2.4).

Nanocrystals (nanostructured, nanophase, and nanocomposite) are materials with separate crystallites or phases, making up their structural base, with size not exceeding 100 nm in one-dimension.

2.1.3 Classification of Dispersive Systems According to Dimension

Dispersive phases in real systems have different forms such as spheres, needles, lamellas, cylinders, and uniaxial formations. Besides, films, membranes, threads, capillaries, various fibers, and pores can form a dispersive system. Due to this, the classification of dispersive systems according to dimensionality is based on the geometry or the number of measurements characterized by dispersive system phase. Their characteristics can depend on those sizes, which determine dispersity. *Dispersity* is an opposite particle size unit in dispersive phase. The size and dispersity of three-dimensional materials can be determined by three self-perpendicular directions (Figure 2.5a). Due to modern classification, *zero-dimensional dispersive systems* include nanopowders (ultra-dispersive) and

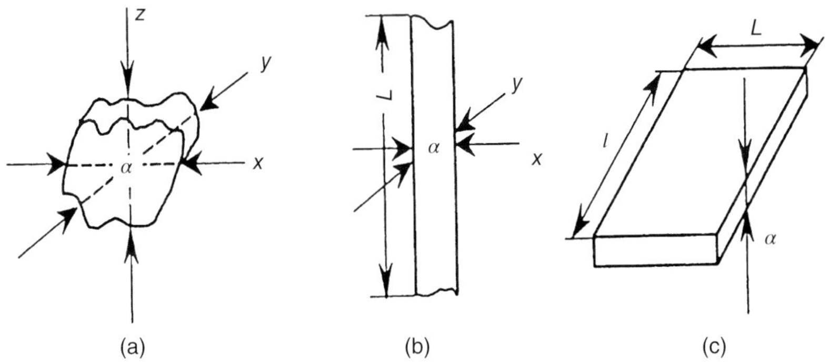

Figure 2.5 Zero-dimensional (a), two-dimensional (b), and one-dimensional (c) phases. (Ryzhonkov *et al.* 2008 [1]. Reproduced with permission of BKL Publishers.)

Table 2.2 Classification of nanomaterials according to their structural features according to Anischik *et al.* 2008 [2].

Nanomaterials		
Nanoparticles	**Nanostructured materials**	
	Consolidated materials	**Nanodispersions**
Nanoclusters	Nanocrystalline materials	Nanopowders
Nanocrystals	Fullerites	Nanosuspensions
Fullerenes	Photon crystals	Nanoemulsions
Nanotubes	Layered nanocomposites	Nanoaerosols
Supermolecules	Nanoaerogels	
Biomolecules		
Micelles	Matrix nanocomposites	Matrix nanocomposites
Liposomes	Nanoporous nanomaterials	Nanoporous nanomaterials

nanoparticles. *Two-dimensional dispersive systems* are characterized by two sizes, determining two mutually perpendicular directions (Figure 2.5b), and L does not affect dispersity. Two-dimensional systems consisting of fibers, threads, and capillaries that have macro length and two other dimensions are measured in nanometers. In the case of one-dimensional substances, only one size can determine dispersity (Figure 2.5c). *One-dimensional materials* include films; membranes; coatings, with thickness in nanometers; and other two dimensions including macroscopical sizes. *Three-dimensional nanosystems* include bulk massive nanomaterials. The classification of nanomaterials according to their structural features by Anischik *et al.* [2] is given in Table 2.2.

Nanomaterials have been divided into two major groups according to their morphology and structures, such as consolidated materials and nanodispersions.

The description and interpretation of the aforementioned nanomaterial types will require quite a large amount of time. Among the types of nanomaterials represented in Table 2.2, in particular of consolidated (or amalgamated) nanomaterials, they have been classified into several groups as represented in Table 2.3 [3].

2.2 Fullerenes

Fullerenes are carbon compounds formed from carbon atoms by sp-bonded zero-dimensional structure. Figure 2.6 shows the fullerene and other carbon compounds as allotropic modifications of carbon. Each type of allotropic modification is characterized by appropriate sp-bonding structure, dimensionality, and morphology. Initial attempts of the fullerene discovery were mentioned by Pacioli (Figure 2.7).

Table 2.3 Classification of consolidated (amalgamted) nanomaterials (according to Gleiter 1997 [3]).

Chemical composition / Shape	Composition and distribution			
	Single-phase	Multi-phase		
		Steady		Matrix
		Identical borders	Non-identical borders	
Lamellar	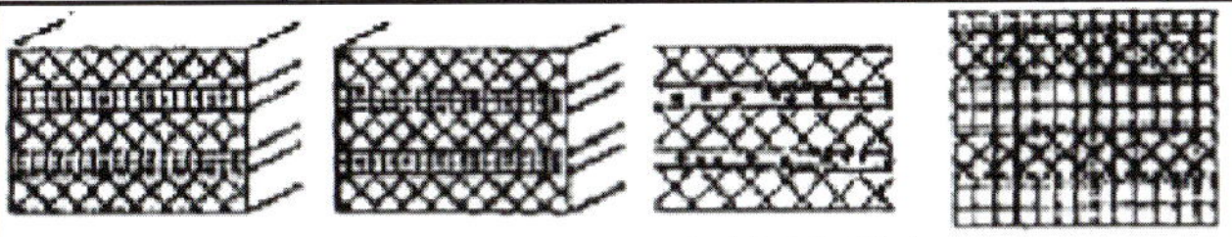			
Columnar	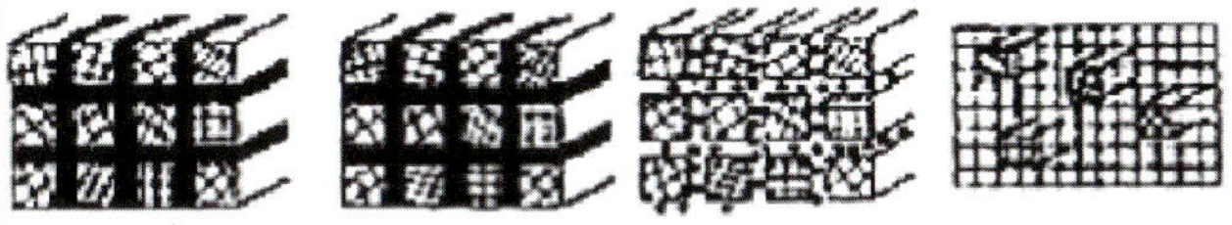			
Uniaxial	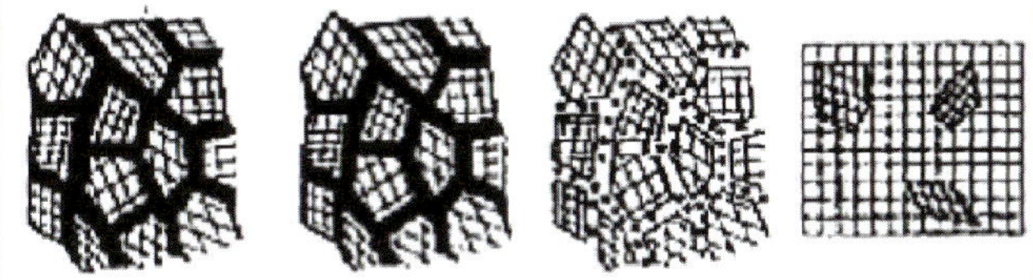			

Source: Glieter. Reproduced with permission of Elsevier.

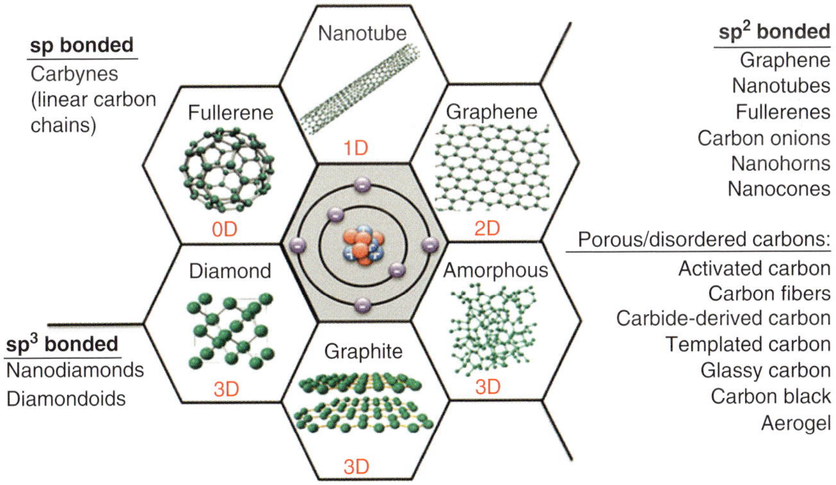

Figure 2.6 The most common carbon materials classified based on their bonding (hybridization of orbitals of carbon atoms) and dimensionality (i.e., the number of dimensions not confined to the nanoscale). Graphite, carbon fibers, glassy carbon, activated carbons, carbon black, and diamond are already widely used in industry as fullerenes and fullerides, carbon onions (multishell fullerenes), nanotubes, whiskers, nanofibers, cones, nanohorns, nanorings, nanodiamonds, and other nanoscale carbons that are being explored for future technologies. Note: 0D, zero-dimensional; 1D, one-dimensional; 2D, two-dimensional; 3D, three-dimensional. (Gogotsi 2015 [4]. Reproduced with permission of Cambridge University Press.)

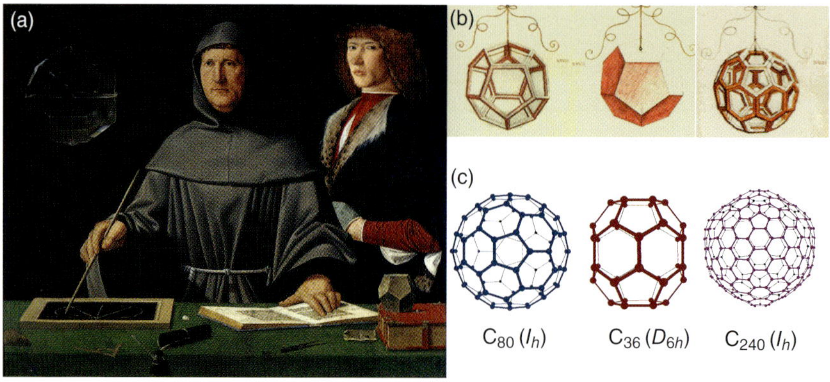

Figure 2.7 (a) Luca Pacioli drawing a construction on a board; in the right corner of the table, there is a dodecahedron resting upon a book bearing Pacioli's initials. A rhombicuboctahedron (a convex solid consisting of 18 squares and 8 triangles) suspends at the left of the painting (source: wikipedia); (b) Geometric models illustrated by Leonardo da Vinci in L. Pacioli's book titled *On the Divine Proportion* (Wikipedia source); (c) Computer models of various fullerenes: C_{80} (I_h), C_{36} (D_{6h}), and C_{240} (I_h). (Reproduced with permission from Glukhova 2014 [5].)

2.2.1 History of Fullerenes

- Fullerenes are a large class of carbon allotropes.
- In 1508 the book of Luca B. Pacioli titled *On the Divine Proportion* was published wherein high-symmetry shapes by Leonardo da Vinci were illustrated (Figure 2.7).
- Later, fullerene was named after Richard Buckminster Fuller, an American engineer and architect who is famous for his geodesic domes built for the 1967 World Exposition in Montreal, Canada.
- In 1985 fullerene C_{60} was synthesized by R. Curl, H. Kroto, and R. Smalley, who were later awarded a Nobel Prize.
- After developing ways for C_{60} synthesis, several types of fullerenes were discovered, such as C_{30}, C_{82}, and C_{96}.
- Fullerenes were recently used for drug delivery and biomedical purposes.

2.2.2 Tetrahedral Fullerenes

Tetrahedral fullerenes such as C_{28}, C_{40}, and C_{76} fullerenes belong to the T_d symmetry group (Tables 2.4 and 2.5) that combines 4 axes of the third order, 3 axes of the second order, 6 symmetry planes, and 24 elements in total. For finding the fullerenes' structural element with this group symmetry, it is necessary to find the smallest part of the tetrahedron, which must be set to re-create the geometry for all of the tetrahedron. This part is a *triangle ABC* (Figure 2.8) [5].

Classification of Tetrahedral Fullerenes

There are several classes of fullerenes, among them, the *three classes* of T_d fullerenes, namely, $A_m a_n$, $A_k b_n$, and $B_k b_n$, are differs by triple of pentagonal

Table 2.4 Compositions of the shells of fullerenes of basic symmetry group.

Group (order)	N_S	$z\theta_3$	Composition	
			Theoretical	Experimental
O_h (48)	$8\theta_3 + 24z$	$n_h + n_\sigma + 2n$	$C_{24}\,(\theta_3 = 0,\ z = 1)$	C_{24} [41]
O (24)	$8\theta_3 + 12z$	$2n$		
		$\theta_3 = 0,1/2,1$		
T_d (24)	$8\theta_3 + 12z$	$n_\sigma + 2n$	$C_{12}\,(\theta_3 = 0,\ z = 1)$	$(C_{28})^{4-}$ [25]
		$\theta_3 = 0,1/2,1$	$C_{28}\,(\theta_3 = 1/2,\ z = 2)$	$(M@C_{28})^{+}$
			$C_{40}\,(\theta_3 = 1/2,\ z = 3)$	M = (U, Hf, Zr) [25] C_{40} [34]
				$C_{36}M_4$ (M = B, P, N) [35, 36]
				$C_{36}M_4$ (M = B, P, N) [37] C_{76}
T_h (24)	$8\theta_3 + 12z$	$n_h + 2n$	$C_{24}\,(\theta_3 = 0,\ z = 2)$	$B_{12}N_{12}$ [42]
		$\theta_3 = 0,1/2,1$		
T (12)	$8\theta_3 + 6z$	$2n$	$C_{20}\,(\theta_3 = 1,\ z = 2)$	
		$\theta_3 = 0,1/2,1$		
D_{4h} (16)	$8z$	$n_\sigma + n'_\sigma + n_h + 2n$		
D_4 (8)	$4z$	$2n$	$C_{20}\,(z = 5)$	
C_{4v} (8)	$4z$	$n_\sigma + n'_\sigma + 2n$	$C_{20}\,(z = 5)$	
D_{2d} (8)	$4z$	$n'_\sigma + 2n$	$C_{4z}\,(z = 6, 9, 21)$	C_{24}, C_{36}, C_{84}
C_{4h} (8)	$4z$	$n_h + 2n$	$C_{20}\,(z = 5)$	
S_4 (4)	$2z$	$2n$	$C_{20}\,(z = 10)$	
C_4 (4)	$2z$	$2n$	$C_{20}\,(z = 10)$	
D_{2h} (8)	$4z$	$n_h + n'_\sigma + n'_\sigma + 2n$	$C_{20}\,(z = 5)$	C_{20} [17]
D_2 (4)	$2z$	$2n$	C_{2z}	C_{40}, C_{44}, C_{56}, C_{64}, C_{76}, C_{80}, C_{84}, C_{92}, C_{100}
C_{2v} (4)	$2z$	$n'_\sigma + n'_\sigma + 2n$	$C_{30}\ (z = 15)$, C_{2z}	C_{26}, $C_{29}Si$ [27], C_{30}, C_{54}, C_{78}, C_{80}, C_{90}
C_{2h} (4)	$2z$	$n_h + 2n$	$C_{20}\ (z = 10)$	C_{20} [17]

(continued)

Table 2.4 (Continued)

Group (order)	N_S	$z\theta_3$	Composition	
			Theoretical	Experimental
D_{6h} (24)	$12z$	$n_h + n'_\sigma + n'_\sigma + 2n$	C_{36} $(z = 3)$, C_{2z}	C_{36} [31], C_{72}, C_{84}, C_{96}
D_6 (12)	$6z$	$2n$	C_{24} $(z = 4)$	C_{24} [43]
C_{6v}	$6z$	$n'_\sigma + n'_\sigma + 2n$		
D_{3h} (12)	$2\theta_3 + 6z$	$n'_\sigma + n_h + 2n$	C_{26} $(\theta_3 = 1,\ z = 4)$	C_{26} [21, 23], C_{26}^{4-} [23] Ti@C_{26} [24]
	$\theta_3 = 0{,}1/2{,}1$			C_{74}, C_{78}
C_{6h} (12)	$6z$	$n_h + 2n$		
C_{3h} (6)	$2\theta_3 + 3z$	$2n_h + 2n$	C_{20} $(\theta_3 = 1,\ z = 6)$	
C_6 (6)	$3z$	$2n$		
D_{3d} (12)	$2\theta_3 + 6z$	$n_\sigma + 2n$	C_{20} $(\theta_3 = 1,\ z = 3)$	C_{20} [17], C_{32} [28, 28, 29]
			C_{32} $(\theta_3 = 1,\ z = 5)$	
D_3 (6)	$2\theta_3 + 3z$	$2n$	C_{20} $(\theta_3 = 1,\ z = 6)$	C_{32}, $C_{30}N_2$ [12], $C_{30}H_2$ [12],
			C_{30} $(\theta_3 = 1,\ z = 10)$	C_{42}, C_{50} [40], $C_{50}CI_{12}$ [45], C_{78}
			C_{50} $(\theta_3 = 1,\ z = 16)$	
C_{3v} (6)	$2\theta_3 + 3z$	$n_\sigma + 2n$	C_{26} $(\theta_3 = 1,\ z = 8)$	$C_{22}N_4$ [24], C_{80}
		$\theta_3 = 0{,}1/2{,}1$		
C_{3i} (6)	$2\theta_3 + 3z$	$2n$	C_{20} $(\theta_3 = 1,\ z = 6)$	
C_3 (3)	$2\theta_3 + 3/2z$	$2n$	C_{20} $(\theta_3 = 1,\ z = 12)$	
C_2 (2)	z	$2n$	C_{20} $(z = 20)$	C_{20} [17]
				C_{34} [21, 30]
			C_{34} $(z = 34)$	
			C_{46} $(z = 46)$	M@C_{46} [12] (M = Ti, Zr, Hf), C_{46}^{4-} [12]
C_s (2)	z	$n_\sigma + 2n$	C_{20} $(z = 20)$	
C_i (2)	z	$2n$	C_{20} $(z = 20)$	C_{20} [17]
C_l(1)	$z/2$	$2n$		

Here and in this table, z is an integer.
Source: Kustov *et al.* 2008 [6]. Reproduced with permission of Springer.

Table 2.5 Compositions of the shells of fullerenes of basic symmetry group [4].

Type	Icosahedron	Dodecahedron	Cube	Octahedron	Tetrahedron
ω	$\frac{5}{6}(3z-1)$	$\frac{5}{6}(\theta_3+3z-1)$	$\frac{2}{3}(\theta_3+3z-1)$	$\frac{2}{3}(3z-1)$	$\frac{1}{2}(\theta_3+3z-1)$
ω	5/3	5/3	4/3	4/3	1
$\theta_3=0$, $z=1$					

Source: Kustov *et al.* 2008 [6]. Reproduced with permission of Springer.

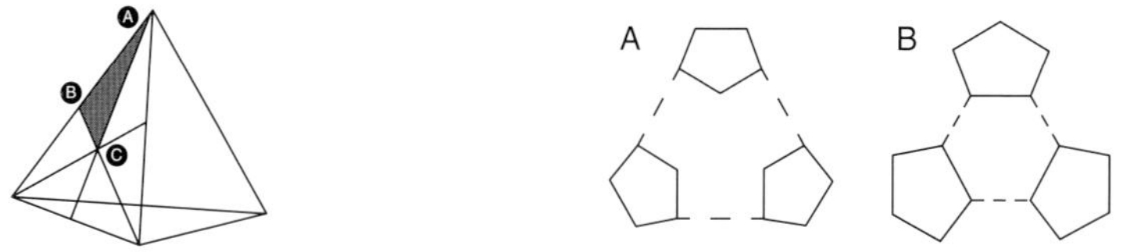

Basic polyhedron: Tetrahedron for the fullerenes with tetrahedral group symmetry

Pentagons may be located within the vertices of the *triangle ABC* or vertices outside (with ribs inside); this allows to distiguish two groups for topological models of the tetrahedral fullerenes: A and B groups

Figure 2.8 Basic elements composing the tetrahedral fullerene [5]. (Reproduced with permission of Glukhova [5].)

orientation, relating to the top (or vertices) A, mid-edge B, and mid-side C, for the basic tetrahedron cells of T_d fullerenes. In this way, the sequences of A_m and B_m are introduced, where m is the number of hexagons between the adjacent pentagons. Between adjacent pentagons, there may be located a few (from zero to infinity) hexagons (for any two adjacent pentagons, due to symmetry, the number of hexagons should be the same). For the configuration of A, hexagons can be zero (denoted as the configuration A_1) and one of hexagons (denoted as the configuration A_2). For the configuration of B, there can be one hexagon (configuration B_1) and two hexagons (configuration B_2). The number of atoms for $A_m a_n$-type fullerenes is determined by the following equation: $N = 4(m^2 + 6mn + 3n^2)$. C_{40} (A_1a_1), C_{76} (A_2a_1), C_{100} (A_1a_1), and C_{120} (A_3a_1) molecules are called $A_m a_n$-type fullerenes. For $m \gg n$ and $n \gg m$, the cluster shape approximates a tetrahedron with rounded vertices. For $m \gg n$, the shape is spheroid. For other relationships between m and n, the outer appearance is intermediate. According to the isolated pentagon rule, a fullerene is stable if its constituent pentagons have no common edges. The isolated pentagon rule is satisfied for fullerenes with $m > 1$; these are fullerenes C_{76} and C_{120}.

The number of atoms in $A_k b_n$-type fullerenes is determined by the following equation: $N = 4(2k^2 + 4kn + n^2)$. C_{28} (A_1a_1), C_{56} (A_1b_2), C_{68} (A_2b_1), C_{92} (A_1b_3), and C_{112} (A_2b_2) are called $A_k b_n$-type fullerenes. The number of atoms in $B_k b_n$-type fullerenes is determined by the following equation: $N = 12(m^2 + 6mn + 3n^2)$. Figure 2.9 shows the three types of fullerene groups described earlier.

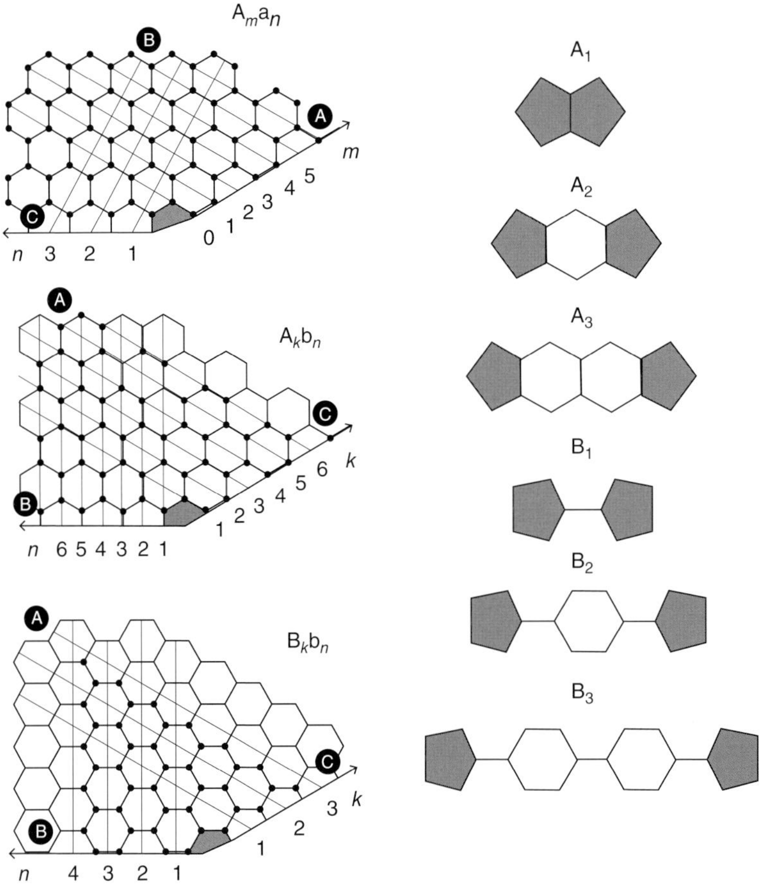

Figure 2.9 Three classes of T_d fullerenes, namely, $A_m a_n$, $A_k b_n$, and $B_k b_n$, differing in terms of triple of pentagonal orientation, related to the top (or vertices) *A*, mid-edge *B*, and mid-side *C*, for the basic tetrahedron cells of T_d fullerenes. (Glukhova 2014 [5]. Reproduced with permission.)

Regarding other fullerene classes, for fullerenes of $A_m b_n$ type, the number of atoms is determined by the formula $N = 4(2m^2 + 4mn + n^2)$. These are fullerenes C_{28} $(A_1 b_1)$, C_{56} $(A_1 b_2)$, C_{68} $(A_2 b_1)$, C_{92} $(A_1 b_3)$, C_{112} $(A_2 b_2)$, and so on. For $m \gg n$, the molecules are nearly octahedral. For $n \gg m$, they are nearly tetrahedral. For the case of $m \approx n$, the form of the molecule is spheroid because pentagons are approximately evenly distributed over the surface of the fullerene. The isolated pentagon rule is satisfied when $m > 1$ and $n > 1$ (C_{112}). The number of atoms in fullerenes of $B_m b_n$ configuration is defined by the formula $N = 12(2m^2 + 4mn + n^2)$. The isolated pentagon rule is satisfied for all fullerenes of this configuration. These fullerenes include C_{84} $(B_1 b_1)$, C_{168} $(B_1 b_2)$, C_{204} $(B_2 b_1)$, and so on. They are similar in shape to fullerenes of type $A_m b_n$ but have greater sphericity. For tetrahedral fullerenes, one can see that they are similar to the graphite layer. Thus fullerene of T_d symmetry group is a convolved graphite layer deformed at the pentagon sites.

Topological Models of Tetrahedral Fullerenes (T_d)

Table 2.6 represents various topological groups of T_d fullerenes, with $n = 1, 2, 3,$ and 4 and $m = 1, 2, 3, 4,$ and 5, for which an appropriate formula and symmetries are given.

According to the previous above, examples for the structures of fullerene are illustrated in Figure 2.10.

Table 2.6 Topological models of fullerenes with T_d (tetrahedral) symmetry.

n / m	Topological model	1	2	3	4
1	$A_m a_n (T_d)$	40	100	184 [1]	292
	$A_m b_n (T_d)$	28	56	92	136
	$B_m b_n (T_d)$	84	168	276	408
2	$A_m a_n (T_d)$	76	160	268	400
	$A_m b_n (T_d)$	68	112	164	224
	$B_m b_n (T_d)$	204	336	492	672
3	$A_m a_n (T_d)$	120	228	360	516
	$A_m b_n (T_d)$	124	184 [2]	252	328
	$B_m b_n (T_d)$	372	552	756	984
4	$A_m a_n (T_d)$	172	304	460	640
	$A_m b_n (T_d)$	196	272	356	448
	$B_m b_n (T_d)$	558	816	1068	1344
5	$A_m a_n (T_d)$	232	388	568	772
	$A_m b_n (T_d)$	284	376	476	584
	$B_m b_n (T_d)$	852	1128	1428	1752

Source: Reproduced with permission from Glukhova [5].

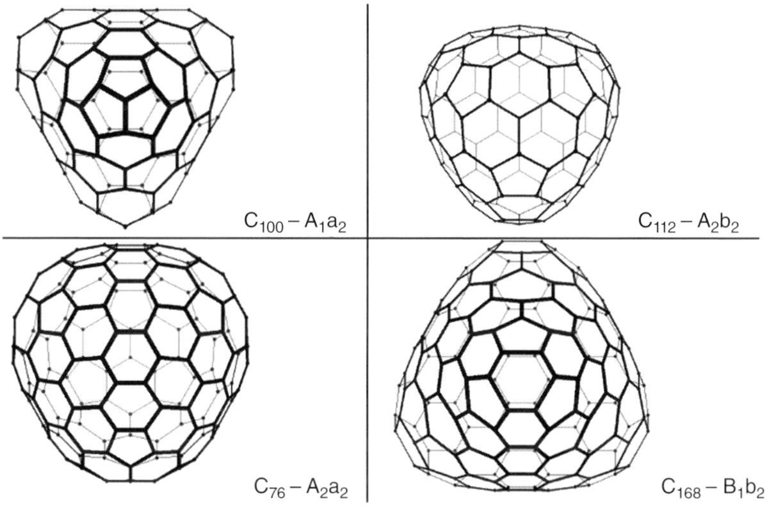

Figure 2.10 Structure of fullerenes according to Table 2.6. (Reproduced with permission from Glukhova 2014 [5].)

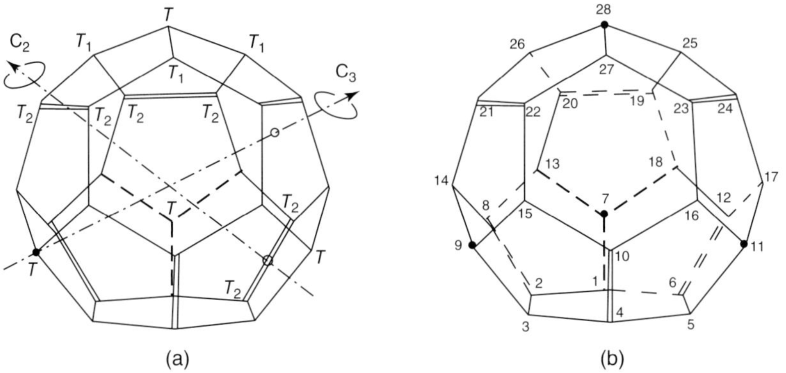

Figure 2.11 C_{28} fullerene: (a) three nuclear bases T, T_1, and T_2; (b) numbering of atom. (Reproduced with permission from Glukhova 2014 [5].)

The expansion of the full 28-dimensional actuated representation in the π-electron approximation will give the following equation [5]:

$$\Gamma^{\pi}_{\text{el}} = 3A_1 + 2E + 5F_1 + 2F_2 \tag{2.1}$$

There are three nuclear bases in fullerene structure – T, T_1, and T_2 – used for determination of atom numbering (Figure 2.11).

Fullerenes can be represented by Eqs. (2.2)–(2.29) [5]:

Normalized functions of degenerated π conditions for fullerenes relevant to irreducible representation of E:

For the basis of atoms A_1,

$$\psi_1(A_1) = \frac{1}{2}(\varphi_7 + \varphi_9 + \varphi_{11} + \varphi_{28}) \tag{2.2}$$

$$\psi_2(A_1) = \frac{1}{2\sqrt{3}}(\varphi_1 + \varphi_3 + \varphi_5 + \varphi_{13} + \varphi_{14} + \varphi_{15} + \varphi_{16} + \varphi_{17} + \varphi_{18} + \varphi_{25} + \varphi_{26} + \varphi_{27}) \tag{2.3}$$

$$\psi_3(A_1) = \frac{1}{2\sqrt{3}}(\varphi_2 + \varphi_4 + \varphi_6 + \varphi_8 + \varphi_{10} + \varphi_{12} + \varphi_{19} + \varphi_{20} + \varphi_{21} + \varphi_{22} + \varphi_{23} + \varphi_{24}) \tag{2.4}$$

Normalized functions of degenerated π conditions for fullerenes relevant to irreducible representation of E [5]:

For the basis of atoms T_1,

$$\psi_1(E) = \frac{1}{2\sqrt{6}}(\varphi_1 - 2\varphi_3 + \varphi_5 - 2\varphi_{13} + \varphi_{14} + \varphi_{15} - 2\varphi_{16} + \varphi_{17} + \varphi_{18} - 2\varphi_{25} + \varphi_{26} + \varphi_{27}) \tag{2.5}$$

$$\psi_2(E) = \frac{1}{2\sqrt{2}}(\varphi_1 - \varphi_5 + \varphi_{14} - \varphi_{15} + \varphi_{17} - \varphi_{18} - \varphi_{26} + \varphi_{27}) \tag{2.6}$$

For the basis of atoms T_2,

$$\psi_3(E) = \frac{1}{2\sqrt{6}}\left(\varphi_2 + \varphi_4 - 2\varphi_6 + \varphi_8 + \varphi_{10} - 2\varphi_{12} + \varphi_{19} + \varphi_{20} - 2\varphi_{21} - 2\varphi_{22} + \varphi_{23} + \varphi_{24}\right) \tag{2.7}$$

$$\psi_4(E) = \frac{1}{2\sqrt{2}}\left(-\varphi_2 + \varphi_4 - \varphi_8 + \varphi_{10} + \varphi_{19} + \varphi_{20} - \varphi_{23} - \varphi_{24}\right) \tag{2.8}$$

Normalized functions of degenerated π conditions for fullerenes relevant to irreducible representation of F_1 [5]:

For the basis of atoms T,

$$\psi_1(F_1) = (-\varphi_7 - \varphi_9 + \varphi_{11} + \varphi_{28})/2 \tag{2.9}$$

$$\psi_2(F_1) = (-\varphi_7 + \varphi_9 + \varphi_{11} - \varphi_{28})/2 \tag{2.10}$$

$$\psi_3(F_1) = (\varphi_7 - \varphi_9 + \varphi_{11} - \varphi_{28})/2 \tag{2.11}$$

For the basis of atoms T_1,

$$\psi_4(F_1) = (-\varphi_1 - \varphi_3 - \varphi_{13} - \varphi_{14} + \varphi_{16} + \varphi_{17} + \varphi_{25} + \varphi_{27})/\sqrt{8} \tag{2.12}$$

$$\psi_5(F_1) = (\varphi_3 + \varphi_5 - \varphi_{13} + \varphi_{15} + \varphi_{16} - \varphi_{18} - \varphi_{25} - \varphi_{26})/\sqrt{8} \tag{2.13}$$

$$\psi_6(F_1) = (\varphi_1 + \varphi_5 - \varphi_{14} - \varphi_{15} + \varphi_{17} + \varphi_{18} - \varphi_{26} - \varphi_{27})/\sqrt{8} \tag{2.14}$$

$$\psi_7(F_1) = (-\varphi_5 + \varphi_{15} + \varphi_{18} - \varphi_{26})/2 \tag{2.15}$$

$$\psi_8(F_1) = (\varphi_1 - \varphi_{14} - \varphi_{17} + \varphi_{27})/2 \tag{2.16}$$

$$\psi_9(F_1) = (\varphi_3 - \varphi_{13} - \varphi_{16} + \varphi_{25})/2 \tag{2.17}$$

For the basis of atoms T_2,

$$\psi_{10}(F_1) = (-\varphi_4 - \varphi_6 + \varphi_{10} + \varphi_{12} + \varphi_{19} - \varphi_{20} - \varphi_{21} + \varphi_{22})/\sqrt{8} \tag{2.18}$$

$$\psi_{11}(F_1) = (\varphi_2 + \varphi_6 - \varphi_8 - \varphi_{12} - \varphi_{21} + \varphi_{22} + \varphi_{23} - \varphi_{24})/\sqrt{8} \tag{2.19}$$

$$\psi_{12}(F_1) = (\varphi_2 + \varphi_4 - \varphi_8 - \varphi_{10} + \varphi_{19} - \varphi_{20} - \varphi_{23} + \varphi_{24})/\sqrt{8} \tag{2.20}$$

$$\psi_{13}(F_1) = (-\varphi_2 - \varphi_8 + \varphi_{23} + \varphi_{24})/2 \tag{2.21}$$

$$\psi_{14}(F_1) = (\varphi_4 + \varphi_{10} - \varphi_{19} - \varphi_{20})/2 \tag{2.22}$$

$$\psi_{15}(F_1) = (\varphi_6 + \varphi_{12} - \varphi_{21} - \varphi_{22})/2 \tag{2.23}$$

Normalized functions of degenerated π conditions for fullerenes relevant to irreducible representation of F_2 [5]:

For the basis of atoms T_1,

$$\psi_1(F_2) = (-\varphi_1 + \varphi_3 + \varphi_{13} - \varphi_{14} - \varphi_{16} + \varphi_{17} - \varphi_{25} + \varphi_{27})/\sqrt{8} \tag{2.24}$$

$$\psi_2(F_1) = (\varphi_3 - \varphi_5 - \varphi_{13} - \varphi_{15} + \varphi_{16} + \varphi_{18} - \varphi_{25} + \varphi_{26})/\sqrt{8} \tag{2.25}$$

$$\psi_3(F_2) = (-\varphi_1 + \varphi_5 + \varphi_{14} - \varphi_{15} - \varphi_{17} + \varphi_{18} - \varphi_{26} + \varphi_{27})/\sqrt{8} \tag{2.26}$$

For the basis of atoms T_2,

$$\psi_4\left(F_2\right)=\left(\varphi_2-\varphi_6-\varphi_8+\varphi_{12}+\varphi_{21}-\varphi_{22}+\varphi_{23}-\varphi_{24}\right)/\sqrt{8} \tag{2.27}$$

$$\psi_5\left(F_2\right)=\left(\varphi_4-\varphi_6-\varphi_{10}+\varphi_{12}-\varphi_{19}+\varphi_{20}-\varphi_{21}+\varphi_{22}\right)/\sqrt{8} \tag{2.28}$$

$$\psi_6\left(F_2\right)=\left(-\varphi_2+\varphi_4+\varphi_8-\varphi_{10}+\varphi_{19}-\varphi_{20}+\varphi_{23}-\varphi_{24}\right)/\sqrt{8} \tag{2.29}$$

2.2.3 Icosahedral Fullerenes

Icosahedral fullerenes are I_h group fullerenes with symmetry group including six fivefold symmetry axes, 10 threefold axes, 15 twofold axes, 15 symmetry planes, and so on, altogether 120 elements including the identical transformation. Let us consider an icosahedron, a polyhedron that gave its name to the symmetry group. It consists of 20 faces (each being a regular triangle), 12 vertices, and 30 edges. The right triangle ABC (Figure 2.12) is the smallest part of the icosahedron used to specify the whole icosahedron by symmetry transformations.

Classification of Icosahedral (I_h) Fullerenes

For the fullerenes with atomic configuration of A_n, the number of atoms is determined by the following equation: $N=20n^2$. For fullerenes with B_n configuration, the equation is $N=60n^2$.

Some of the topological models for A_n and B_n fullerenes are given in Table 2.7, and the representatives of this fullerene class are shown in Figure 2.13.

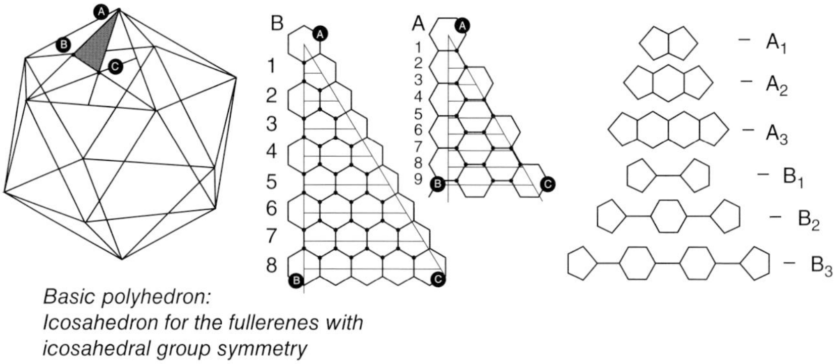

Figure 2.12 Basic elements composing the icosahedral fullerene. (Reproduced with permission from Glukhova 2014a [5].)

Table 2.7 Topological models of fullerenes with I_h (icosahedral) group symmetry.

n	n Topological	1	2	3	4
—	$A_n\left(I_h\right)$	20	80	180	320
—	$B_n\left(I_h\right)$	60	240	540	960

Source: Reproduced with permission from Glukhova [5].

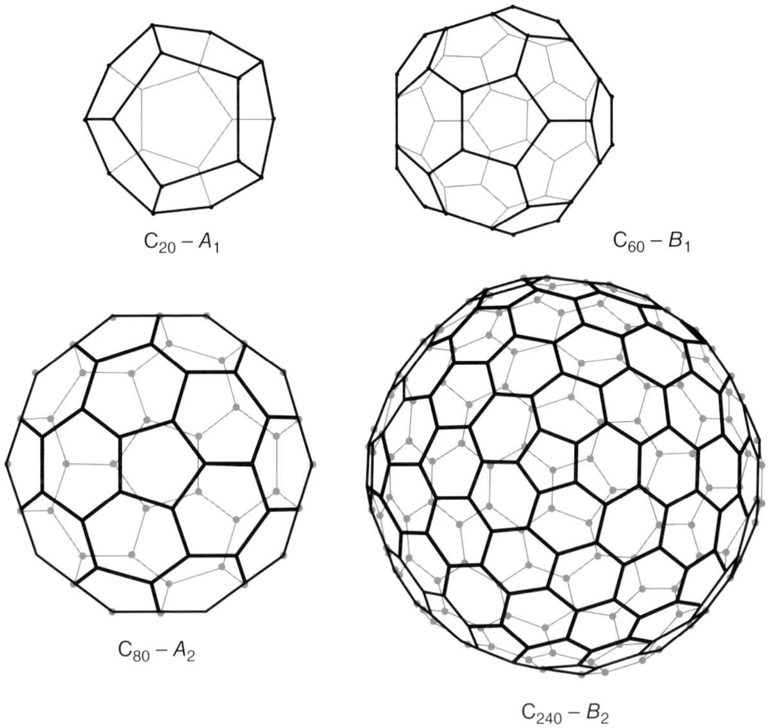

Figure 2.13 Structure of icosahedral fullerenes according to topological models as given in Table 2.7. (Reproduced with permission from Glukhova 2014 [5].)

Belonging to the multishell fullerene structure $C_m@C_n$, the C_{240} fullerene has icosahedral symmetry I_h. As for C_{20}, there is no firm opinion about the symmetry of this fullerene in literature nowadays. Therefore, it was considered that C_{20} belongs to group D_{3d} symmetry as in some other works. Taking into account these assumptions necessary for further analysis, numerical values of geometry and energy parameters of fullerenes C_{240} and C_{20} (in the ground state) were calculated. The molecule C_{540} is the outer shell of nanoparticles $C_{60}@C_{540}$; it has icosahedral symmetry I_h. The molecule C_{60} has a structure of a truncated icosahedron. It consists of 12 pentagons and 20 hexagons [10].

The electronic representation of π-system icosahedral fullerene C_{60} (I_h) can be presented by the following equation [5]:

$$\Gamma_{\text{el}}^{\pi} = A_g + F_{1g} + 2F_{1u} + F_{2g} + 2F_{2u} + 2G_g + 2G_u + 3H_g + 2H_u \tag{2.30}$$

Classification of Multilayered Fullerenes

1) *Centered (double-layered) fulleren*es, stability of which is characterized by the following properties:
   a) The negative value of the enthalpy reaction corresponds to the exothermic reaction.

b) The negative value of van der Waals energy (negative value denotes attraction of layers, whereas positive shows repulsion, as well as the deformation of fullerene strain cells).
c) The interlayer gap ≥3 Å (value corresponding to distance between the layers of graphite).

The interaction of atoms belonging to different shells is simulated by the *Lennard-Jones potential* [5]:

$$E_{\mathrm{VDV}} = \sum_{k=1}^{N_{\mathrm{p}}} \frac{A}{\sigma^6} \left(\frac{1}{2} y_0^6 \frac{1}{\left(r_k/\sigma\right)^{12}} - \frac{1}{\left(r_k/\sigma\right)^6} \right) \tag{2.31}$$

where k is the counter for interacting pairs of carbon atoms, which belongs to different layers of nanoparticle; r_k is the distance between atoms of the kth pair; N_{p} is the number of pairs (e.g., $N_{\mathrm{p}} = 4800$ for nanocluster $C_{20}@C_{240}$); $\sigma = 1.42$ Å – length between the C—C bond; $y_0 = 2.7$; and $A = 24.3 \times 10^{-79}$ J m^6 that are empirically selected parameters.

2) *Fullerenes with non-central effect,* characterized by topology of multi-well potential interaction and calculation to reveal the regularities of movement for internal fullerene in the field of holding potential of the external shell, $C_m@C_n$. In Figure 2.14a–f, the basic structures of the following fullerenes with non-central effect are illustrated:
   a) Tetrahedron – During the displacement of C_m toward vertices
   b) Polyhedron – During the displacement of C_m toward middle edges of the tetrahedron

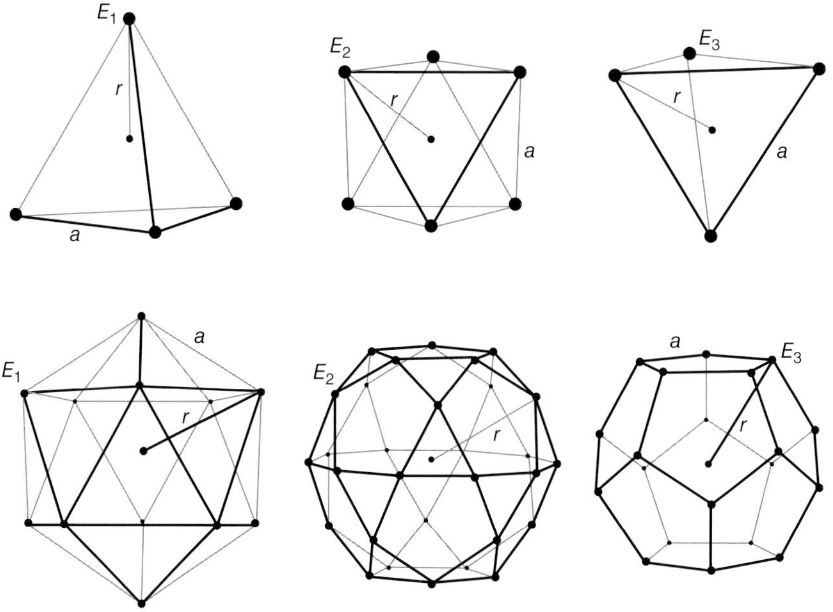

Figure 2.14 Fullerenes with non-central effect (Reproduced with permission from Glukhova 2014a [5].)

c) Tetrahedron – During displacement of C_m in the direction of face centers of tetrahedron
d) Icosahedron – During the displacement of C_m toward the peaks
e) Roklar – During the displacement in the direction of midpoint edges of the icosahedron
f) Pentagonal dodecahedron – During the displacement in the direction of face centers of an icosahedron

Fullerenes with non-central effect are subdivided according to position and interactions between the inner and outer shells:

Fullerenes with Non-central Effect and Tetrahedral Outer Layer

The molecule C_{228} is the outer shell of nanoparticles $C_{28}@C_{228}$, and it has tetrahedral symmetry T_d. The positioning of C_{28} fullerene in a field of trapping potential for C_{228} fullerene corresponds to the interactions of energies E_1, E_2, and E_3 for $C_{28}@C_{228}$ nanocluster layers. Three orientations of fullerene C_{28} in the field of fullerene C_{540} retaining potential, corresponding to the interaction between layers of nanocluster $C_{28}@C_{228}$ energies d_1, d_2, and d_3, are presented in Figure 2.15. The position of the fullerene m near one of the basic icosahedrons with 12 vertices corresponds to the ground state of the nanocluster $C_m@C_n$ with icosahedral outer shell. The basic icosahedron forms the base of the fullerene

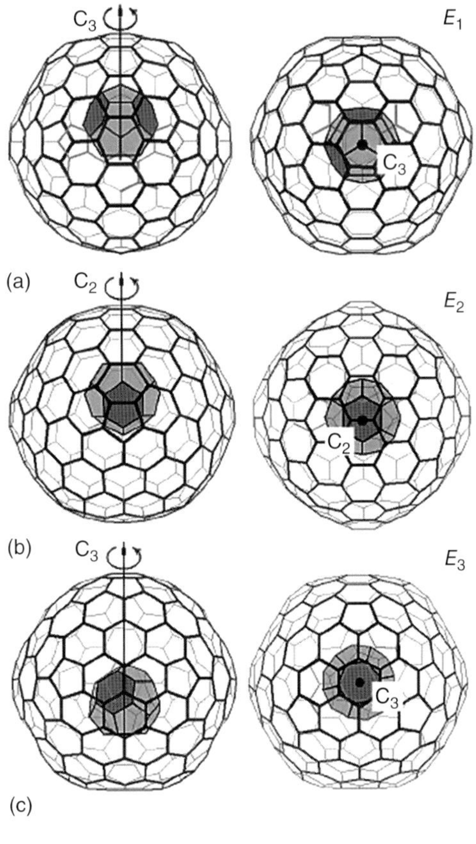

Figure 2.15 Fullerenes with noncentral effect and tetrahedral outer layer. Position of the C_{28} in the field of fullerene C_{228} retaining potential (a) for interaction between nanoparticle layers energy E_1 and (b) for energy E_2, and (c) for energy E_3. (Reproduced with permission from Glukhova 2014 [5].)

skeleton. The interaction energy δ_1 between fullerene shells of the nanoclusters corresponds to this m orientation. The potential wells with energy δ_1 form icosahedron. The fullerene C_m may be situated in any of the vertexes of this icosahedron with equal probability. Thirty potential wells with higher energy δ_2 form roklar in the space. These wells are located near the middle of the edges of the basic fullerene icosahedron. Twenty identical potential wells with even greater energy δ_3 form a pentagonal dodecahedron. These wells are located in the face centers of the basic icosahedron [5].

Nanoparticles of $C_{20}@C_{240}$

In the ground state of nanoparticle $C_{20}@C_{240}$, corresponding to 50 K, the fullerene C_{20} is situated near the center of one of the fullerene C_{240} 12 regular pentagons, that is, the fullerene C_{20} is displaced from the center in the direction of the fifth-order symmetry axis of the external shell. δ_1 is the energy of interaction between the fullerene layers of the nanoparticle corresponding to this state of the fullerene C_{20}. The fullerene C_{20} may be located in any of the vertexes of this icosahedron with equal probability. Besides the 12-deep potential wells with energy δ_1, there are also 30 identical potential wells with greater energy δ_2 located near the middle of the icosahedron edge of fullerene C_{240} cage and 20 identical potential wells with greater energy δ_3 ($\delta_3 > \delta_2 > \delta_1$) near the center of the icosahedron face [7].

Nanoparticles of $C_{60}@C_{540}$

Three orientations of fullerene C_{60} in the field of fullerene C_{540} retaining potential, corresponding to the interaction between layers of nanocluster $C_{60}@C_{540}$ energies δ_1, δ_2, and δ_3, are presented. In the ground state of nanoparticle $C_{60}@C_{540}$, the fullerene C_{60} is located near the center of one of the fullerene C_{540} 12 regular pentagons. Also, as for the case of $C_{20}@C_{240}$, there are 30 identical potential wells with greater energy δ_2 located near the middle of the icosahedron's edge of fullerene C_{540} cage and 20 identical potential wells with greater energy δ_3 near the center of the icosahedron's face. The models of two-shell fullerenes $C_{20}@C_{240}$ and $C_{60}@C_{540}$ were considered. The feature of such fullerenes is that, at low temperatures, the internal fullerene will move in a certain way: between the potential wells [7].

Fullerenes with Non-central Effect and Outer Icosahedral Layer

The molecule C_{540} is the outer shell of nanoparticles $C_{60}@C_{540}$; it has icosahedral symmetry I_h. Positioning of fullerene C_{60} in a field of trapping potential for C_{540} fullerene corresponds to the interactions of energies E_1, E_2, and E_3 for $C_{60}@C_{540}$ nanocluster layers. The three orientations of fullerene C_{60} in the field of the fullerene C_{540} retaining potential corresponding to the interaction between layers of nanocluster $C_{60}@C_{540}$ energies d_1, d_2, and d_3, are presented in Figure 2.16. In the ground state of nanoparticle $C_{60}@C_{540}$, the fullerene C_{60} is located near the center of one of the fullerene C_{540} 12 regular pentagons [7].

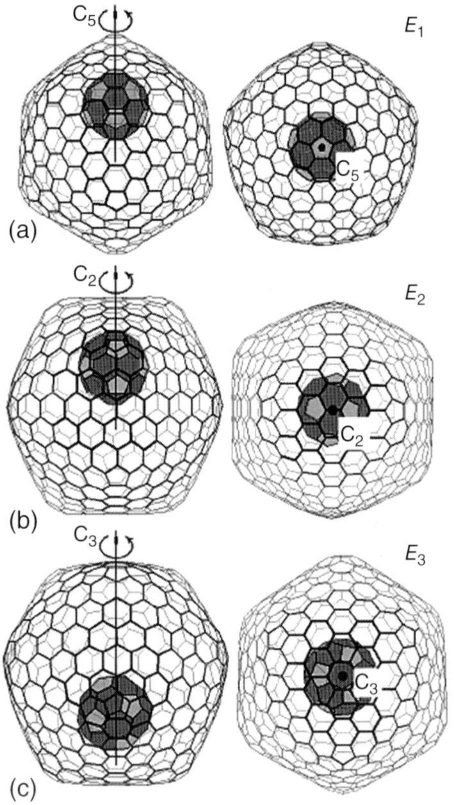

Figure 2.16 Fullerenes with non-central effect and icosahedral outer layer. Position of the C_{60} in the field of fullerene C_{540} retaining potential (a) for interaction between nanoparticles layers energy E_1, (b) for energy E_2, and (c) for energy E_3 (Glukhova *et al.* 2014 [7]. Reproduced with permission of John Wiley and Sons.)

2.2.4 Physical Properties of Fullerenes

Fullerenes exhibit several properties, including semiconducting bandgap, ionization potential, binding energy, enthalpy, and minimum and maximum bond length. These physical parameters for fullerene C_{28} with tetrahedral symmetry group, for icosahedral fullerenes, and for the double-layer centered fullerenes are represented in Tables 2.8–2.10.

In conclusion, the classification of multilayer fullerenes allows the notifying of topology of the surface layers energy cooperation, stability, chemical activity, thermodynamical properties, and so on. Classification of multilayer fullerenes allows description of properties of each layer of multilayer clusters; systematization of double-layered fullerenes completely defines layer interaction and positioning of its inner component in relation to the outer shell. Thus, further investigation and search of classification features for multilayer fullerenes with the number of more than three shells is not required. Cluster with any number of layers can be consistently regarded as a set of two-layer fullerenes, by analogy of the double-layer fullerenes, and can be judged based on its properties [10].

Table 2.8 Physical parameters of fullerene C_{28}.

C_n	E_g (eV)	IP (eV)	E_b (eV)	$\Delta H^0_{f(C_n)}$ (kcal mol^{-1} atom^{-1}	Min/max. bond length
$C_{40}(A_1a_1)$	1.57	6.88	6.74	15.85	1.44/152
$C_{100}(A_1a_2)$	1.24	6.90	7.00	10.36	1.40/1.52
$C^1_{184}(A_1a_3)$	1.00	6.82	7.09	7.83	1.41/1.47
$C_{76}(A_2a_1)$	1.0	6.50	7.01	9.53	1.39/1.47
$C_{160}(A_2a_2)$	0.81	6.54	7.09	8.00	1.40/1.46
$C_{268}(A_2a_3)$	0.65	6.54	7.00	9.68	1.40/1.55
$C_{228}(A_3a_2)$	1.35	7.09	7.15	6.47	1.38/1.47
$C_{172}(A_4a_1)$	0.10	7.05	6.88	12.74	1.39/1.46
$C_{28}(A_1b_1)$	2.18	7.06	6.54	20.54	1.44/1.52
$C_{112}(A_2b_2)$	1.14	6.83	7.06	8.58	1.41/1.47
$C_{164}(A_2b_3)$	0.55	6.97	6.96	10.91	1.40/1.70
$C_{224}(A_2b_4)$	0.12	6.59	7.14	6.67	1.40/1.47
$C^2_{184}(A_3b_2)$	0.72	6.49	7.13	6.92	1.39/1.47
$C_{168}(B_1b_2)$	1.37	6.86	6.58	19.57	1.38/2.01
$C_{204}(B_2b_1)$	1.12	6.86	7.08	9.67	1.40/1.46

Source: Reproduced with permission from Glukhova [5].

Table 2.9 Energy and metric parameters of I_h fullerenes of classes A_n and B_n.

C_n	E_g (eV)	IP (eV)	E_b (eV)	$\Delta H^0_{f(C_n)}$ (kcal mol^{-1} atom^{-1})	Min/max. bond length (Å)	Max. angle θ (°)
$C_{20}(A_1)$	3.52	6.39	6.20	32.32	1.425	20.9
$C_{80}(A_2)$	2.20	6.72	7.02	9.52	1.42/1.46	10.6
$C_{180}(A_3)$	1.45	7.33	7.04	9.03	1.39/1.43	9.5
$C_{60}(B_1)$	2.03	7.62	7.00	10.03	1.40/1.49	11.6
$C_{240}(B_2)$	1.30	7.06	7.17	6.00	1.40/1.47	10.6
$C_{540}(B_3)$	0.90	6.84	7.17	5.97	1.40/1.47	10.6

Source: Reproduced with permission from Glukhova 2014 [5].

Symmetry of Fullerene

Fullerene has high symmetry characterized by rotations around an axis. There are three kinds of rotation axes for C_{60}.

Important Applications of Fullerenes

- Medical (antiviral and antioxidant activity, biological activity)
- Potential scaffold for photodynamical therapy
- Water purification, biohazard protection
- Photodetector performance

Table 2.10 Energy and metric parameters of the double-layer centered fullerenes.

$C_n@C_m$	Distance between layers (Å)	E_{VdV} (eV)	$E_{atom}(C_n@C_m)$	$\Delta H_{formation}$ (kcal mol^{-1})
$C_{240}@C_{540}$	3.90	−11.403	−43.22	−265
$C_{60}@C_{240}$	3.50	−4.571	−43.17	−108
$C_{28}@C_{184}$ [2]	3.55	−2.317	−43.091	−92
$C_{28}@C_{168}$	3.72	−2.111	−42.61	−68
$C_{20}@C_{160}$	3.36	−1.814	−43.063	−116
$C_{28}@C_{160}$	3.26	−1.574	−43.071	−86
$C_{20}@C_{184}$ [2]	3.83	−1.547	−43.084	−35
$C_{20}@C_{168}$	3.75	−1.451	−42.584	−33
$C_{80}@C_{240}$	3.06	−1.266	−43.16	−21

Source: Reproduced with permission from Glukhova 2014 [5].

2.3 Carbon Nanotubes

Carbon nanotubes are cylindrical structures with diameter from 1 to several 10th of nanometers. They are sheets of graphite folded in a cylindrical shape with size ranging from 1 to 3 nm in diameter and 100–1000 nm in length. Usually, the thickness of a nanotube is 1.3–1.4 g cm^{-3}. The term nanotubes can also be referred to the term of *carbon tubular nanoclusters*. In further, the types of nanotubes and tubular nanoclusters will be described in the following text.

2.3.1 Types and Classification of Carbon Nanotubes

Generally nanotubes can be divided into two groups based on their structure or chiral vector position and the number of layers:

According to structure or position of a chiral vector: a single-walled nanotube's structure is represented by a pair of indices (n and m), which are called *chiral vectors* (Figure 2.17). According to the position of chiral vector, nanotubes can have zigzag, armchair and chiral conformations. As it is seen from Figure 2.17, a_1 and a_2 are the vectors defining the direction for zigzag(n, o); the dashed line drawn below the vector $C_h = na_1 + ma_2$ defines the direction for armchair(n, n) types of carbon nanoclusters [9].

T and $C_h = na_1 + ma_2$ are the vectors defining the directions for the *chiral* type of carbon nanoclusters. According to this criterion, two groups of carbon nanotubes exist, achiral and chiral (Figure 2.17, right side):

Zigzag-Type Carbon Nanoclusters

Calculation of coordinates in zigzag-type tubular carbon nanoclusters can be achieved by using Eqs. (2.32)–(2.36) from three-parameter method represented in Figure 2.18:

$$X_k = R \times \cos \alpha_k, \quad Y_k = R \times \sin \alpha_k \tag{2.32}$$

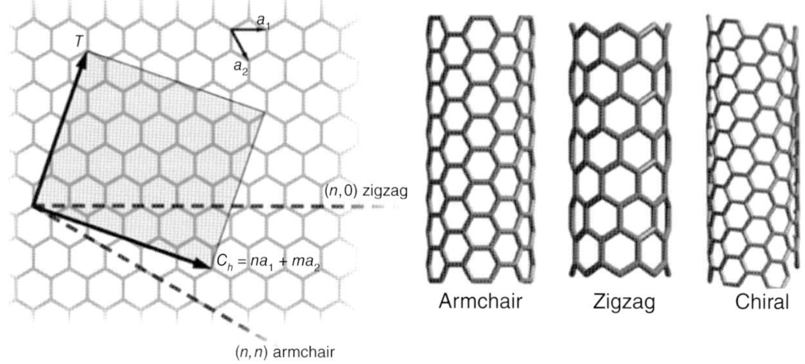

Figure 2.17 Position of a chiral vector in sp²-bonded carbon structures; carbon nanotubes. (Adapted from Kanoun *et al.* [8].)

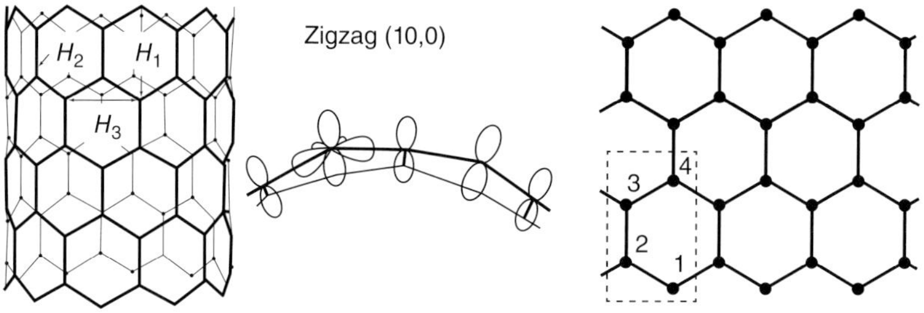

Figure 2.18 Calculation of coordinates for zigzag-type carbon tubular nanoclusters: (a) location of H_1, H_2 and H_3 nanocluster radius components; (b) location of atoms in the hexagonal carbon ring segment. (Reproduced with permission from Glukhova 2014 [15].)

where $R = n{\cdot}H_3/2\pi$ is nanocluster radius, α is the angle appropriate for atom and number of atom in segment, calculating by the use of equations given below, $k = 1 \ldots 4$ is the number of atom in segment. Z coordinate and α angle for atom in segment are calculated by using the following equations:

$$Z_1 = i \times (H_1 + H_2), \quad a_1 = j \times \frac{2\pi}{n} \tag{2.33}$$

$$Z_2 = i \times (H_1 + H_2) + \frac{H_1 - H_2}{2}, \quad a_2 = (j \times 2 - 1) \times \frac{\pi}{n} \tag{2.34}$$

$$Z_3 = i + \frac{1}{2} \times (H_1 + H_2), \quad a_3 = (j \times 2 - 1) \times \frac{\pi}{n} \tag{2.35}$$

$$Z_4 = i \times (H_1 + H_2) + H_1, \quad a_4 = j \times \frac{2\pi}{n} \tag{2.36}$$

where $i = 0\ (M/2 - 1)$ – segment number along Z axis, and $j = 0\ (n - 1)$, segment number in radius.

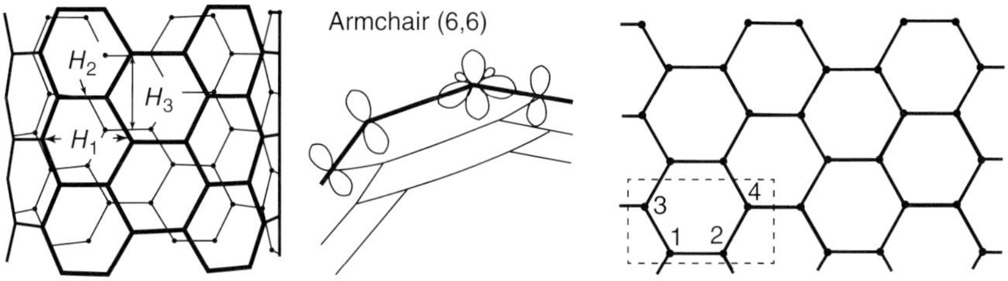

Figure 2.19 Calculation of coordinates for armchair-type carbon tubular nanoclusters: (a) location of H_1, H_2 and H_3 nanocluster radius components; (b) location of atoms in the hexagonal carbon ring segment. (Reproduced with permission from Glukhova 2014 [15].)

Armchair-Type Carbon Nanoclusters

Calculation of coordinates for armchair-type tubular carbon nanoclusters (Figure 2.19) can be done by following Eqs. (2.37)–(2.40).

$X_k = R \cdot \cos \alpha_k$, $Y_k = R \cdot \sin \alpha_k$, where $R = m \cdot (H_1 + H_2)/2\pi$, which is the nanocluster radius; α is the angle appropriate for atom and number of atoms in segment, calculated using the equations below; and $k = 1 \ldots 4$, which denotes the number of atoms in segment. *A* coordinate and α angle for atom in segment are calculated by using the following equations:

$$Z_1 = i \times H_3, \quad a_1 = j \times \frac{2\pi}{m}, \quad Z_2 = i \times H_3 \tag{2.37}$$

$$a_2 = \left[j + \frac{H_2}{H_1 + H_2} \right] \times \frac{2\pi}{m}, \quad Z_3 = \left(i + \frac{1}{2} \right) \times H_3 \tag{2.38}$$

$$a_3 = \left[j - \frac{H_1 - H_2}{2 \times (H_1 + H_2)} \right] \times \frac{2\pi}{m}, \quad Z_4 = \left(i + \frac{1}{2} \right) \times H_3 \tag{2.39}$$

$$a_4 = \left[j + \frac{H_2}{H_1 + H_2} - \frac{H_1 - H_2}{2 \times (H_1 + H_2)} \right] \times \frac{2\pi}{m} \tag{2.40}$$

Above structures were obtained by calculation of CTN coordinates by three-parameter method of the atomic frame by *O. Glukhova et al.*

According to the number of layers: single-walled nanotubes (SWNTs) and multiwalled nanotubes (MWNT). SWNT consist of a single layer, with a length up to 1 cm. MWNT are those carbon structures, composed of several layers (also called "Russian matryoshka" structure).

Classification for Topological Models of Achiral Tubular Nanoclusters

Zigzag nanotubes and armchair-type carbon nanotubes are classified according to several criteria, given above, and the number of hexagonal carbon atom lattices (m, n) that are located parallel to the horizontal surface, σ_h (Figures 2.20 and 2.21). In both cases, the hexagonal carbon lattices are denoted by *D*. However, the number of hexagonal carbon atom lattices for zigzag- and armchair-type carbon nanotubes is marked by indices $6h$, $5h$, $8d$, and $7d$ and indices $4h$, $5h$, $5d$, and $6d$, *respectively, of D.* In nanotube, vertical axis surface, σ_y, is marked as C_6, C_5, C_8, and C_7 for the number of hexagonal carbon atom lattices in a carbon nanotube (6, 0), (5, 0), (8, 0), and (7, 0), respectively. On the other hand, in armchair-type

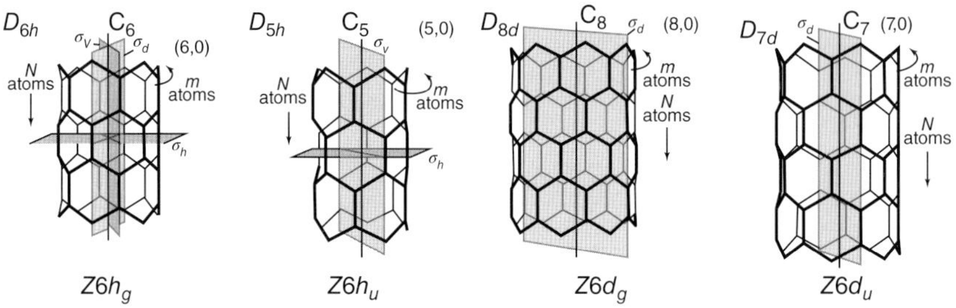

Figure 2.20 Classification of achiral-type (zigzag) tubular carbon nanoclusters. (Reproduced with permission from Glukhova 2014 [5].)

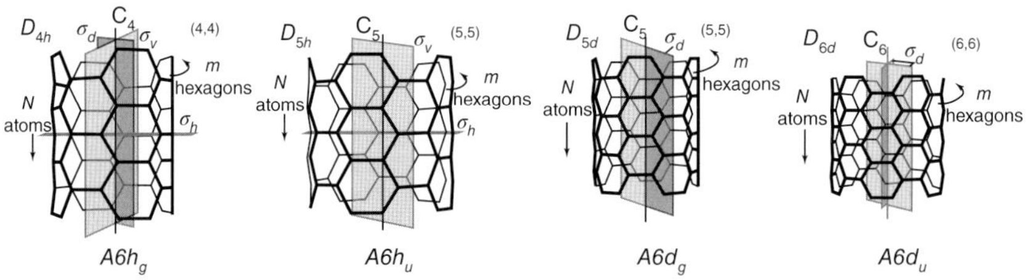

Figure 2.21 Classification of achiral-type (armchair) tubular carbon nanoclusters. (Reproduced with permission from Glukhova 2014 [5].)

carbon nanotubes, vertical axis surface σ_y, marked as C_4, C_5, C_5, and C_6, corresponds to carbon nanotube (4, 4), (5, 5), (5, 5), and (6, 6), respectively. N means the number of individual carbon atoms situated horizontally along the hexagonal carbon atom lattices. Zigzag-type and armchair-type carbon nanoclusters are indicated by Z and A, respectively. 6h indicates six hexagonal carbon atoms, composing the single lattice, while indices g and u indicate the even and odd numbers, respectively, for hexagonal carbon atom lattices in a carbon nanotube.

2.3.2 Mechanical Properties and Physical Parameters of Carbon Nanotubes

Mechanical properties of carbon nanotubes include their linear elastic parameters, nonlinear elastic instabilities, buckling (folding), inelastic relaxation, yield strength, and fracture mechanism. Fracture phenomenon involves microscopic, mesoscopic, and macroscopic modeling. Also, their relative simplicity and atomically precise morphology offer the opportunity to address the validity of different macroscopic and microscopic models of fracture mechanical response [10].

Some of the physical parameters such as length, atomic energy, enthalpy, binding energy, ionization potential, and semiconducting bandgap for various topological models of tetrahedral and icosahedral fullerenes are given in Tables 2.11 and 2.12.

Table 2.11 Parameters of $A6d_u$, $A6h_u$, $A6d_g$, and $A6h_g$ armchair topological model nanoclusters.

Number of atoms	Length (Å)	E_{atom} (eV atom^{-1})	$\Delta H^0_{f(C_n)}$ (kcal mol^{-1} atom^{-1})	E_b (eV)	IP (eV)	E_g (eV)
Nanocluster (3,3) $d = 4.10$ Å						
30 ($A6h_u$)	4.78	−42.30	26.85	6.26	6.74	0.76
48 ($A6d_u$)	8.50	−42.52	21.59	6.49	6.57	0.49
156 ($A6d_u$)	30.67	−42.82	14.84	6.78	6.34	0.27
540 ($A6d_u$)	101.91	−43.05	22.08	6.47	6.13	0.05
Nanocluster (4,4) $d = 5.52$ Å						
96 ($A6d_g$)	13.4	−42.80	15.16	6.77	6.27	0.24
168 ($A6h_g$)	24.5	−42.94	12.13	6.90	6.20	0.16
664 ($A6h_g$)	100.9	−43.07	9.02	7.04	6.10	0.04
Nanocluster (5,5) $d = 6.84$ Å						
50 ($A6h_u$)	4.88	−42.39	24.67	6.36	6.30	0.20
390 ($A6h_u$)	46.42	−43.09	10.52	7.87	6.15	0.01
Nanocluster (6,6) $d = 8.36$ Å						
96 ($A6d_g$)	8.51	−42.75	16.37	6.72	6.36	0.45
168 ($A6d_g$)	15.92	−42.95	11.76	6.92	6.25	0.28
252 ($A6h_g$)	24.50	−43.04	9.64	7.01	6.18	0.25

Source: Reproduced with permission from Glukhova [5].

Table 2.12 Parameters of $Z6d_u$, $Z6h_u$, $Z6d_g$, and $Z6h_g$ zigzag topological model nanoclusters.

Number of atoms	Length (Å)	E_{atom} (eV atom^{-1})	$\Delta H^0_{f(C_n)}$ kcal mol^{-1} atom^{-1})	E_b (eV)	IP (eV)	E_g (eV)
Nanocluster (9,0) $d = 7.20$ Å						
36 ($Z6h_u$)	2.51	−42.37	25.11	6.34	7.03	1.91
54 ($Z6d_u$)	4.94	−42.24	28.13	6.24	6.94	0.34
144 ($Z6h_u$)	15.50	−42.85	14.09	6.81	6.56	0.00
180 ($Z6h_u$)	19.72	−42.92	12.49	6.89	6.56	0.00
198 ($Z6d_u$)	21.84	−42.95	11.80	6.92	6.56	0.00
288 ($Z6h_u$)	32.42	−43.03	9.96	6.70	6.56	0.00
414 ($Z6d_u$)	46.63	−43.08	8.81	7.05	6.56	0.00
Nanocluster (6,0) $d = 4.84$ Å						
24 ($Z6h_g$)	2.73	−42.13	30.59	6.1	6.23	0.25
60 ($Z6d_g$)	9.18	−42.48	22.65	6.45	6.62	0.08
72 ($Z6h_g$)	11.31	−42.58	20.37	6.54	6.62	0.17
120 ($Z6h_g$)	19.80	−42.77	15.92	6.74	6.63	0.35
252 ($Z6d_g$)	43.21	−42.92	12.49	6.89	6.57	0.28
264 ($Z6h_u$)	45.33	−42.93	12.35	6.89	6.55	0.26

Source: Reproduced with permission from Glukhova [5].

Case Study 1: Comparison of Structural Characteristics between Carbon Nanotubes and Fullerenes

- Carbon nanotube structure was described previously by Wilder *et al.* [16]. According to this study, carbon nanotubes can be thought of as graphitic sheets with a hexagonal lattice that have been wrapped up into a seamless cylinder. Electronic and bandgap properties were described depending on their structural features.
- Depending on the number of sheets, carbon nanotubes are classified as SWCNT and MWCNT.
- The direction of vectors in hexagonal carbon lattice determines the types of carbon nanotubes, such as zigzag, armchair, and chiral nanotubes.
- Open structures of fullerene were studied by Prato and reported in the [11]. According to this study, there are several structures of fullerene molecules, such as open types, three- to six-membered rings, structures with hole, and heterofullerenes.
- Linking two fullerene molecules results in the formation of clusters with different structures and energies, which was studied by Krylova *et al.*, and reported in the [12]. According to this study, right angles between the C—C bonds are energetically unfavorable, and the reduction in the energy of clusters in the process of relaxation is connected with the optimization of valence angles, which leads to a reduction in the symmetry of clusters.

Control Questions

1) Define dispersive systems and types of dispersive systems.
2) Describe classification of dispersive systems according to their size.
3) Describe classification of dispersive systems according to their aggregate states.
4) Discuss classification of dispersive systems according to their dimensions.
5) Define fullerenes and their structural characteristics.
6) Describe the history of fullerenes.
7) Tell about the classification of fullerenes and criteria on which the classification was based.
8) Define tetrahedral fullerenes and their characteristics.
9) Describe icosahedral fullerenes and their characteristics.
10) Define multilayered fullerenes and their difference from other fullerene types.
11) Describe the difference between fullerenes with non-central effect and other fullerene types.
12) Tell about the physical properties of fullerenes.
13) Define carbon nanotubes and tell about their difference from fullerenes.

14) Describe the types of nanotubes according to the position of achiral vector.
15) What is the difference between zigzag, armchair, and chiral nanotubes?
16) Classify carbon nanotubes according to the number of layers.
17) Tell about mechanical properties of carbon nanotubes.
18) What kind of physical parameters are carbon nanotubes exhibiting?

References

1 Ryzhonkov, D.I., Levina, V.V., and Dzidziguri, E.L. (2008) *Nanomaterials, BINOM*, BKL Publishers, Moscow.

2 Anischik, V.M., Borisenko, V.E., Jdanok, S.A., Tolochko, N.K., and Fedosyuk, V.M (2008). *Nanomaterialy i nanotehnologii*, ISBN 978-985-476-618-8, National Academy of Science, Belorussia Republic.

3 Gleiter, H. (1997) Nanostructured materials. *Acta Metall. Sin.*, **33** (2), 165–174.

4 Gogotsi, Y. (2015) Not just graphene: the wonderful world of carbon and related nanomaterials. *MRS Bull.*, **40** (12), p. 1110–1121.

5 Glukhova, O.E. (2014) Carbon Nanoclusters, Structure, Classification, Size Effects, Lectures, http://nanokvazar.ru/uploads/files/learning/glukhova_1_1 .pdf (accessed 30 December 2016).

6 Kustov, E.F., Nefedov, V.I., Kalinin, A.V. *et al.* (2008) *Russ. J. Inorg. Chem.* **53**: 1384. doi:10.1134/S0036023608090076.

7 Glukhova, O.E., Kolesnikova, A.S., Slepchenkov, M.M., and Shunaev, V.V. (2014) Moving of fullerene between potential wells in the external icosahedral shell. *J. Comput. Chem.*, **35**, 1270–1277.

8 Glukhova, O.E. (2012) *Classification of the Achiral Tubular Nanoclusters, Carbon Nanotubes: Synthesis and Properties*, Nanotechnology Science and Technology, Nova Science Publishers, pp. 319–336.

9 Kanoun, O. *et al* (2014) Flexible carbon nanotube films for high performance strain sensors. *Sensors*, **14**, 10042–10071.

10 Glukhova, O.E., Druzhinin, A.A., Zhbanov, A.I. and Rezkov, A.G. (2005) Structure of High-Symmetry Fullerenes. *Journal of Structural Chemistry*, Vol. **46**, No. 3, pp. 501–507.

11 Glukhova, O.E. and Terentév, O.A. (2006) Theoretical study of the dependences of the young's and torsion moduli of thin single-layer carbon zigzag and armchair nanotubes on the geometric parameters. *Phys. Solid State*, **48** (7), 1411–1417.

12 Dresselhaus, M.S., Dresselhaus, G., and Avouris, P. (2001) *Carbon Nanotubes, Synthesis, Structure, Properties, and Applications*, Springer-Verlag, ISBN: 978-3-540-41086-7.

13 Prato, M. (1997) Fullerene chemistry for materials science and applications. *J. Mater. Chem.*, **7** (7), 1097–1109.

14 Krylova, K.A., Baimova, Y.A., Dmitriev, S.V. *et al* (2016) Calculation of the structure of carbon clusters based on fullerene-like C_{24} and C_{48} molecules. *Phys. Solid State*, **58** (2), 394–401.

15 Glukhova, O.E. (2014) Carbon Nanoclusters, Structure, Classification, Size Effects, Lectures, http://nanokvazar.ru/uploads/files/learning/glukhova_1_2.pdf (accessed 30 December 2016).

16 Wilder, J.W.G. *et al* (1998) *Nature*, **391**, 59–62.

Further Reading

Brinkmann, G. and Dress, A.W.M. (1997) A constructive enumeration of fullerenes. *J. Algorithms*, **2**, 345–358.

Choudhary, V. and Gupta, A. (2011) Polymer/carbon nanotube nanocomposites, in *Carbon Nanotubes – Polymer Nanocomposites* (ed. S. Yellampalli), InTech, doi: 10.5772/18423.

Maniwa, Y., Kataura, H., Matsuda, K., and Okabe, Y. (2003) A one-dimensional Ising model for C70 molecular ordering in C70-peapods. *New J. Phys.*, **5**, 127.1–127.5.

Pichler, T., Liu, X., Knupfer, M., and Fink, J. (2003) Electronic properties of intercalated single-wall carbon nanotubes and C60 peapods. *New J. Phys.*, **5**, 156.1–156.23.

Online Sources

Glukhova Research Group. http://nanokvazar.ru/en (accessed 30 December 2016).

MPI-FKF http://www2.fkf.mpg.de/andersen/fullerene/symmetry.html#top (accessed 30 December 2016).

3

Nanocomposite Materials and Their Physical Property Features

Translated materials from the original work of Ryzhonkov, D.I., Levina, V.V. and Dzidziguri, E.L. were used in this chapter.

Success is getting what you want; happiness wants what you get.
Andrew Carnegie, industrialist (1835–1919)

3.1 Nanocomposite Materials

Nanocomposite materials are those materials consisting of several materials different in composition or shape in a macro scale in order to obtain specific properties or characteristics of the final material. A large variety of metal oxide mesocrystals with their interior particle [1] are represented in Figure 3.1. The formation of these nanomaterials depends on the physical and chemical properties of the initial precursors [2].

3.2 Size Dependence as Nanomaterial Property

Size dependence is the change in any property of a solid material during the sequential decrease of its size. First of all, it relates to the commensurability of material geometric sizes with specific range (or length) of its physical properties, for example, the mean free path of charge carriers, de Broglie wavelength, and the diffusion path length. The change in material property might be a result of the increase in surface effects. Size effects can be described in classical and quantum approximations [2].

In *classical* consideration, macroscopic properties and material characteristics are determined by macroscopic mass, charges, and currents within material volume and atomic sizes. As an example of classical size effect, oscillation phenomenon during electrical conductivity can be observed in strong magnetic field, and in case when material size is comparable with conducting electrons' orbital diameters. Orbit, depending on the field quantity, might be included or not within the sample. In this case, there is an oscillation of electrical conductivity during the change in magnetic field value. Also, classical size effects occur in nanomaterials. It was found that nearly all mechanical and physical properties of a material

Nano- and Biomaterials: Compounds, Properties, Characterization, and Applications,
First Edition. Zhypargul Abdullaeva.

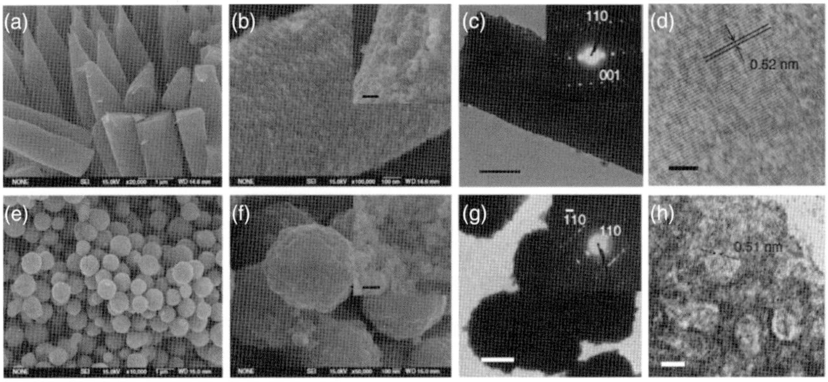

Figure 3.1 Pure metal oxide mesocrystals. (a, b) FESEM images of ZnO. Inset of the panel (c) shows the interior particles at the broken part. Scale bars: 1 mm and 100 nm for (a) and (b), respectively. (c) TEM image of ZnO. Scale bar: 500 nm. (d) HRTEM image of ZnO. Scale bar: 5 nm. (e, f) FESEM image of CuO. Inset of the panel (f) shows the interior particles at the broken part. Scale bars: 1 mm and 100 nm for (e) and (f), respectively. (g) TEM image of CuO. Scale bar: 500 nm. (h) HRTEM image of CuO. Scale bar: 5 nm. SAED patterns (insets of TEM images) show the single-crystal diffraction. (Reprinted by permission from Macmillan Publishers Ltd: [Nature Communications, 5, 3038] Bian 2014 [1]. Reproduced with permission of Nature Publishing Group.)

change as a result of a decrease in its linear sizes. In particular, the hardness of nanomaterials increases to the extent that the size of separate grains becomes nanosized. For dispersive materials, there is significant change in resistivity, magnetic properties, coefficient of volume expansion, and so on. The appearance of quantum size effects is observed when the geometric size of the material (small particles, diameter of wires, film thickness) becomes comparable with de Broglie wavelength of λ – electrons [2]:

$$\lambda = h/mv \tag{3.1}$$

where h is Planck's constant, m is the electron mass, and v is the electron speed. In metal nanoparticles, quantum size effect is bound with distance change between the energetic levels of the electron. As the number of conducting electrons in a particle decreases, the distance between energetic levels increases, becoming comparable with heat energy. Considering the number of atoms in isolated system as N, the distance δ between energy levels will be equal to [2]

$$\delta \sim E_F/N \tag{3.2}$$

where E_F is the Fermi energy, which can be comparable with the heat energy, E_{heat}. This allows to determine the particle size, during which quantum size effects come out. For metals, the Fermi energy is near to 10 eV, at the temperature of 300 K, $\delta = E_{heat} \approx 0.025$ eV. $N \approx 400$ atoms, which agree with the particle diameter of 2 nm.

3.3 Thermodynamical Features of Nanomaterials

One of the distinctive features for nano condition is the existence of large grain boundaries, or the surface of a material. As it is known from classical thermodynamics, the change in the internal energy of system dU is determined by the amount of heat δQ and work δA:

$$dU = \delta Q - \delta A \tag{3.3}$$

Transmitted to the system, the amount of heat is determined by the function of $T\,dS$, where T is temperature and dS is entropy change. Work done by the nanomedium system can be defined by two ways: firstly, the outer pressure forces pdV, where p is the pressure and dV is the volume change, and secondly, by the surface tension during formation of a new surface with S area equal to $-\sigma ds$, where δ is the surface tension; an increase in surface area increases the energy of the system. The total equation to calculate the inner energy change for dispersive system is the following:

$$dU = T\ dS - p\ dV + \sigma\ ds \tag{3.4}$$

Let us determine the Helmholtz and Gibbs free energies for nanomediums. In thermodynamics, the Helmholtz function is defined as $F = U - TS$, and its differential is accordingly equal to

$$dF = dU - T\ dS - S\ dT \tag{3.5}$$

Substituting dU from Eq. (3.4), the following equation can be obtained:

$$dF = p\ dV + \sigma\ ds - S\ dT \tag{3.6}$$

By this way, at constant temperature conditions, the differential for the Helmholtz function is determined by the following formula:

$$dF = p\ dV + \sigma\ ds \tag{3.7}$$

The Gibbs function according to the first law of thermodynamics is defined as $G = H - TS$, where H is the enthalpy (equal to $H = U + pV$). Accordingly, the Gibbs function differential will be equal to

$$dG = dU + p\ dV + V\ dp - T\ dS - S\ dT \tag{3.8}$$

With Eq. (3.4), the following equation is derived:

$$dG = -S\ dT + V\ dp + \sigma\ ds \tag{3.9}$$

Consequently, under constant pressure and temperature conditions, because of the increase in surface area, the increase in Gibbs free energy in nanomediums will be equal to

$$dG = \sigma\ ds \tag{3.10}$$

The approximations obtained showed that in equal conditions, nanomediums possess large energy value of $\sigma s\ ds$ compared with those of bulk materials. In other words, at constant temperature and pressure conditions, the energy of nanomediums is reduced due to the reduction of surface area. Therefore, dispersive phase tending to decrease its own energy must spontaneously aggregate. It can be summarized that the difference of the properties of nanomaterials from that of the bulk materials at a significant level is caused by the increase in surface as a result of the decrease in its linear sizes.

3.4 Phase Equilibrium Changes in Nano-sized Systems

Studies showed that in nanosized materials there are distinctive phase conditions compared with the bulk materials. Large experimental data materials, which had been collected recently, showed changes in phase conditions in nanomaterials: transfer in the melting temperature and polymorphic changes, stabilization of equilibrium states, and phase formations, which are not observed in the bulk materials. In the first approximation, phase condition changes can be explained by the following way: if phase 1 and phase 2 exist in the bulk material and phase 1 is stable at dependent temperature, that is, $F_v^1 < F_v^2$ (where F_v is the volume for free energy), in consideration of free energy, the following condition might be realized:

$$F_v^1 + F_s^1 > F_v^2 + F_s^2 \tag{3.11}$$

where F_s is the surface for free energy. In this case, phase 2 will be stable. Thus, for solid nanomaterial, equilibrium boundary with liquid and gas must shift to low-temperature regions, as in the dotted line in Figure 3.2.

The equilibrium state of solid phase depends on the radius and can be defined by a balance between forces that tend to widen and press the nanoparticle. It is clear that the resulting inward force is determined by the sum of the outer pressure p_{outer} and surface tension. Let us imagine that the particles have a spherical shape. In this case, the surface energy is equal to $4\pi r^2\sigma$. To determine the surface tension energy, the necessary work will be calculated for stretching the given surface to dr. It is equal to $d(\sigma s)$ or $8\pi\sigma r\ dr$. From another point of view, the inner pressure of the particle will prevent its pressing. If the inner pressure is p_{inner}, the outer force for nanoparticle with r radius is equal to

$$4\pi r^2 p_{\text{inner}} = 4\pi r^2 p_{\text{outer}} + 8\pi r\sigma \tag{3.12}$$

And after transitions,

$$p_{\text{inner}} - p_{\text{outer}} = \Delta p = 2\sigma/r \tag{3.13}$$

The as-obtained equation is called *Laplace* equation, showing that the pressure inside the curved surface is always larger than the outer pressure. This difference falls down to zero if the curve radius became unlimitedly large, that is, in the case of a flat surface. Nanoparticles exhibit very large curve radius; that is why their pressure differences are also large. First of all, solid nanoparticles are not always in

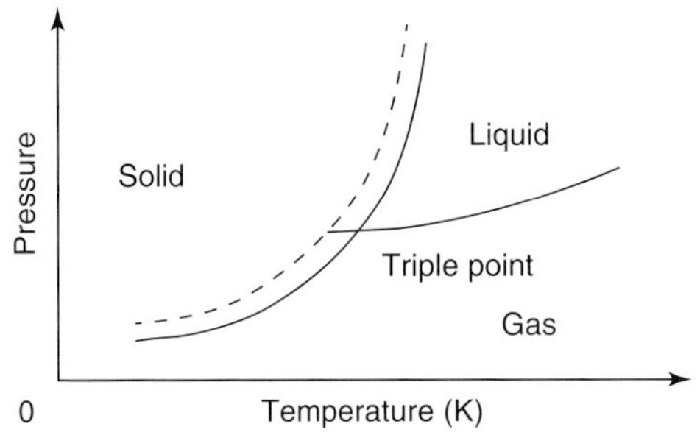

Figure 3.2 Phase diagram of a substance: straight line – phase equilibrium boundaries for large crystal material; dotted line – phase equilibrium boundaries for nanomaterials (Reproduced with permission of BKL Publishers).

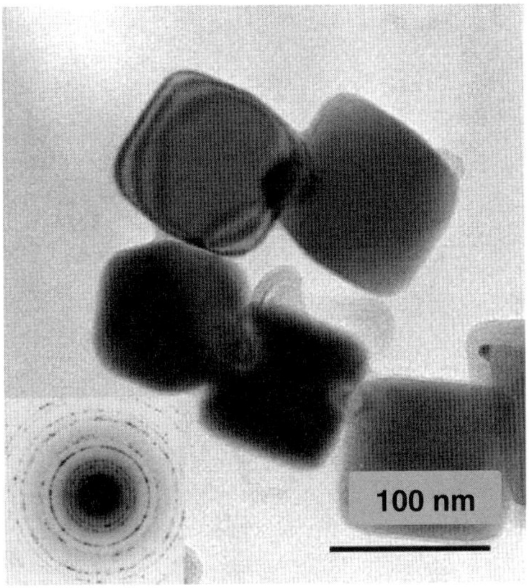

Figure 3.3 TEM image of the cobalt oxide nanoparticles (Reproduced with permission of BKL Publishers).

spherical shape. Often, they have a polygonal structure (see Figure 3.3), showing the particle with flat surface.

3.5 Melting Temperature Changes in Nanomaterials

According to the laws of thermodynamics, the substance should melt and crystallize at the same temperature. But this law refers only to the condition when liquid is in equilibrium state. In practice, under such conditions, liquid crystallizes at significantly cool temperatures. Liquid never becomes solid at thermodynamically stable temperature. To initiate the crystallization process, energetical fluctuations that tend toward cooling should occur. But the melting temperature of bulk material will remain within the tabulated value. For nanosized crystals however, it was observed that they can melt at lower temperatures than their tabulated values. The following definition can be made: the smaller the size, the lower the melting temperature of nanomaterials is. In other words, two nanoparticles of the same substance but with different radii will melt in different temperatures.

By melting the surface energy of material will decrease by about 10%. This means that half of the released surface energy can be utilized to melt that material. The amount of the released energy ΔW_s is equal to the product of materials surface S and change of surface energy during melting $\Delta\sigma$: $\Delta T = T_m - T$, where T_m is the tabulated melting temperature and T is the real melting temperature of nanomaterial.

3.5.1 Polymorphic Characteristic Changes in Nanosystems

It is well known that every system tends to decrease its own energy. As nanomaterials have high surface energy, it is preferable to form low surface energy phases and more packed (tight) lattice, that is, low amount of ω per one atom. For example, from well-known crystal lattices of metals (FCC and BCC), FCC has advantages due to its smaller specific volume and surface energy. That is why during the decrease of nanomaterial size, FCC lattice will remain stable, but BCC lattice will undergo phase transitions with significant possibility. So, stability of grain of close-packed structure should shift toward the region at cold temperatures. This is the result of polymorphic transformation temperature changes, fixation of metastable conditions, or phase formations, which are not characteristics of bulk materials. For example, in pure Fe, stabilization of γ-phase is much difficult, because the allotropic transformation temperature is notably high −911 °C. In the nano state, the electrolytic appearance of γ-Fe particles with particle diameter of 20 nm was seen. Fe nanopowder with a size of 20–40 nm, obtained by gas pyrolysis, contained 70.6% of FCC phase, and the rest was α-Fe. In the nanocrystal layer, obtained by radiation of bulk metal using high-current electron beam, the γ-Fe grains with average particle size of 30 nm were also detected.

At low temperature, catalytic reduction of Mo from the Mo_2O_3 formation of FCC phase lattice was experimentally found, while at high temperatures, usual BCC phase Mo forms.

However, some unexpected results are found. During research, the formation of nano-Co with BCC structure instead of stable FCC structure was observed. This fact is explained by stabilization of BCC phase in thin sheets with thickness of several hundreds angstrom and by surface tension with substrate. More thick layers of BCC-Co might be stabilized by imperfections in structure. Also it was found that Ni powder with size less than 4 nm, obtained by reduction of sodium hydroxide (NaOH) using the Ni(II) salt in organic solvent, represented a FCC phase.

3.6 Structure of Nano-sized Materials

The structure of nano-sized materials has been studied and reported by various groups in the field of nanoscience and nanotechnology. Here, the dependence of crystal lattice on material size is described. Nanomaterial research showed opposite effect of the diameter on the structural characteristics of materials. Decrease in crystal lattice (inter-atom distance) was observed in a number of experiments. The reason for the structural changes in nanomaterials is not fully determined. However, several hypotheses exist. The first is the most famous opinion explaining the change in crystal lattice $\Delta a/a$ as a result of excess *Laplace pressure* leading to pressure of material's inner layers.

For maximal exclusion of factors affecting the structure of materials, several experiments were conducted on Fe, Co, Ni, Cu, Mo, and W metals, which were obtained by chemical dispersion methods. Final product in this method can be achieved through synthesis during continuous reduction at increased temperatures. As a result, the material structure has time for relaxation. That is why nanopowders obtained by this method have more equal structure, maximally free from inner stress, deformation, and defects (Figure 3.4). In addition, this is one of the genuine methods for nanomaterial synthesis. Experimental results showed that crystal lattice of metal nanopowders does not depend on particle radius (see Table 3.1).

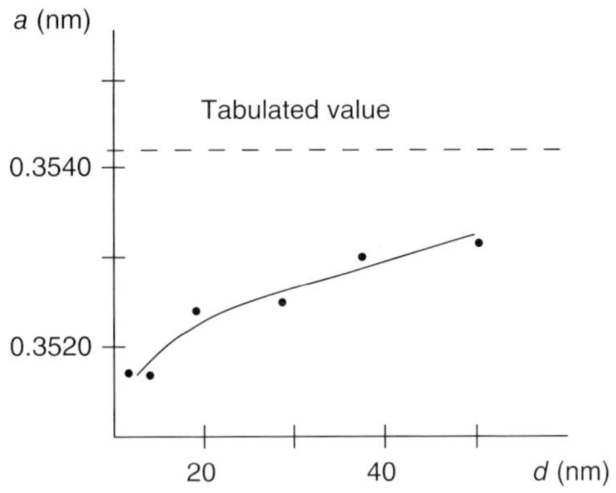

Figure 3.4 Size dependence in the Co nanoparticle lattice parameter (Reproduced with permission of BKL Publishers).

Table 3.1 Crystal lattice and average crystallite size for Ni nanopowders [2].

Metallization T (°C)	Conditions Time (min)	Lattice period, a (nm)	Average crystallite size (nm)
200	60	0.35188	22
250	60	0.35188	34
260	60	0.35192	36
300	60	0.35192	49
360	60	0.35192	49
500	60	0.35192	49
500	180	0.35192	49
650	60	0.35185	52
650	120	0.35185	48
650	200	0.35185	56

According to another hypothesis, shortening in inter-atomic distances in nanoparticles might be due to change in crystal lattice. As it is known, in FCC structure, 12 closer atoms will form coordinate polyhedron, named as cubic octahedron (Figure 3.5). In this geometric figure, all directions are not equal. Deformation of cubic octahedron into icosahedron will occur by insignificant atomic transformations: decrease in distance from center to top for 1.052 times and breaking of cube borders in diagonals. Breaking line became icosahedron base, shortening to 1.952 times. After deformation, each top vertex of the formed icosahedron matches well with five true polyhedrons. Packing thickness in icosahedron is 89%. That is why possessing an icosahedron structure is more reasonable for nanomaterials. Calculations showed that particles consisting of 150–300 atoms should have an icosahedron structure. And only larger formations will change their structure to FCC. Obviously, in particles with 5 nm in size, fifth-order structure was observed experimentally. Works are done on the following nanomaterials: Al–Cu, Au–Cu, Al–Mn, Mg–Zn, Pd–U–Si, and other double- and triple-component alloys. It should be noted that theoretical

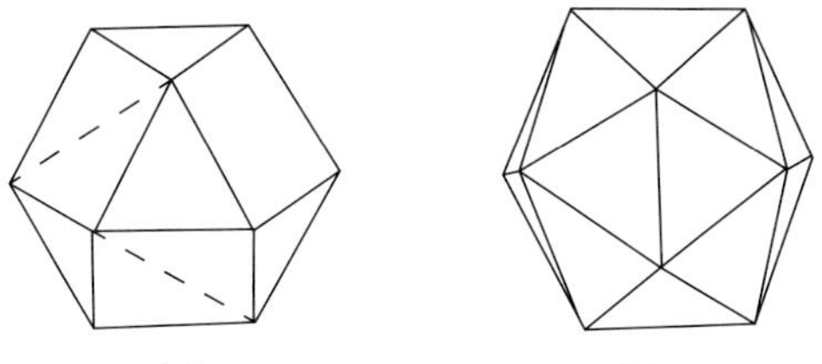

Figure 3.5 Coordinate polyhedrons. (a) Cubic octahedron; (b) icosahedron (Reproduced with permission of BKL Publishers).

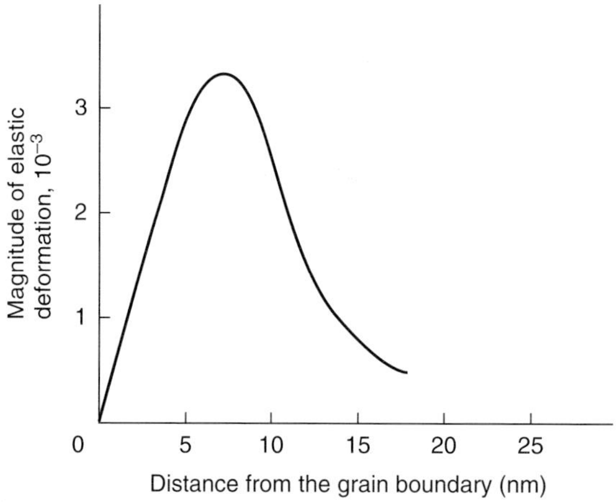

Figure 3.6 Field distribution of internal stress depending on the distance from grain boundary (Reproduced with permission of BKL Publishers).

calculations predict possibility of keeping the pentagonal symmetry in larger particles with size of 10–13 nm. Change in symmetry can explain the decrease of lattice period in nanomediums, because inter-atomic distances in icosahedron are less than in FCC structure for 1.052 times. But, in most cases, nanomaterials have lattice structure under bulk condition. And, in this lattice structures, a decrease in lattice periods is seen.

Another theory explains the distortion of lattice structure, due to the formation of *surface relaxation* of nanomaterials. Atoms from the surface layer have few neighboring atoms, located on one side. Such atomic structure disturbs equilibrium and symmetry in the distribution of forces and changes the ordering in surface regions. Further, this can cause shear and angular deformations in inter-atomic region on the entire volume of nanoparticle and result in the change in inter-atomic distances. For metals this inter-atomic distance is equal to 1–1.5 nm. Thus, atoms of the surface layer form the surface "volume" in the form of a sphere, with thickness of five inter-atomic distances.

The above results were confirmed for materials exposed to intensive plastic deformation. Estimation showed that the distribution of elastic deformation depending on the grain boundary distance is heterogeneous. Figure 3.6 shows the curve with a maximum in border region and exponential slump at 10 nm distance.

Also, there is a hypothesis explaining the decrease of lattice periods in nanomaterials, thermal vacancy formation, and growth of their quantity during the decrease of particle size. The concentration of vacancies in the crystal lattice at pre-melting temperatures is less: $c_0 \approx 10^{-3}$–10^{-4}.

3.7 Crystal Lattice Defects in Nanomaterials

The previous chapter discussed the vacancy dislocations that are not characteristic of nanomaterial structures. As HRTEM observation results showed, the main defects exhibited in nanomaterials are singular (Figure 3.7) or multiple twinning plane (Figure 3.8), cleaving nanoparticle by its diameter as well as its straight counterparts, forming the tertiary or quinary joints (Figure 3.9).

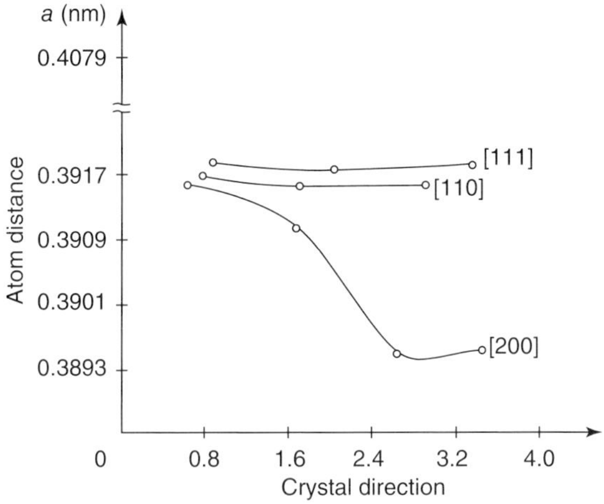

Figure 3.7 Change in atom distance in various crystallographic directions from the center to the edge of 1047th atomic Au (gold) particle (Reproduced with permission of BKL Publishers).

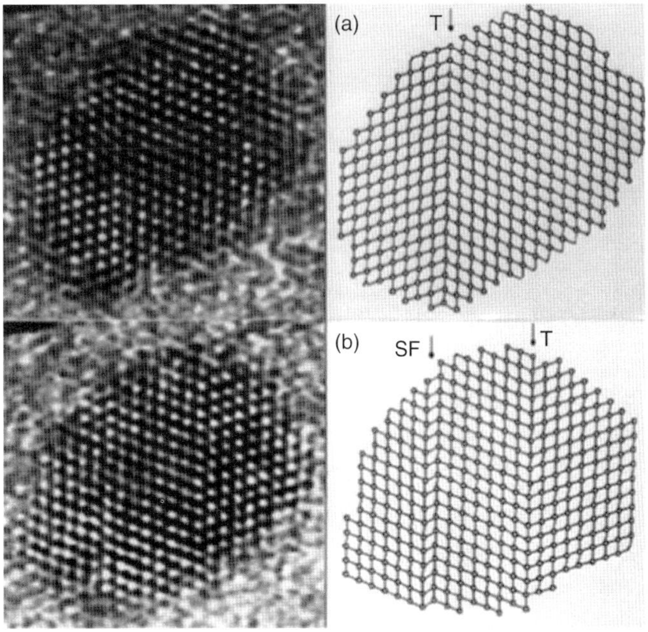

Figure 3.8 Microphotography and schematics of Ag nanomaterial, containing one (a) and two (b) surface counterparts (Reproduced with permission of BKL Publishers).

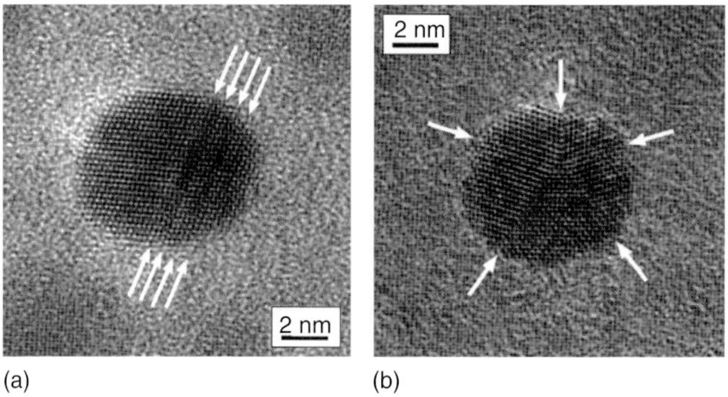

Figure 3.9 Microphotographs of silver nanoparticle: (a) containing the multiple-twin planes; (b) containing the multiple joints of its straight counterparts (Reproduced with permission of BKL Publishers).

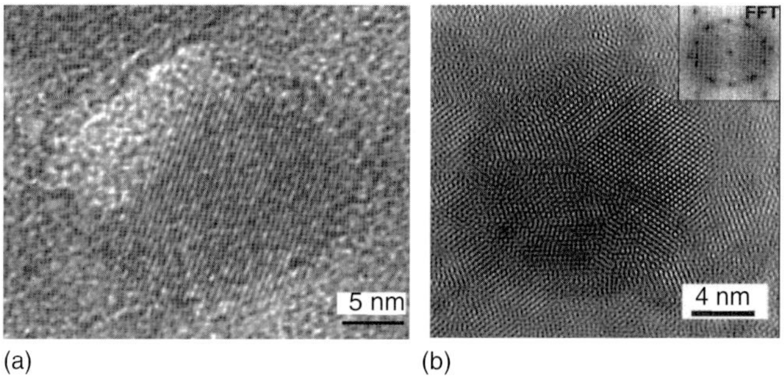

Figure 3.10 Microphotographs: (a) monocrystal Si particle; (b) nanoparticle with block structure (Reproduced with permission of BKL Publishers).

It was observed that nanoparticles smaller than 20 nm are always monocrystals (Figure 3.10a) or have a block structure without large angular borders (Figure 3.10b).

3.8 Microdistorsions of Crystal Lattice in Nanomaterials

As nanoparticles are synthesized in non-equilibrium state, they exhibit high level of microdistorsions in their crystal lattice. In particular, in nanomaterials obtained by intensive plastic deformation, microdistorsions of $(\Delta a/a) = 10^{-1}$–10^{-2} order were observed, whereas in metal nanopowders, synthesized by chemical dispersion method, microdistorsions were less than $(\Delta a/a) = 10^{-4}$, which corresponds to the value of a given property in annealed large crystal materials. From these facts, it can be assumed that the level of microdistorsions in a crystal lattice can be a result of synthesis of nanomaterial but not the property characterizing exactly the nanomaterial structure. For example, during annealing of samples through intensive plastic deformation, a significant decrease in microdistorsion level will occur (see Figure 3.11), but grain size will remain stable.

Under various synthesis conditions, structural changes in metal nanopowders obtained by chemical dispersion method were observed. Figure 3.12 represents

Figure 3.11 Change in microdistorsions in nanomaterials, obtained by intensive plastic deformation, depending on the annealing temperature (Reproduced with permission of BKL Publishers).

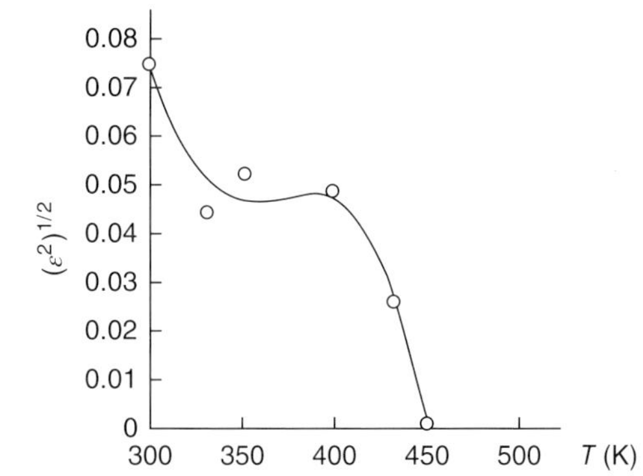

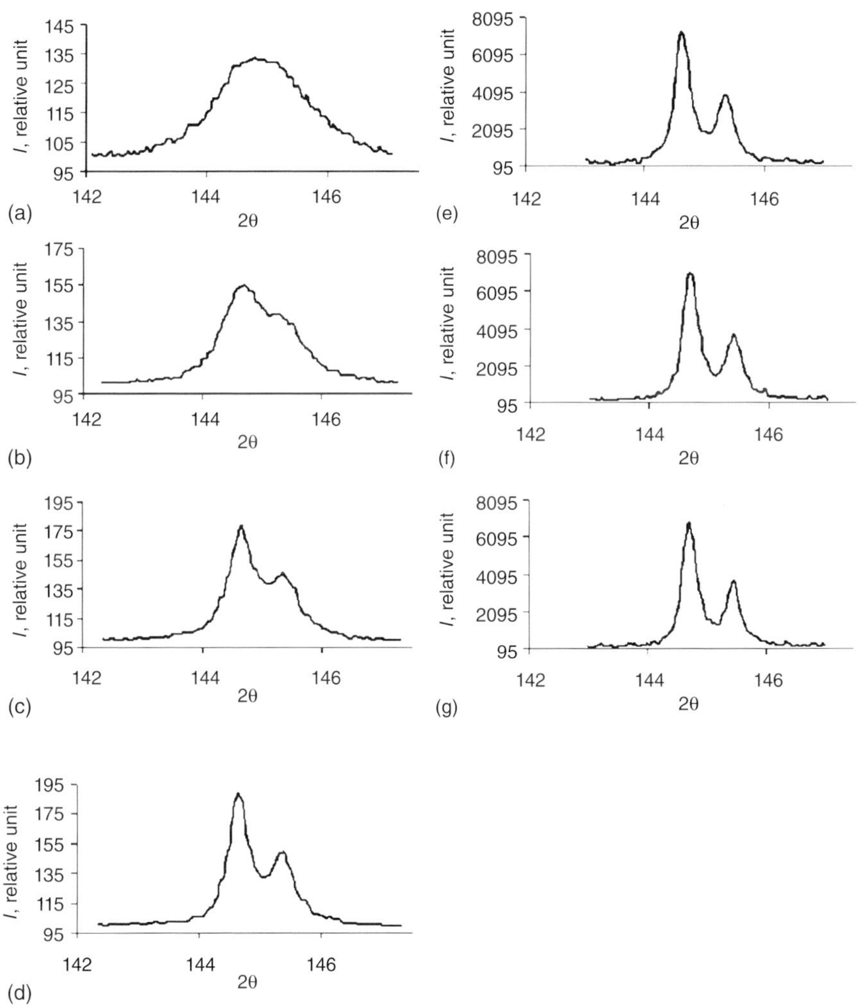

Figure 3.12 Diffractograms of FCC (222) phase Ni, reduced at various temperatures during 1 h: (a) 200 °C; (b) 250 °C; (c) 300 °C; (d) 360 °C; (e) 500 °C; (f) 650 °C; and (g) 650 °C with reduction time of 200 min (Reproduced with permission of BKL Publishers).

Table 3.2 Results of diffraction profile broadening analysis for metal nanopowders.

Sample	Metallization	Conditions	β_2/β_1	$\cos\theta_1/\cos\theta_2$ mass	$\text{tg}\,\theta_2/\text{tg}\,\theta_1$ mass
	Reduction temperature (°C)	Curing time (min)			
Fe	470	65	0.8	2.9	5.8
W	740	60	0.98	1.8	3.6
Cu	140	120	1.5	2.8	5.6
Ni	260	60	2.6	2.85	5.7
Mo	700	120	1.31	1.8	3.6

Source: Ryzhonkov *et al.* 2008 [2]. (Reproduced with permission of BKL Publishers).

large angular peaks for Ni nanopowders obtained at various temperatures within 1 h. As it is seen from the figure, increase in temperature at reduction time leads to the narrowing of intensity maximums and division of α-doublet, which indicates a decrease of microdistorsion in materials structure.

X-ray diffraction is one of the methods for studying microdistorsions. As it is known, if the physical broadening ratio of two diffraction levels from one surface of β_2 and β_1 is equal to the tangents of appropriate diffraction angles of θ_2 and θ_1, the broadening of diffraction lines by microdistorsions is

$$\beta_2/\beta_1 = \text{tg}\theta_2/\text{tg}\theta_1 \tag{3.14}$$

In such case, when relation of broadenings is close to inverse ratio of cos, the broadening of diffraction lines will result by dispersity:

$$\beta_2/\beta_1 = \cos\theta_1/\cos\theta_2 \tag{3.15}$$

During the study of physical broadening diffraction maxima for nanometals obtained by chemical dispersion method, peculiarity, which is impossible from the kinematic theory of dispersion, was observed: the ratio of two broadening diffraction levels from one surface in the given samples (Table 3.2) is much less than inverse ratio of cos.

The given results do not have satisfactory explanation in the present time.

3.9 Consolidation of Nano-sized Powders

In most nanomaterial-obtaining methods, powders are a final product. In some materials, it is difficult and sometimes impossible to create nanostructures in large volume. To obtain bulk materials from nanopowders, first of all, different variants of pressing method are used. However, for practical purposes, compact products consisting of nano-sized morphological elements are usually in demand, hence the necessity in obtaining consolidated products from nanopowders. This can be achieved by using different technological processes: pressing, sintering, rolling, and extrusion.

In practice, an increase in the dispersity of powders is followed by a significant decrease in their compactability during pressing. This is related to an increase in adhesive and autohesive activity and a tendency toward aggregation with a decrease in particle size.

The pressing of nanopowders essentially depends on particle size distribution, specific surface area, surface condition, presence of adsorbents, defects, and agglomeration. Therefore obtaining bulk materials from nanopowders is an independent task. *Pressing* is defined as technological formation of powder with different shapes, sizes, and thicknesses under pressure. All pressing methods can be divided into two groups: statistical and dynamical. The two groups vary:

- According to the process temperature: cold and hot pressing
- According to the character of loading stress: single axial, double axial, and comprehensive (isostatic)

In case of necessity, together with pressing, other processing types are used. For example, static cold pressing is often combined with sintering, which in turn can be isothermal and non-isothermal. To increase process effect, during consolidation of nanopowders, ultrasound, microwave, electric impulse, plasma, laser, and radiation can be applied. For example, dynamical pressing might be magneto-impulsive, detonative, and electro-hydraulic. Static *single-axial* pressing can be expressed schematically (Figure 3.13).

Powder is inserted inside a press-form, which is located in a vacuum chamber. After pumping, the pressing is conducted in vacuum. By this method, nanopowder mixture ($Dy_2O_3 + TiO_2$) is compacted. The double-axial press-forms are used for compacting products, which have the height to transverse dimension ratio of more than one. In this case, force is applied to the upper or lower punches, or construction includes mobility of the matrix.

Isostatic shaping is based on nanopowder consolidation in hydrostatic compression conditions. Several kinds of this method were developed. As an example, hydrostatic pressing given in Figure 3.14 is discussed.

To conduct this process, elastic or resin shell is filled with powder, which is inserted in the working chamber. The apparatus will be closed hermetically in order to provide the required pressure inside the chamber. Liquid (oil, water, or glycerin) comprehensively and equally presses the powder, thus providing shape to the product.

Gas static pressing is one of the shaping methods by comprehensive pressing, in which interaction is generated by gas (helium, argon, and so on) (Figure 3.15).

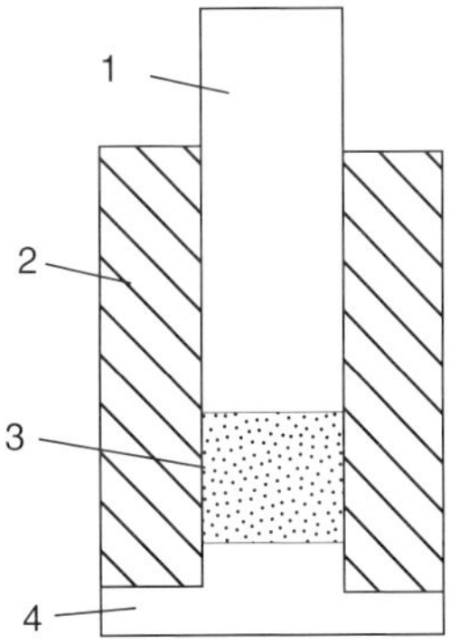

Figure 3.13 Schematics of the press-form: 1 – upper punch; 2 – matrix; 3 – pressing powder; 4 – lower punch (Reproduced with permission of BKL Publishers).

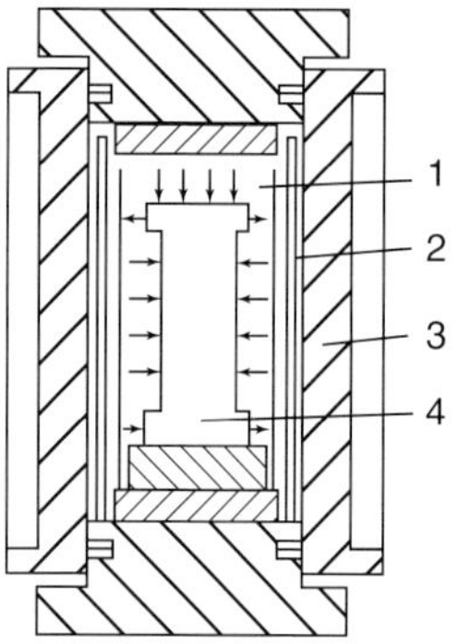

Figure 3.14 Schematic for shaping of nanopowder by hydrostatical pressing: 1 – heater; 2 – insulating layer; 3 – working chamber; 4 – sample of powder shell (Reproduced with permission of BKL Publishers).

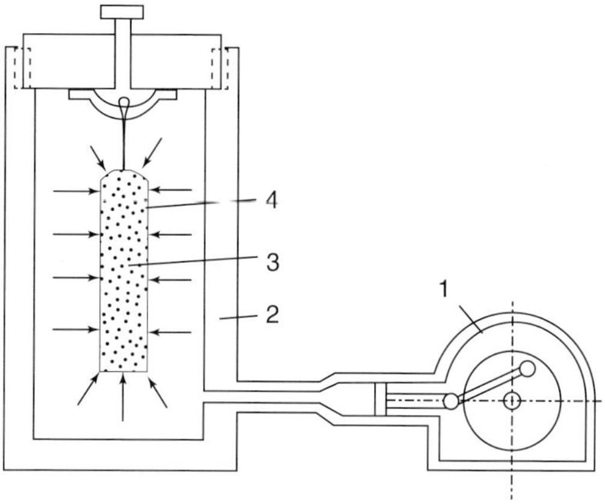

Figure 3.15 Working chamber equipment for gas static shaping of nanomaterials: 1 – high-pressure pump; 2 – insulating layer; 3 – powder; 4 – elastic shell (Reproduced with permission of BKL Publishers).

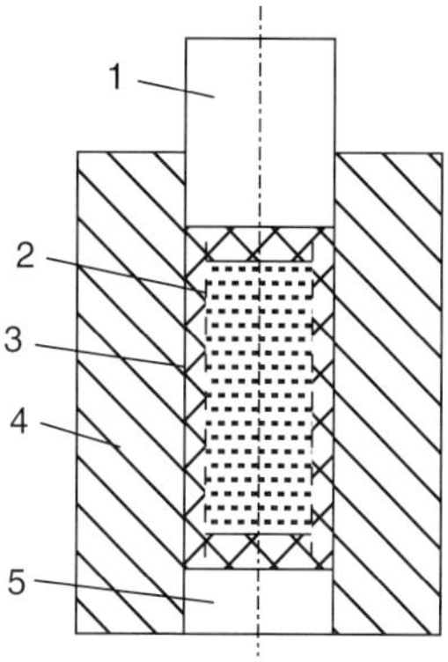

Figure 3.16 Schematic of isostatic pressing in elastic shell: 1 – pressing punch; 2 – powder; 3 – elastic shell; 4 – matrix of press shape; 5 – lower punch (Reproduced with permission of BKL Publishers).

As a rule, rather than powder, a sample preliminarily obtained undergoes such pressing process.

Pressing in elastic shells is one kind of isostatic pressing. In this method, elastic shells filled with initial powder are inserted in one-sided or double-sided press-form. Paraffin, wax, gelatin, epoxy resins, or resin mass is used as material for shell preparation (Figure 3.16).

Dynamical pressing is based on the use of shock waves, the source of which might be a hydraulic discharge from a high-voltage battery capacitor, with a gap in water between two electrodes, magnetic impulse field, pressed hot gases and liquids, and detonating materials.

Dynamic pressing methods for nanopowders effectively overcome the particle adhesion and coupling forces caused by fast movement of powder medium. This allows greater thickness of the final material than that of static methods at the same pressure level. Also, under an impulse load, the higher pressures are realized, which gives an opportunity to use less expensive equipment, unlike in static methods. Moreover, using soft compression waves with gradual rise and fall of pressure allows exclusion of microcracks and reaching of maximal close packing of particles.

In *magneto-impulse pressing*, the diamagnetic effect of pushing the conductor from the magnetic impulse field is used. Mechanical impulse force will be generated inside the press-form resulting from interactions between magnetic impulse inductor fields and conducting surface hub. An inductor is a flat spiral made of copper tape and is part of impulse generator circuit. An electrical circuit concentrator is ejected from the magnetic field zone and compresses the powder. An impulse is several microseconds and pressure is 1–2 GPa. Figure 3.17 presents schematic of magneto-impulse pressing. Here the press-form is inserted into a vacuum chamber. Vacuum is conducted until enough pressure at 1 Pa. The height of powder laying is 3–15 mm, with an initial relative thickness of 0.2–0.4. In case of necessity, heating powder up to 300–600 °C for 1.5 h or cold pressing at room temperature is conducted.

The pressing type should be good for obtaining solid metals. For example, ceramics, obtained by impulse pressing method, possess highly mechanical properties.

Using liquid transferring medium during a hydrodynamic method, pressure impulses are generated, which are limited by amplitude values of the order of 0.5 GPa under severe operating conditions of detonating cameras.

Use of detonation energy in shock wave compaction is successfully applied for obtaining of metallic, amorphous, and composite materials.

Experiments showed that to obtain composite nanomaterials, in particular ceramic nanomaterials, it is important to combine pressing with further *high-temperature sintering*.

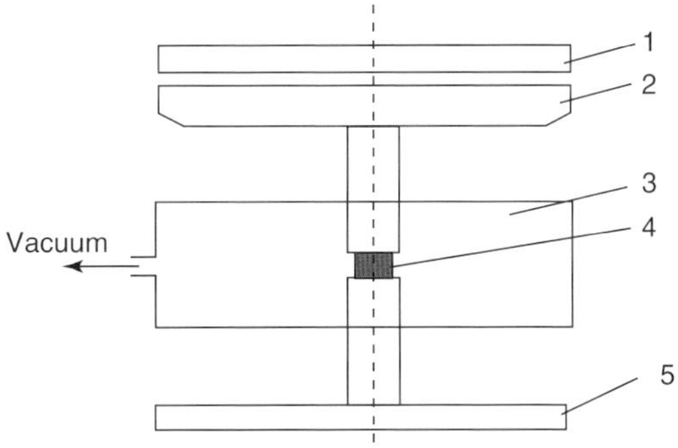

Figure 3.17 Schematic of isostatic pressing in elastic shell: 1 – inductor; 2 – hub; 3 – vacuum chamber; 4 – specimen; 5 – support (Reproduced with permission of BKL Publishers).

Sintering is heating applied to powder under a temperature lower than the melting temperature of the main component to provide mechanical, chemical, and physical properties in the obtained material. The sintering of powders should be performed in conditions when an increase in the grain size of a material is minimal or does not occur completely. In compacts at high pressure, about 0.7 times more than of X-ray, and T_{melt} of 0.5, the sintering occurs fast.

By sintering method the following nanosystems were obtained: Ni–Al and Al_2O_3–ZrO_2. Pressing with further sintering consolidate the nanodiamond composite: metals such as Nb, W, Ta, Mo, Ni, and Co; carbides such as TiC, NbC, NiC, and WC; and carbide-metal and aluminum oxide composites.

Sintering of not only powders but also their small dopants in traditional compounds significantly changes the properties of the final product. Such addition of small amount of nanomaterial to the mixture of micron-sized powders increases the mechanical property of high-current pieces. This effect is achieved through single cold pressing technology and sintering without any additional strengthening methods.

Hot pressing is a compacting method at high temperature conditions. The powder is hot-pressed at high temperature that exceeds the recrystallization temperature of the main component.

In the given process, pressing and sintering are combined in same operation, which results in a decrease in pressure to 10 times several than cold pressing. With increase in temperature, deformation resistance of materials significantly decreases. At the same time, duration of aging under pressure is considerably increasing, which is necessary for sintering process flow. However, due to the presence of an external pressure, the entire process is shortened. Temperatures for hot pressings are selected based on the nature of the sintering material. Usually, they are equal to 0.50–0.9T_{melt} of the main component.

Hot pressing is useful for compacting items made from refractory metal nanopowders. The as-obtained compacts from Ta and Nb have porosity of less than 1% and strain hardness of 2–2.5 times higher than that of a molded material.

In boron carbide, several WC–Co compositions were obtained by hot pressing. Microhardness and yield strength of these pressings exceeded appropriate values for materials made from traditional hard alloys. Thickness of obtained samples was equal to 97–99% from the theoretical value.

Vibrational interaction is used during filling and tapping of nanopowder in press shape or in the shaping process, which decreases the pressing pressure and increases the thickness of complex shaped items. The loading of vibration gives great results in the consolidation of materials with less plasticity, for example, metal carbides and borides. The positive effect of the vibration on the consolidation process is related to the destruction of interparticle bonds. Aside from this, by giving the high mobility to particles, vibrational interaction promotes their dense packing and a few pressure, providing blockage in this position. Vibrational interaction might be combined with single axial, isostatic, cold, and hot pressings.

To obtain nanopowders with high thickness, ultrasound is used. The use of ultrasound destroys particle agglomerates, which provides an effective consolidation of material in the initial stage of pressing and decreases interparticle and wall frictions and elastic aftereffect in pressing 3–4 times. At the end, there are internal current decrease in pressing, increase in hardness, and plastic deformation starting from border displacement to the region of high pressures, providing more uniform thickness of compact, decrease in grain size, and increase in microhardness and impact elasticity.

Ultrasound interaction is more effective during the pressing of items made from ceramic oxide nanopowders. In the course of compacting items, at the same time with mechanical pressing of powder blend, there is a possibility of impulse thermal interaction loading. Impulse heating is carried out with an electrical current of less than 10^{-4} s, providing some amount of time to shape the item in a heated condition, and practically excludes growth of its structural components.

In combination of electrical impulse interaction, bulk items from copper nanopowders were obtained, with hardness 10 times higher than pressed micron-sized particles. It was observed that the hardness of copper nanopowders increased by aging time at room temperature.

The process of nanopowders flatting in many ways differs from the processing of compact materials, thus having a number of common features. Schematics of powder flatting are given in Figure 3.18. Initial material is directed from the loading device to the region between two shafts, rotating toward each other. By the friction force, powder is interesting in constipation and compacting into a strip. Consolidation is possible due to the existence of a gap between single particles that provides junction of particles and their mutual fixation in the packed condition. By the given method, an intermediary layers for diffusion welding of dissimilar materials are obtained from nanomaterials. Nanopowders of Fe, Co, Ni, Cu, Mo, W, and their combined compositions are used as initial materials.

To obtain consolidated nanomaterials, in most cases, *extrusion* can be applied. There are several types of extrusion: mouthpiece pressing, hydro extrusion, and gas extrusion.

Mouthpiece pressing is called pressing method, based on punching powder through the hole, determining shape and size of the cross section of an obtaining

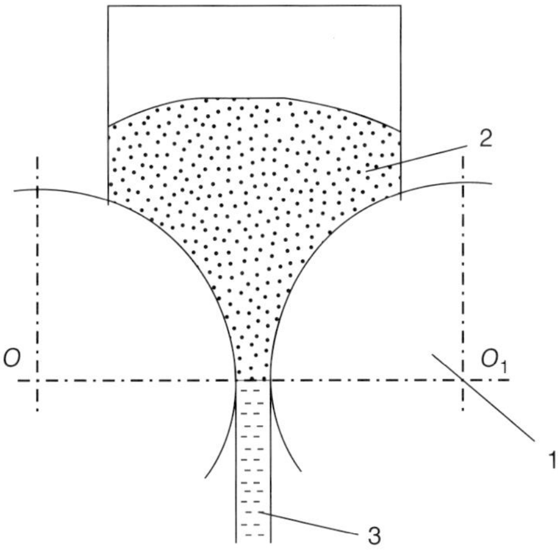

Figure 3.18 Schematic of powder flatting: 1 – shaft; 2 – powder in loading device; 3 – obtaining billet (Reproduced with permission of BKL Publishers).

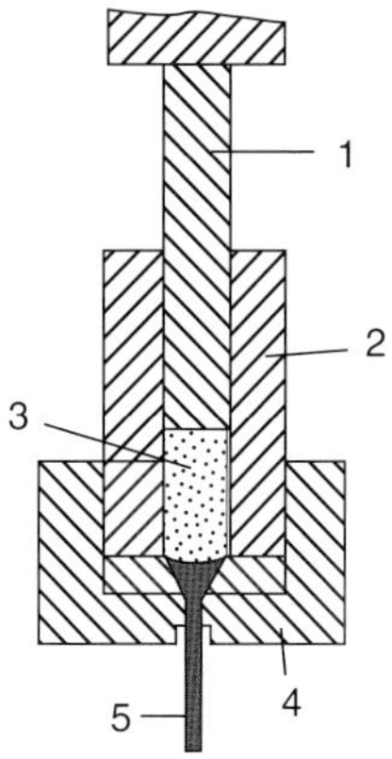

Figure 3.19 Schematic of nanopowders by mouthpiece pressing: 1 – punch; 2 – steel cup; 3 – powder; 4 – matrix; 5 – obtaining billet. (Reproduced by permission of BKL Publishers).

billet. Press-shape for mouthpiece pressing is presented in Figure 3.19. Material porosity is obtained after a given pressing is often close to null.

By mouthpiece pressing, an item made from poorly compressible materials, such as refractory metals and hard alloys, are obtained. By this method nanocrystalline nickel and iron rods are with increased mechanical properties.

Case Study 1: Applications of Composite Nanomaterials Due to Their Improved Mechanical Properties

- Composite nanomaterials exhibit a variety of mechanical properties, such as size distribution, thermodynamical properties, phase equilibrium changes, melting temperature and polymorphic change characteristics, and so on. Due to these properties, composite nanomaterials can be applied in energy saving, electronic, magnetic device manufacturing, and biomedicine.
- New application opportunities for composite nanomaterials were determined and reported [3]. According to this study, nanocomposites are determined as a high-performance material, exhibiting unusual property combinations and unique design possibilities. With an annual growth rate of about 25% and fastest demand to be in engineering plastics and elastomers, the potential of composite nanomaterials is so striking that they are useful in several areas ranging from packaging to biomedical applications. In this chapter, three types of matrix nanocomposites are presented, which underlay the need for these materials as well as their processing methods and some recent results on their structure, properties, potential applications, and perspectives. Possible uses of natural materials such as clay-based minerals, chrysotile, and lignocellulosic fibers were highlighted in this study. Environmentally friendly applications of nanocomposite materials offer new technology and business opportunities for several sectors of the aerospace, automotive, electronics, and biotechnology industries.

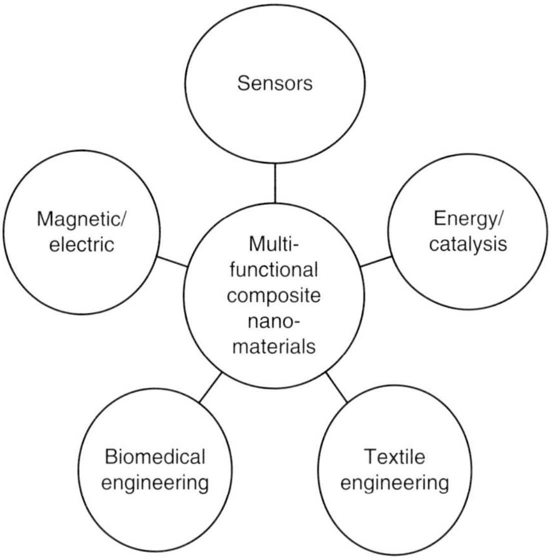

Figure 3.20 Characterization of nanocomposites based on their applications [4].

- The applications of multifunctional composite nanomaterials were studied by Sahay *et al.*, [4]. The characterization of nanocomposites based on their applications is illustrated in Figure 3.20. Nanocomposites are a new generation of novel materials, which are formed by mixing one or more dissimilar materials at the nanoscale in order to control and develop new and improved structures and properties.

Control Questions

1) Describe the main characteristics of nanocomposite materials.
2) Describe size dependence as a nanomaterial property.
3) Describe the relation of energy types with size changes in nanomaterials.
4) Enumerate the thermodynamical features of nanomaterials.
5) Which kind of phase changes will occur in nanomaterials?
6) Describe the relation of Laplace equation with pressure changes in nanomaterials.
7) What kind of melting temperature changes occur in nanomaterials?
8) What is the difference between melting temperature of bulk and nanosized materials?
9) Describe the polymorphic characteristics changes in nanosystems.
10) Define the main characteristics related to the structure of nanosized materials.
11) Describe the relation between the atomic distance and change in crystal lattice of nanomaterial.

12) Describe the features of surface relaxation and its effect on nanomaterial structure.
13) Describe the crystal lattice defects in nanomaterials.
14) The role of HRTEM in studying of the crystal lattice defects in nanomaterials.
15) What kinds of crystal lattice microdistorsions are existing in nanomaterials?

References

1 Bian, Z. *et al.* (2014) *Nat. Commun.*, **5**, 3038.
2 Ryzhonkov, D.I., Levina, V.V., and Dzidziguri, E.L. (2008) *Nanomaterials, BINOM*, BKL Publishers, Moscow.
3 Camargo, P.H.C., Satyanarayana, K.G., and Wypych, F. (2009) Nanocomposites: synthesis, structure, properties and new application opportunities. *Mat. Res.*, **12** (1), 1–39.
4 Sahay, R. *et al* (2014) Synthesis and applications of multifunctional composite nanomaterials. *Int. J. Mech. Mater. Eng.*, **9**, 25.

Further Reading

Chiu, F., Chen, C.C., and Chen, Y. (2014) Binary and ternary nanocomposites based on PVDF, PMMA, and PVDF/PMMA blends: polymorphism, thermal, and rheological properties. *J. Polym. Res.*, **21**, 378.
Huang, B., Cao, M., Nie, F., Huang, H., and Hu, C. (2013) Construction and properties of structure- and size-controlled micro/nano-energetic materials. *Def. Technol.*, **9** (2), 59–79.
Iyer, R.S. and Sastry, S.M.L. (1999) Consolidation of nanoparticles—development of a micromechanistic model. *Acta Mater.*, **47** (10), 3079–3098.
Kattan, N., Hou, B., Fermín, D.J., and Cherns, D. (2015) Crystal structure and defects visualization of Cu_2ZnSnS_4 nanoparticles employing transmission electron microscopy and electron diffraction. *Appl. Mater. Today*, **1** (1), 52–59.
Lee, J.S., Choi, J.P., and Lee, G.Y. (2013) Consolidation of hierarchy-structured nanopowder agglomerates and its application to net-shaping nanopowder materials. *Materials*, **6**, 4046–4063.
Mangal, R., Srivastava, S., Narayanan, S., and Archer, L.A. (2016) Size-dependent particle dynamics in entangled polymer nanocomposites. *Langmuir*, **32** (2), 596–603.
Minglu, L., Yuanyu, M., Hsinwei, W., and Wang, R.Y. (2015) Metal matrix–metal nanoparticle composites with tunable melting temperature and high thermal conductivity for phase-change thermal storage. *ACS Nano*, **9** (2), 1341–1351.
Piloyan, G.O., Bortnikov, N.S., and Boeva, N.M. (2013) The determination of surface thermodynamic properties of nanoparticles by thermal analysis. *J. Mod. Phys.*, **4**, 16–21.

Vasanthan, N., Ly, H., and Ghosh, S. (2011) Impact of nanoclay on isothermal cold crystallization kinetics and polymorphism of poly(L-lactic acid) nanocomposites. *J. Phys. Chem. B*, **115** (31), 9556–9563.

Online Source

Nanowerk. http://www.nanowerk.com/spotlight/spotid=23934.php (accessed 17 January 2017).

4

Mechanical Characteristics of Dispersive Systems

Translated materials from the original work of Ryzhonkov, D.I., Levina, V.V. and Dzidziguri, E.L. were used in this chapter.

Actions speak louder than words.

Proverb

4.1 Dispersion Characteristics of Nanomaterials

The most important characteristic for nanomaterials is the particle size of powder or the grain size of bulk material. In most cases, nanomaterials can be polydisperse systems consisting of grains or particles with various coarsenesses. Size scattering highly changes the physical–chemical properties of material. Hence, its *particle size distribution composition* is the primary size characteristic, except for average sizes, which is defined as the composition of particles or grains dependent on size intervals in relation to their total quantity.

Other size characteristics of nanomaterials include their specific surface area (for nanopowders) that determines the average size for aggregates; average particle size or grain size and average size of coherent scattering region; and size distribution of particles, grains, and crystal lattices.

4.1.1 Specific Surface Area

Specific surface area is an important characteristic of nanomaterial that determines the activity of the physical–chemical process, most technological properties, interaction with environmental medium, and so on.

A specific surface area holds 1 g (or kg) of a certain substance, and its value is designated as $S_{specific}$, with the unit being m^2/g or m^2/kg. $S_{specific}$ is significant in cases wherein the surface is exactly "working" in the technological process, for example, in catalysis. The specific surface area of materials such as zeolite and activated carbon might reach 400–500 m^2/g, and traditional powder samples are characterized by values of 0.05–2 m^2/g. Specific surface area of powders is determined by several factors: dispersity, shape, phase composition, and surface condition of particles and their aggregation.

Nano- and Biomaterials: Compounds, Properties, Characterization, and Applications,
First Edition. Zhypargul Abdullaeva.

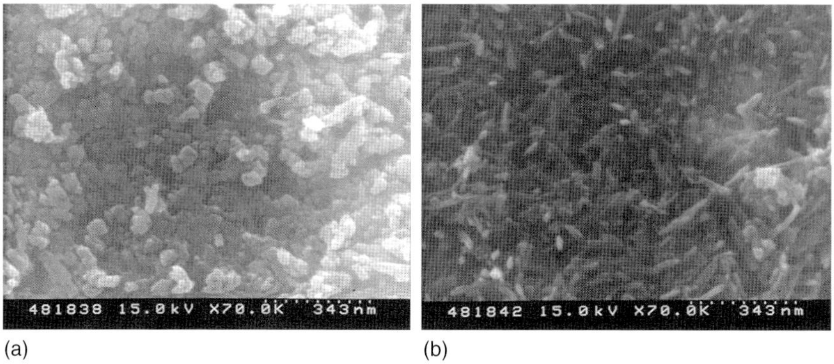

Figure 4.1 Micrographs of (a) spherical and (b) needlelike iron hydroxide nanopowder. (Ryzhonkov *et al.* 2008 [1]. Reproduced with permission of BKL publishers.)

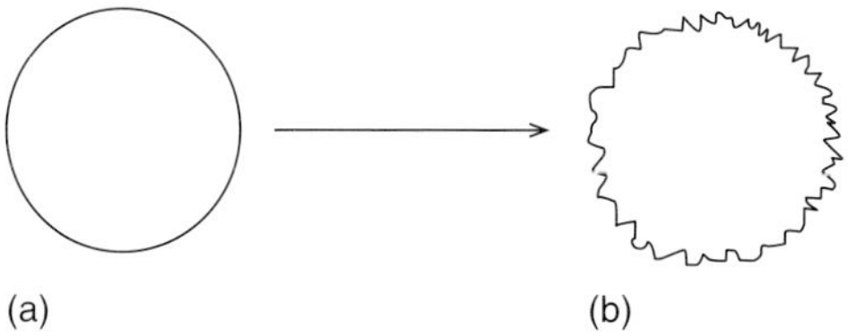

Figure 4.2 Maturity of nanoparticle surface: (a) spherical particle with smooth surface; (b) particle with advanced surface and shape close to spherical (Ryzhonkov *et al.* 2008 [1]. Reproduced with permission of BKL publishers.)

A decrease in particle diameter under equal conditions increases S_{specific}. Spheroidization decreases specific surface area, because a sphere has minimal surface at a given dispersity of material. Accordingly, a change in particle shape during size preservations leads to an increase in S_{specific}. For example, the specific surface areas of spherical (Figure 4.1a) and needlelike (Figure 4.1b) iron hydroxide are equal to 78 and 121 $\mathrm{m^2/g}$, respectively. In turn, as-called sophistication of surface (Figure 4.2) can significantly increase the specific surface area of material.

A change in phase composition, for example, formation of oxide film on the surface of metal nanopowders, might increase S_{specific} from 7–8 to 50–70 $\mathrm{m^2/g}$. Metallization, in contrast, can sharply decrease the specific surface area of powders (Table 4.1).

High-level powder aggregation is caused by intensity of nanosized systems to decrease their surface energy. In the case of magnetic metals, the tendency to form aggregates is further increased, which leads to a growth of their average sizes. These processes decrease the specific surface area of material.

As for the aggregation level of equiaxed particles, the average number of particles in agglomerate n is used, which can be determined by the following equation [1]:

$$n = \left(D_{\mathrm{a}}\rho_{\mathrm{a}}/D_{\rho}\right) \tag{4.1}$$

where D_{a} and D are the average sizes of agglomerates and initial particles, respectively, and ρ_{a} and ρ are agglomerate and material thickness, respectively.

4.1.2 Size Distribution in Nanomaterials

Except for average size, in general, the properties of nanopowders are mostly determined by the behavior of particle assembly. Large size distribution averages

Table 4.1 Specific surface area and average aggregate size of Fe, Co, Ni, and Cu nanopowders.

Sample	Reduction conditions		Specific surface area ($m^2 g^{-1}$)		Average aggregate size of metal nanopowders
	Temperature (°C)	Curing time (min)	Initial hydroxide	Metal nanopowder	
Fe	460	70	52.6	6.1	126
	200	60		7.59	89
Ni	250	60	101.0	2.93	230
	300	60		1.74	386
	360	60		0.66	1022
Co	300	60	66.6	4.8	140
	200	60		5.08	133
Cu	260	60	45.7	2.59	259
	300	60		2.26	296

Source: Ryzhonkov *et al.* 2008 [1]. Reproduced with permission of BKL publishers.

the material properties and can grade the features of nanostate. In relation to this, in practice, obtaining powders with narrower particle size distribution is often required.

The formation of particles can occur through one of the following mechanisms: In *diffusionless* mechanism, the rate of particle growth is determined by interphase boundary processes (adsorption, heterogeneous chemical reaction, dissolution, etc.). If this is realized efficiently, the linear dimensions of forming material are proportional to the length of its growth. In *diffusional* mechanism, transferring atoms of various components to significant distances is required to support particle growth. Particle growth is proportional to diffusion speed (in some cases, proportional to convection speed) of atoms on the surface of forming material. In this case, the particle radius is proportional to the square root of growth time. The *coagulative* mechanism involves the collision of particles of various sizes with each other and their adhesion. This process can be accompanied by fast recrystallization or fusion or viscous flow *coalescence* (similar to liquid drops). It can be assumed that fast rate of coalescence in nanomaterials is related to an excess in surface energy, which leads to a decrease in the melting temperature of small particles and formation of liquid-like film on their surfaces. Moreover, products of chemical reaction, formation of particles with different compositions, complex morphology of particles, and necessity of diffusion for components of condensed phase have a complicating influence on the type of distribution.

If conditions of high temperature (usually higher than 2/3 T_s, where T_s is the melting temperature of bulk material) and strong interaction between particles are realized simultaneously, then *coalescence* occurs, wherein particles fuse for a more or less continuous period of time. As a result, their initial shape disappears and a single particle with a more stable configuration forms. At higher temperatures, the coalescence of solid nanoparticles occurs immediately, similar to the fusion of two liquid drops. Such phenomenon is called *liquid-like coalescence.*

If nanoparticles have an unstable shape and very rough surface as a result of diffusion processes occurring under surface tension forces, each particle shrinks, becomes round, and acquires a more stable shape. This process is called *autocoalescence.* In this case, if the process temperature is low (less than $1/3\ T_s$) and the change in shape of particles is inhibited, *coagulation* occurs as a result of particle engagement. During this process, in contrast to coalescence, the change in shape of initial particles is insignificant.

Particle size distribution function has its own features during the formation of nanomediums through various mechanisms. If coagulation growth is inhibited, atomic mass transfer and surface boundary phase processes will play an important role.

Theoretical investigations and experimental data have shown that for experimental points described by normal distribution,

$$f(D) = \left(\sqrt{2\pi}\,\sigma_a\right)^{-1} \exp\left[-\left(D - \overline{D}\right)^2 / \left(2\sigma_a^2\right)\right] \tag{4.2}$$

As in the case of particle formation, layer growth through adsorption of new atoms will dominate. However, particle size distribution under real conditions might never be truly Gaussian and can be described as more or less symmetrical in histograms. For this, the term normal distribution is usually used.

Normal distribution is determined by possibilities of continuous random variable, which is described by the density

$$f(x) = (\sigma)^{-1} \exp\left[-(x-a)^2 / \left(2\sigma^2\right)\right] \tag{4.3}$$

where a is the mathematical expectation of the random value and σ is its average square deviation. *Normal curve* (or *Gaussian curve*) in a graph denotes normal distribution thickness (Figure 4.3). Variation of the mathematical expectation value does not change the shape of normal curve but just moves it along the Ox axis: to the right if "a" is increasing and to the left if "a" is decreasing.

Different matters arise during a change of σ parameter (Figure 4.4): With an increase in dispersion, the ordinate of normal curve decreases and the curve itself becomes more sloping, like it is pressed toward the Ox axis. With a decrease in σ, the normal curve becomes more "peaked" and stretches toward the positive direction of Oy axis.

If, during the formation of nanoparticles, the coagulation process dominates in all growth stages, the curve will have a long "tail" toward the large size direction.

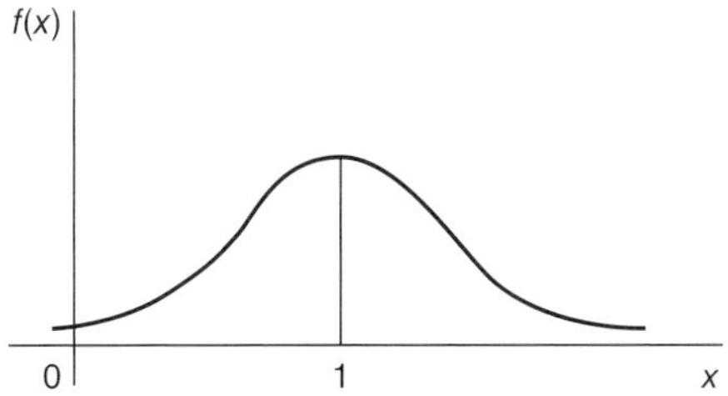

Figure 4.3 Graph illustrating normal distribution thickness. (Ryzhonkov *et al.* 2008 [1]. Reproduced with permission of BKL publishers.)

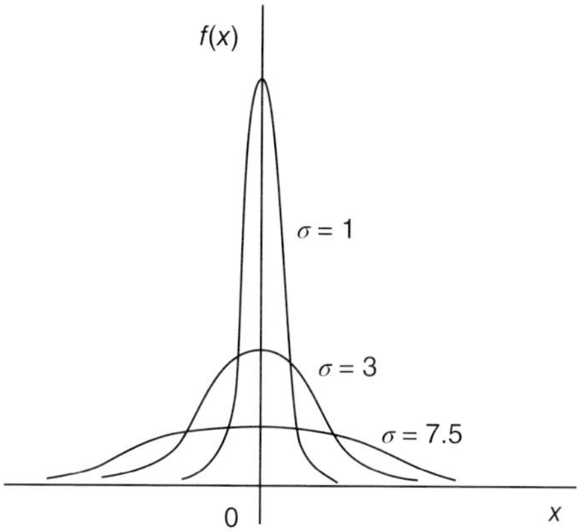

Figure 4.4 Influence of average square deviation on normal distribution curve. (Ryzhonkov *et al.* 2008 [1]. Reproduced with permission of BKL publishers.)

Such relation is described by logarithmic-normal law:

$$f(D) = \left(\sqrt{2\pi}\,\mathrm{In}\sigma_g\right)^{-1} \exp\left[-\left(\mathrm{In}D - \mathrm{In}\overline{D}\right)^2 / \left(2\mathrm{In}^2\sigma_g\right)\right] \tag{4.4}$$

where D is diameter, D_a is average arithmetical diameter, D_g is average geometrical diameter, σ_a is standard arithmetical deviation, and $\ln \sigma_g$ is standard geometrical deviation.

In practice, the size distribution often exists as an average of the aforementioned two laws, because small particles always grow through the layer connection of new atoms and then through coagulation. As studies have shown, normal distribution is a characteristic of particles with a size of ≤10 nm. Deviation of experimental data from this law occurs for larger particles. In such way, the probability of logarithmic-normal distribution is high for particles with a large average size. If conformity to the given law is fully explained by the coagulation process, it can be concluded that growth mechanism plays an important role in particles with a large average size, and for nanoparticles, except the smallest, normal distribution is least likely, logarithmic-normal distribution is more likely, and finally the distribution of intermediate form is much more likely.

There are a number of examples regarding how the acquisition process of particles can influence their distribution. Recently, the precipitation process of nanomaterials from the gas phase has been mostly studied. Experimental data showed that the size distribution of aerosol particles in the precipitation process can be described as superposition of normal and logarithmic-normal distributions. Depending on precise experimental data, one of the aforementioned processes can dominate and therefore determines the particle size distribution. Moreover, it was found that, under specific experimental conditions, it is possible to obtain the particle size distribution function, which, at first sight, resembles the Gaussian distribution. For example, quasi-Gaussian distributions were obtained for Al particles with an average size of 5–40 nm by sedimentation of Al powder on the substrate, which was located at a strictly determined distance from the evaporator. Inversely, strongly asymmetric logarithmic-normal distributions were observed under conditions wherein particles were collected at a significant distance from the evaporation source. In other experiments, it was impossible to fully describe the particle size distribution for V, Sn, and Pd obtained by sedimentation from the steam phase in the inert gas medium by normal or logarithmic-normal laws. Moreover, size distribution of β-Co particle with a size of 6 nm, formed during arc spraying of anode, agrees with statistical model for crystal growth, in which the main process is particle coalescence.

Nanoparticles obtained by plasma chemical process can also have a logarithmic-normal distribution, which certifies the significant role of coagulation. For example, the logarithmic-normal distribution better describes the size distribution of W particles obtained by plasma chemical synthesis method (Figure 4.5).

Particle growth as a result of coagulation was also detected in insular (or isolated) films and the general rule for metal film formation was further described. Initially, the nucleus will form on the surface of the substrate. Next, caused by

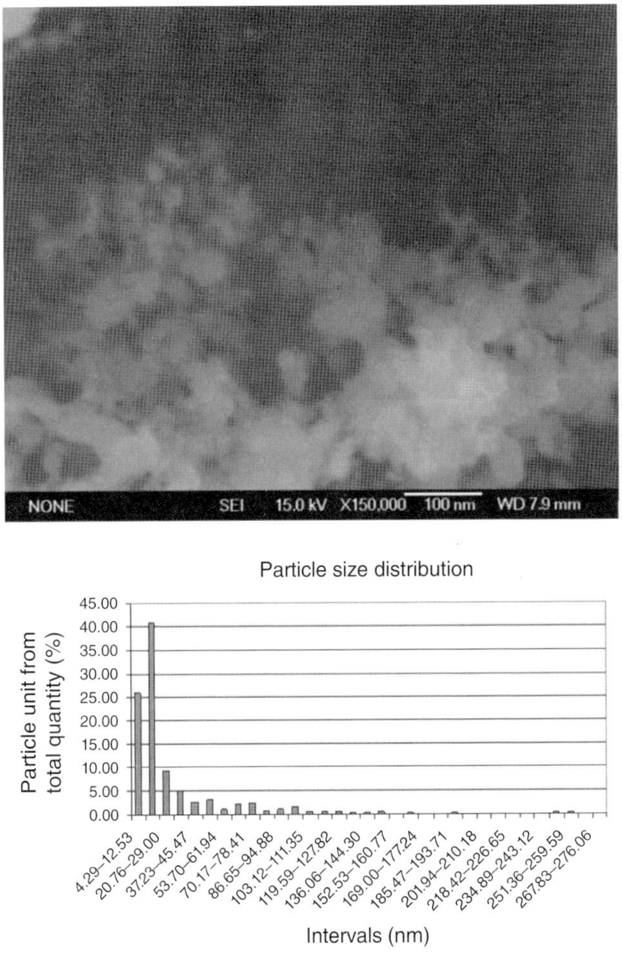

Figure 4.5 Micrograph and particle size distribution histogram for W, obtained by plasma chemical method. (Ryzhonkov *et al.* 2008 [1]. Reproduced with permission of BKL publishers.)

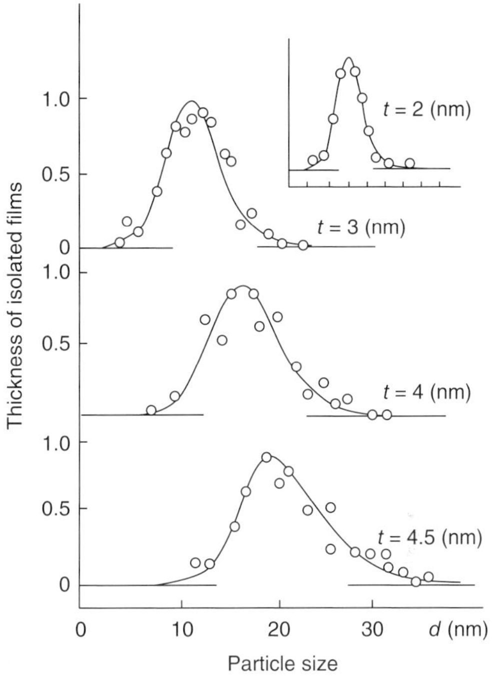

Figure 4.6 Size distribution of Al nanoparticles depending on the thickness of isolated films. (Ryzhonkov *et al.* 2008 [1]. Reproduced with permission of BKL publishers.)

surface diffusion or striking, the growth of particles will occur when each separate atom joins together. And finally, depending on the surface condition and thickness of nuclei, the isolated film might enter the phase in which the dominating growth mechanism is particle coagulation process.

Coalescence and diffusion transfer process of mass through two-dimensional steam determine the resultant distribution of insular films. As a result, for these samples, logarithmic-normal distribution often well describes the experimental data. The most studied distributions (Figure 4.6) are the distribution functions of isolated films, formed in a short time distance and during the significant diffusion transfer of atoms. An increase in process time will lead to coalescence during the growth of isolated films, resulting in a wider and more asymmetric distribution. Particle growth in vacuum forms a narrower size distribution than sedimentation in the inert gas phase. A wider size distribution is realized when metal drops in initial phase and in particle growth stage are present.

In general, the size distribution of metallic nanoparticles obtained by chemical dispersion method has an asymmetric shape with a tail toward the large size regions (Figure 4.7). Formation of large particles can be determinedly decreased through variation of process conditions.

In nanomaterials obtained through the plastic deformation method, the main means for which nanostructure is formed is crushing of initial grains. In this case, mechanisms of nanostructures obtained by evaporation–condensation processes or chemical sedimentation method are completely different. However, as it turns out, particle size distribution obeys similar laws. For example, in copper,

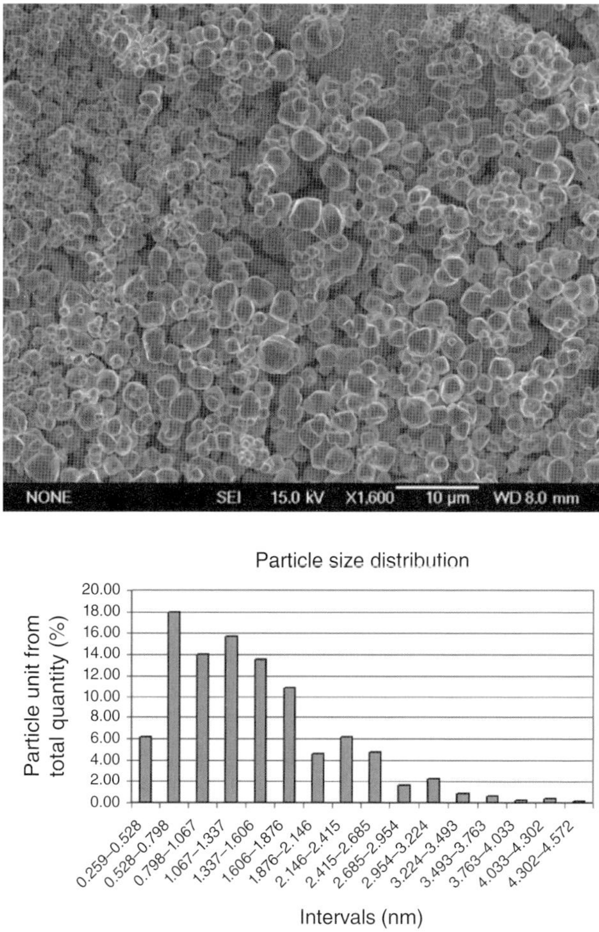

Figure 4.7 SEM image and size distribution of the wolfram nanoparticles. (Ryzhonkov *et al.* 2008 [1]. Reproduced with permission of BKL Publishers.)

obtained by equal-channel angular pressing, grain size distribution was described by logarithmic-normal law.

Region of coherent scattering is related to temperature and reduction time and was studied on metal nanopowders obtained through chemical dispersion method. Figure 4.8a shows the coherent region distribution curve for Fe BCC phase samples, reduced at various temperatures for one hour. As it can be seen in the figure, an increase in metallization temperature leads to consolidation (or enlargement) of coherent region distribution and narrowing of size distributions. For example, a change of metallization temperature from 400 to 440 °C (Figure 4.8a, curves 1 and 2, respectively) leads to a decrease in average crystallite size to 17 nm during insignificant narrowing of the distribution curve. At 470 °C, consolidation of the coherent region distribution occurs (2 nm in average), as well as narrowing of the distribution curve (Figure 4.8a, curve 3). Reduction at 515 °C (Figure 4.8a, curve 4) leads to a further narrowing of the

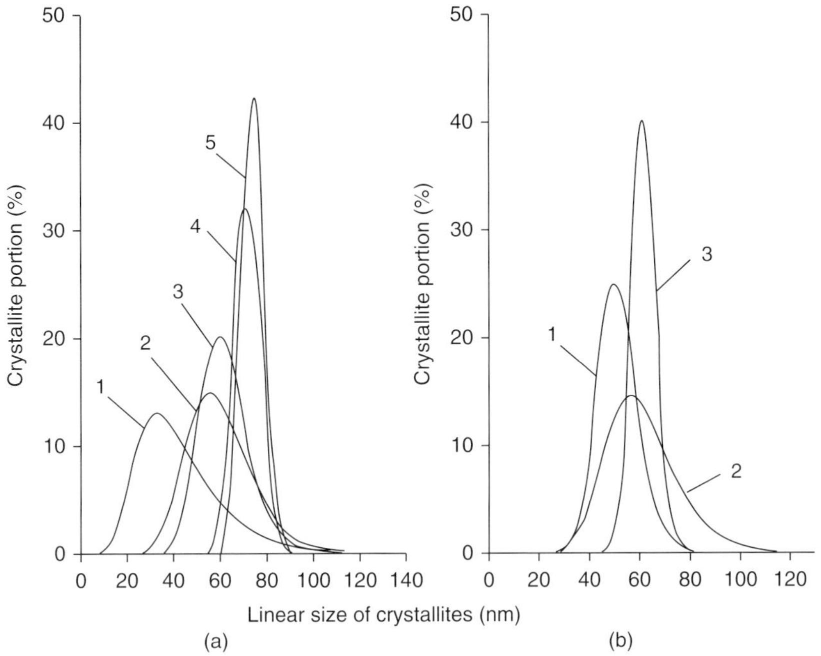

Figure 4.8 Coherent region distribution curves for Fe nanopowders, obtained by hydroxide reduction: (a) at different temperatures; (b) at 440 °C during different time. (Ryzhonkov *et al.* 2008 [1]. Reproduced with permission of BKL publishers.)

distribution curve during an increase in average size to about 10 nm. A further increase in metallization temperature up to 300 °C almost does not lead to an increase in average coherent region distribution (Figure 4.8a, curve 5). At 800 °C the neatly monodisperse Fe powder with a size of 75 nm can be obtained.

The influence of metallization time at 440 °C on the particle size distribution is shown in Figure 4.8b. Reduction for 10 min does not allow completion of the metallization process. As a result, coherent region distribution for α-Fe phase will have an average size of 51 nm and a narrow size distribution. During more prolonged reduction, the average crystallite size and size distribution curve will increase at the same time. In a sample reduced for 60 min (Figure 4.8b, curve 2), the size of coherent region distribution increases to 9 nm and the size distribution is significantly wide. If the metallization process is conducted at 440 °C for 90 min, the monodisperse powder with coherent region distribution growth to only 1 nm can be obtained.

Interrelation of nanomaterial size characteristics is an important issue in the synthesis of nanopowders and study of their structures and sizes. As an example, the size characteristics of Fe nanopowders obtained by chemical dispersion will be described. Main determination methods such as specific surface area measurement, electron microscopy, and X-ray diffraction were applied. $S_{specific}$ and calculated average sizes of Fe nanoaggregates are listed in Table 4.2. Results showed that an increase in reduction temperature from 400 to 500 °C leads to a

Table 4.2 Specific surface area, average aggregate size, and CDR particles of Fe, reduced at various temperatures.

Hydroxide	Reduction temperature (°C)	$S_{specific}$ ($m^2 g^{-1}$)	D_{BET} (nm)	$D_{elec.micros.}$ (nm)	$D_{Scherer}$ (nm)	$D_{Selyakov}$ (nm)
Fe	400	8.1	94	72	43	41
Fe	450	6.4	124	115	60	58
Fe	500	4.0	194	181	70	67
Fe	400	9.0	84	81	46	45
Fe	450	6.7	117	111	47	45
Fe	500	4.2	186	109	43	44

Source: Ryzhonkov *et al.* 2008 [1]. Reproduced with permission of BKL publishers.

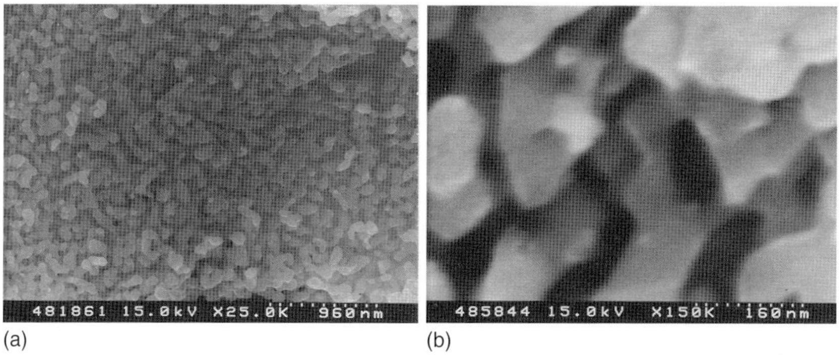

Figure 4.9 Micrographs of Fe nanopowder. (Ryzhonkov *et al.* 2008 [1]. Reproduced with permission of BKL publishers.)

two times decrease in $S_{specific}$ values and, accordingly, an increase in the average size of aggregates.

From electron microcopy results shown in Figure 4.9a, Fe nanopowders have a shape close to spherical. In all powders obtained under different conditions, particles are collected into large aggregates, which, by joining together, form porous structures. Each particle is joined together to its neighboring particles by contact necks. Material and pore sizes in dimensional porous structures are equal.

At high magnification, the shape of particles can be seen as close to spherical (Figure 4.9b) and is, in fact, polygonal. The surface of each angle is similar to flat surface. It can be assumed that the contact between particles is initially determined by planes. During isothermal aging, polygon angles in contact necks are flattened by diffusion.

Average particle size based on the electron microscopy results $D_{elec.micros.}$ is presented in Table 4.2. From the obtained data, it can be seen that the size of Fe nanopowder reduced at 450 and 500 °C is almost the same and Fe nanopowder is 1.5 times larger than those synthesized at 400 °C, wherein, with an increase in temperature, the aggregate sizes, estimated from the specific surface area, steadily

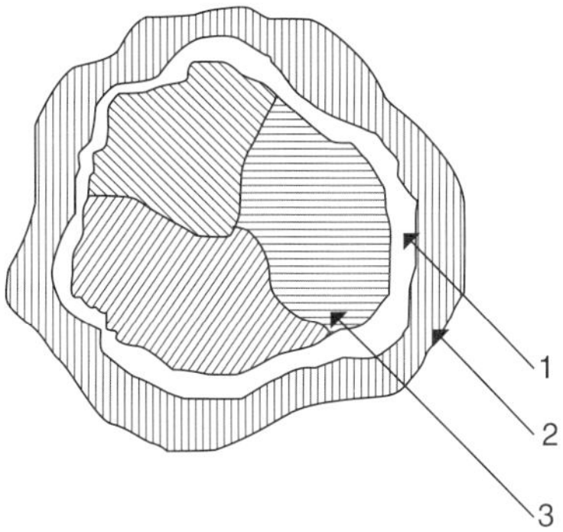

Figure 4.10 Schematic of nanoparticle structure: 1 – unpacked layer; 2 – oxide layer; 3 – crystallite (coherent region distribution). (Ryzhonkov *et al.* 2008 [1]. Reproduced with permission of BKL publishers.)

increase. Apparently, after reaching a definite size, particles will not grow further. Aggregation process will continue at this time, resulting in an increase in D_{BET}.

Estimation of the average size for coherent region distribution of Fe nanopowder, obtained by X-ray diffraction analysis $D_{Scherer}$ and $D_{Selyakov}$, gave similar results (Table 4.2).

As seen from the table, outer particle sizes and coherent region distributions, according to electron microscopy analyses, are not similar, which can be explained by the following reasons: Firstly, the surface of the metallic nanoparticles is always in oxidized form, with significant thickness of the oxide film. Secondly, each separate particle can consist of several coherent region distributions. And finally, nanoparticles can have a surface layer whose structure is different from the structure of the coherent region distribution (Figure 4.10).

Comparison of $D_{elec.micros.}$ and crystallite sizes in this case shows that each particle might constitute several coherent region distributions. An increase in reduction temperature allows the growth of coherent region distribution of average size. The quantity of coherent region distributions in a particle has influence on the physical–chemical properties of nanomaterial in general.

Thus, experimental results showed that change in size of Fe nanopowders by $S_{specific}$ value during electron microscopy and X-ray diffraction analyses led to three different characteristics for nanomaterials, namely, aggregate size, single particle diameter, and coherent region distribution diameter. All of the obtained sizes have their own physical and technological definitions in relation to full characteristics of nanopowder.

4.1.3 Surface, Boundaries, and Morphology of Nanomaterials

In each contacting medium, dynamical, electronic, and magnetic properties such as elemental composition, chemical condition, and atomic and electronic structures are different from volume properties. The thickness of layer depends on the nature of touched surfaces and outer conditions and is determined by length, a physical characteristic.

Surface is the border between two contacting mediums. Interphase boundaries allow a number of surface phenomena that have significant influence on nanosystem properties. This is in relation with an increase in nanomaterials surface area and surface curving due to interactions with other surfaces.

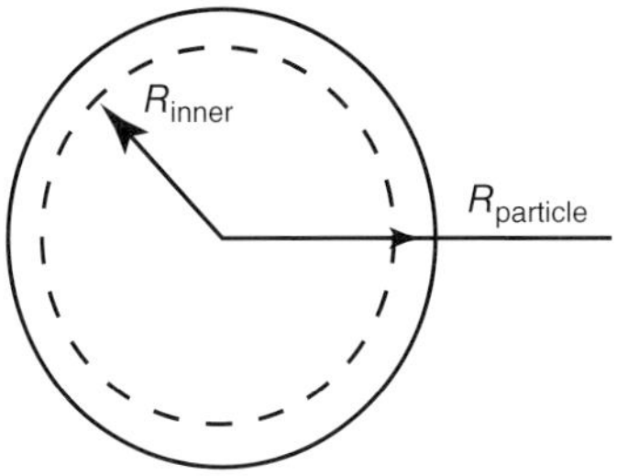

Figure 4.11 Scheme of nanoparticle. (Ryzhonkov *et al.* 2008 [1]. Reproduced with permission of BKL publishers.)

Amount of surface in nanomaterials is characterized by a decrease in size of structural components and growth of surface atom quantity at the grain boundaries. For example, the shape of particle with radius R_{particle} is spherical. As mentioned previously, the influence of atoms on each other can extend up to five interatomic distances. Let us assume that the thickness of surface layer consists of five atomic layers, which is equal to 1 nm. So $R_{\text{particle}} - 1 = R_{\text{inner}}$ (Figure 4.11). Initially, let us evaluate particle size, in which the surface layer volume is equal to 0.1% of the total volume, that is, $V_{\text{surface}} = 0.001V_{\text{particle}}$. As it is known, particle volume is equal to $V_{\text{particle}} = 4\pi R^3{}_{\text{particle}}/3$, and the inner region volume is equal to $V_{\text{inner}} = 4\pi R^3{}_{\text{inner}}/3$. In such way, the surface volume will be equal to

$$\Delta V = 4\pi r\left(R^3_{\text{particle}} - R^3_{\text{inner}}\right)/3 \tag{4.5}$$

Because the $\Delta V = 0.001V_{\text{particle}}$, $0.001V_{\text{particle}} = 4\pi r\left(R^3_{\text{particle}} - R^3_{\text{inner}}\right)/3$.

After transformations, we will obtain $0.001R^3_{\text{particle}} = R^3_{\text{particle}} - R^3_{\text{inner}}$

$$R^3_{\text{inner}} = 0.999\,R^3_{\text{particle}}$$

In this case, initial condition of $R_{\text{inner}} = R_{\text{particle}} - 1$. Taking into consideration Eq. (4.5), we will obtain $R_{\text{particle}} = 2999$ nm. Calculation results for other surface layers are presented in Table 4.3, which shows that 50% surface layer volume corresponds to a diameter of 10 nm. In fact, the terms surface and volume are conditional in such case.

Table 4.3 Evaluation values for particle radius and portion of surface atoms.

Surface layer volume (%)	Particle radius (nm)
0.01	29 999
0.10	2 999
1.00	299
10.00	29
50.00	5

Source: Ryzhonkov *et al.* 2008 [1]. Reproduced with permission of BKL publishers.

As shown previously, nanostructures and nanomaterials have a large amount of surface atoms for volume unit. Such significant increase in the relation between surface atoms and volume atoms in nanomaterials explains the change in materials' physical–chemical properties caused by alterations in their sizes at a nanometer scale.

4.1.4 Grain Boundaries in Nanomaterials

Bulk materials contain a large amount of grain boundaries in their structure, which influence physical–chemical and mechanical properties. Grain boundaries, in comparison with neighboring grains, are unpacked two-dimensional defects, with interatomic region distance not exceeding 0.5–1 nm.

Influence of boundaries on grains in the nanomaterials is much more significant, even for substances composed of single-type atoms, the model of double-structured component: grain-forming crystals and grain boundary regions are considered (Figure 4.12).

The structure of crystals is considered absolute when the grain boundary regions are characterized by low atomic thickness and changed interatomic distances. In the case of the aforementioned model, two opinions exist. First, based on electronic microscopy, grain boundaries are narrower than they should be in the model. Grain width in the nanomaterial is composed of 1–2 nm interatomic distance, that is, close to that in large crystal materials (Figure 4.13). Second, grain boundaries are characterized by high thickness of various defects: stairs, facets, and dislocations. But their existence is closely bound with elastic distortions in the crystal itself, at least close to borders. Also it should be noted that most of grain boundaries in the bulk materials are large angle simultaneous borders.

Nowadays, for nanomaterials obtained by intensive plastic deformation, the model based on unequal grain boundary performance is considered.

Unequal condition of grain boundaries is characterized by two features, namely, excess energy and the existence of long-lasting elastic stresses. The sources of elastic fields are grain boundary dislocations and their complexes.

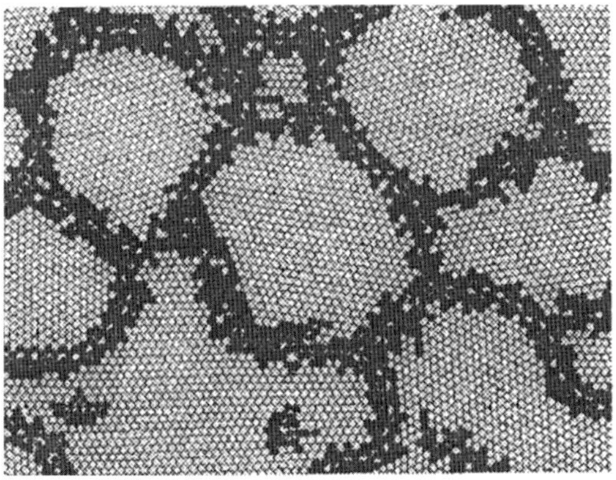

Figure 4.12 Atomic model of nanomaterial, modeled using the Morse potential. Atoms at the grain boundaries are marked with black. (Ryzhonkov *et al.* 2008 [1]. Reproduced with permission of BKL publishers.)

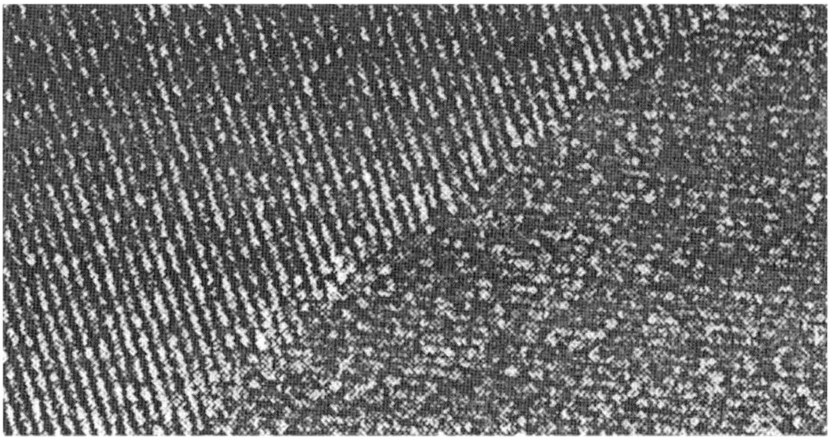

Figure 4.13 Micrograph of grain boundary in the nanoparticle, obtained by intensive plastic deformation. (Ryzhonkov *et al.* 2008 [1]. Reproduced with permission of BKL publishers.)

4.1.5 Morphology of Nanodisperse Particles

Minimal condition of surface free energy must certainly follow the equilibrium form of disperse particles. In particular, equilibrium or energetically beneficial surface shape of liquid drop should be spherical. But if the particle has a crystalline structure, then its equilibrium shape is polygonal (Figure 4.14).

A more beneficial shape of a tiny particle can be determined by Wolf's rule, which means that equilibrium facet should consist of surface areas, in accordance with crystallographic surfaces with few index values. At the same time, with an increase in surface indexes, square of appropriate areas will decrease. In real nanoparticles, the shape is far from equilibrium and depends on how they were obtained. In most cases, powders, obtained by evaporation–condensation method, are spherical (Figure 4.15a). Grinding of ball mill (Figure 4.15b) results

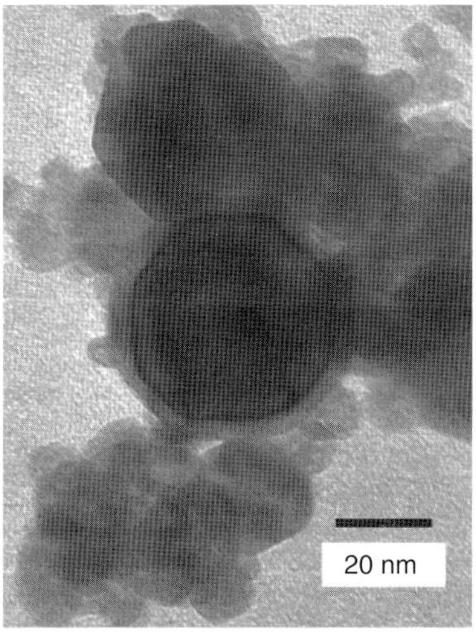

Figure 4.14 TEM image of iron nanoparticles. (Ryzhonkov *et al.* 2008 [1]. Reproduced with permission of BKL publishers.)

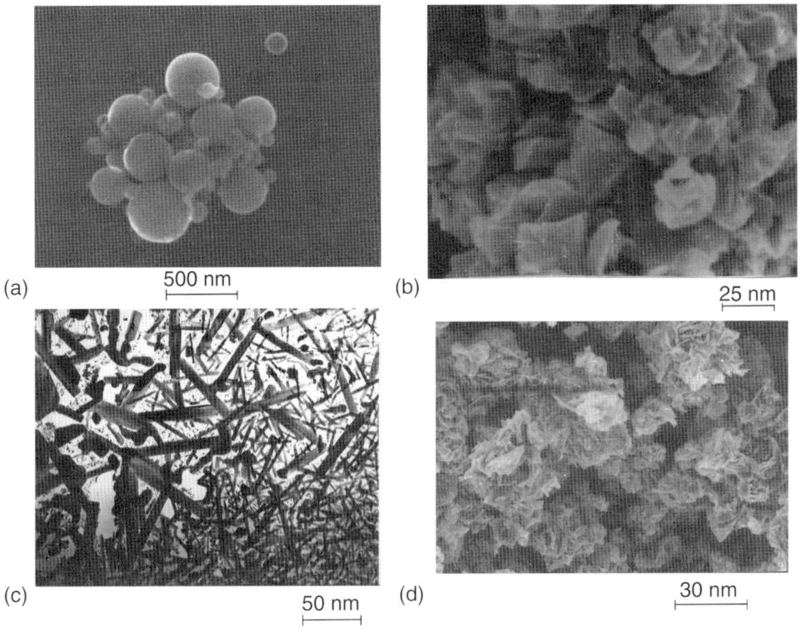

Figure 4.15 Micrographs of nanoparticles: (a) aluminum; (b) cobalt after ball milling; (c) iron oxide; (d) nickel oxide. (Ryzhonkov *et al.* 2008 [1]. Reproduced with permission of BKL publishers.)

in particles with inappropriate fragmental shape. In the case of chemical methods, formation of particles with needlelike (Figure 4.15c) and flaky (Figure 4.15d) shapes is possible.

In intensive plastic deformation methods, the grain shape of nanomaterials can be determined by the following technological features: geometrical rig, processing regime, deformation level, and initial microstructure with phase composition of specimen. For example, during equal-channel angular pressing, depending on the specimens' rotating angle at the next passage (refer to Figure 1.5 in Chapter 1), spherical or ellipsoidal grains can be formed (Figure 4.16).

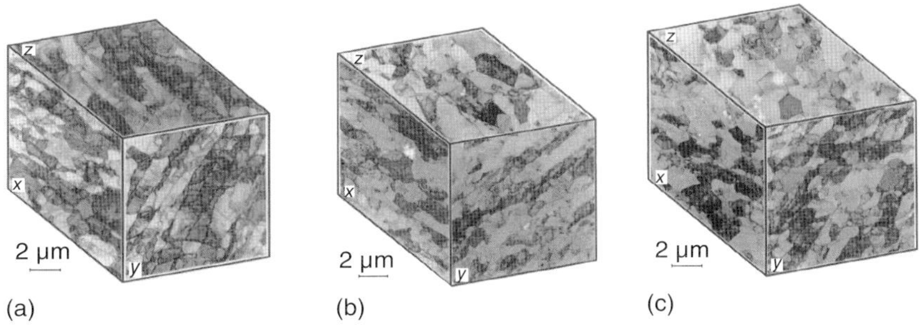

Figure 4.16 Microstructure of aluminum: (a) after passage during equal-channel angular pressing; (b) after four passages during equal-channel angular pressing through way A; (c) after four passages through way B. (Ryzhonkov *et al.* 2008 [1]. Reproduced with permission of BKL publishers.)

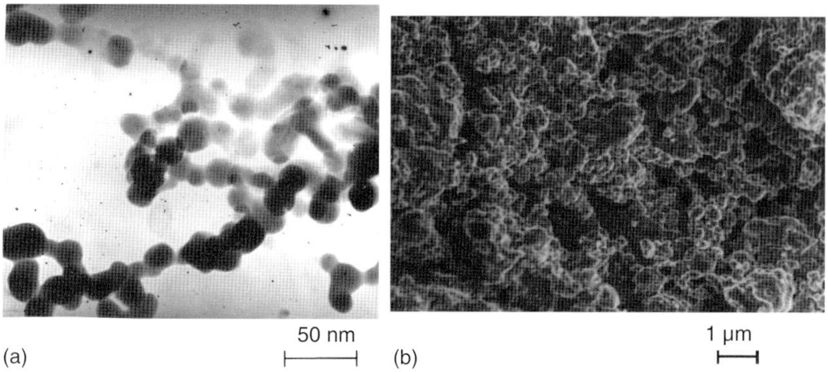

Figure 4.17 Micrographs of nanoparticles: (a) wolfram; (b) aluminum oxide. (Ryzhonkov *et al.* 2008 [1]. Reproduced with permission of BKL publishers.)

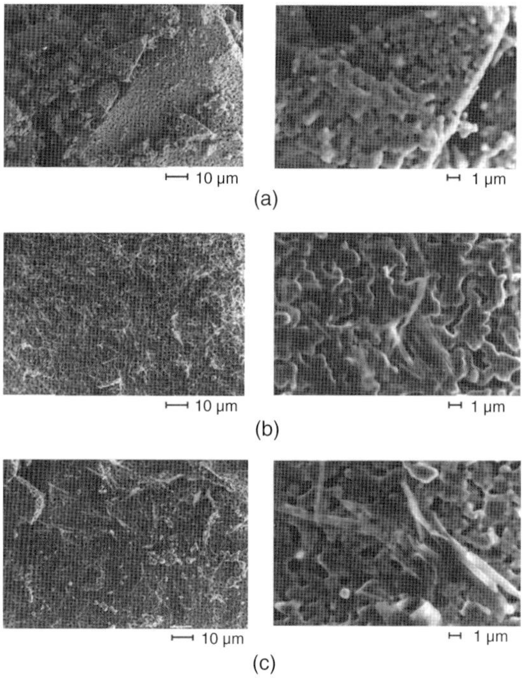

Figure 4.18 Micrographs of copper nanoparticles reduced at 650 °C during various times: (a) 60 min; (b) 120 min; (c) 200 min. (Ryzhonkov *et al.* 2008 [1]. Reproduced with permission of BKL publishers.)

Agglomeration tendency of nanosized objects is especially noticeable for powders. Nanoparticles can form chains (Figure 4.17a) or porous bulk structures (Figure 4.17b), the latter demonstrating high thermal stability.

Conducted studies showed that aging of Ni nanopowder at 650 °C for 60, 120, and 200 min (Figure 4.18) practically does not have an influence on the average size of aggregates and pores in the porous bulk structures.

4.2 Electrical Properties of Nanomaterials

A change in the electrical properties of nanomaterials and in electronic conductance behavior can be due to a decrease in their sizes. Phase dimensionality, surface morphology, aggregation of particles, structure disorders, and grain boundary thickness can have an impact on the properties of nanomaterials.

4.2.1 Change in Length of Electron Free Path in Nanomaterials

The length of electron free path l is determined by distance in which an electron covers between two sequential scattering interactions. Its value results from the interaction of electrons, moving to the outer electrical field, with ionic lattice frame. Based on experimentally determined values of specific conductivity, in various large crystalline materials, l is equal to 6–100 nm, which is equivalent to 3–100 interatomic distances.

In classical theory, the following equation was derived for specific electrical conductivity of metals λ:

$$\lambda = \left(ne^2/m\right) \cdot (l/v) \tag{4.6}$$

where n is electron conductivity concentration, e is electron charge, m is electron mass, and v is electron speed.

Hence, with a decrease in electron free path, electrical conductivity of material should decrease. In the material, the size of which is greatly larger than the electron free path, the interaction between electron wave and surface can be neglected. However, because of the commensurability of electron free path and structural component sizes, their borders should be considered as an additional source of electron free path scatterings. Hence, changes in the electrical properties of bulk materials can be expected, while in thin films and threadlike crystals, thickness or diameter is less than the length of electron free path. Nowadays, most conductivity theories on nanosized thin films and whiskers are developed mathematically. Let us look at a model: electrons move upon colliding with thin film surface, with thickness of h, that is, fluctuating between planes I and II (Figure 4.19).

Electrons after scattering start to move toward the direction of plane I from an arbitrary point O on plane II. Let us also assume that the movement directions of electrons after and before collision are independent of each other and electrons are uniformly distributed in the half space. If an average length of electron free path in monocrystal metal at a given temperature is equal to l_0, as from relation $\cos h$, the angle $> \varphi_0$ can realize the electron free path length corresponding to bulk material. However, the electron free path length will shorten in electrons scattered at an angle less than $\varphi_0 = h/l$. Thus, the average length of

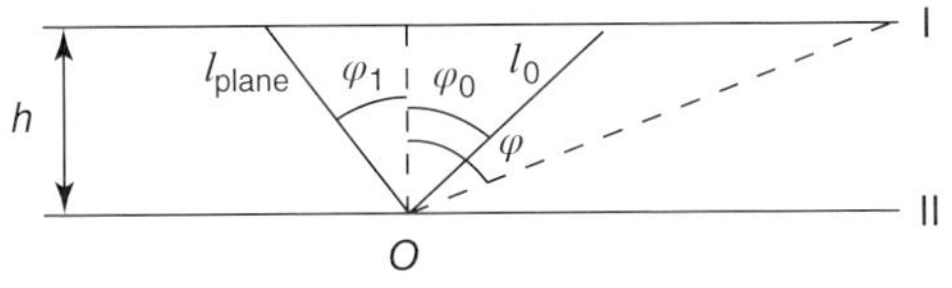

Figure 4.19 Schematic of electron movement in thin film. (Ryzhonkov *et al.* 2008 [1]. Reproduced with permission of BKL publishers.)

electron free path in film l_{plane} will decrease compared with l_0 in accordance with the relation

$$l_{plane} = h\left(1 + \ln\left(l_0/h\right)\right) \tag{4.7}$$

This equation can only be withdrawn under the condition of electron collision with planes I and II. If we remove this limit and accept $h < l_0$, then the equation for electron free path in thin film will be

$$l_{plane} = 3/4h\left(0.4228 + \ln\left(l_0/h\right)\right) \tag{4.8}$$

Let us focus on another point. In transfer models of thin films and whiskers, various cases are allowed: electrons can be mirrored and scattered diffusively, that is, uniformly in all directions, independent of their initial falling direction onto the specimen surface. For realization of various conditions, mirroring parameter is accepted and behavior diversity of all electrons is included in the change of mirroring parameter from zero (when the surface is considered absolutely rough) to unit (when it is considered absolutely mirrored).

As already mentioned, during the expression of previous equations, it was assumed that scattering from the film surface is not completely diffusive. This scattering is possible when the materials' surface deviates from ideal due to atom disorder, presence of impurities, adsorption centers, and change in electronic structure of surface. During diffusion scattering, nonelastic scattering to spontaneous angles is of high importance; that is, charge carriers leave the surface at speeds independent of initial speeds. A change of charge carriers in forming impulse leads to a change in conductivity.

In the case of ideal surface, mirror scattering is realized and surface scattering does not have an influence on conductivity because the energy loss does not occur.

Thus, dependence of electron free path length on the thickness of thin film is observed only in full or partial diffusion scattering from the surface. Only in this case will electron wave fully or partially lose its velocity component of directed movement by projecting from the surface. This will result in the energy scattering and hence the decrease in the average length of free path.

A study on the dependence of electrical resistance on temperature showed that mirroring parameter on the grain boundary for copper is equal to 0.468 and 0.506 at 100 and 275 K, respectively, and is equal to 0.24 for large crystal copper, which is twice less. This result is caused by the difference in length, width, and grain structure of nanocrystal and large crystal copper.

During acceptance of mirroring parameter η in the model, the equation of electron free path length transforms to

$$l_{plane} = 3/4h\left(0.4228 + \ln\left(l_0/h\right)\right)(1+\eta)/(1-\eta) \tag{4.9}$$

Based on experimental data, the length of electron free path in nanocrystal copper at a grain size of 7 nm was equal to 4.7 nm.

4.3 Electrical Conductivity in Nanomaterials

Electrical conductivity in nanomaterials is determined by several competitive factors. As shown earlier, in the equilibrium state, crystal lattice of nanomaterials is free of vacancy and dislocations. This should lead to an increase in conductivity of nanostructures, compared with large crystal materials.

In nanomaterials, the influence of grain boundaries should not be neglected, as it apparently contributes to conductivity change. Grain size in nanocrystals becomes commensurable with the length of conductivity electron free path and hence with a decrease in specific electrical conductivity of nanomaterials, compared with large crystal materials.

In this case, when scattering on surface and in volume is statistically independent, the following equation holds true:

$$1/l = 1/l_0 + 1/l_s \tag{4.10}$$

where l_0 and l_s are average lengths of electron free path during scattering in volume and on surface, respectively.

Let us assume that the length of electron free path is commensurable with diameter of threadlike crystal or thickness of ribbon $l_s \approx d$ (or $l_s \approx h$) and $\rho_0 = m\upsilon_F/\left(n_0 e^2 l\right)$. It is possible to obtain the following size dependencies for specific electrical conductivity:

$$\rho = \rho_0 \left(1 + l_0/l_s\right) = \rho_0 \left(1 + l_0/h\right) \tag{4.11}$$

$$\rho = \rho_0 \left(1 + l_0/d\right) \tag{4.12}$$

where h is film thickness, d is diameter of threadlike crystal, ρ_0 is resistance for monocrystal material, and υ_F is electron velocity on the Fermi level.

In other words, with a decrease in material's linear sizes, its specific electrical resistance values increase. This conclusion was proved by a large number of experimental data. Significant increase in value ρ with decrease in grain size was observed in nanodisperse Cu, Pd, Fe, Ni, Ni–P, Fe–Cu, Si–B, and Ni–Al.

Temperature dependencies of electrical resistance for nanostructured copper with a size of 7 nm are presented in Figure 4.20. Usual copper wire data in graph is given for comparison.

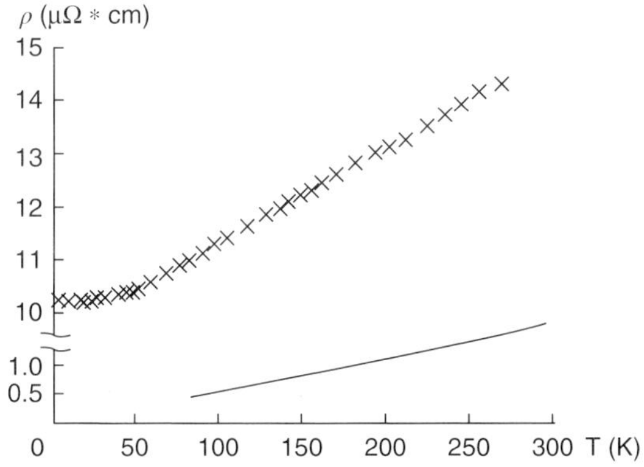

Figure 4.20 Temperature dependence of electrical resistance for nanostructured copper. Data for large crystal copper wire is shown by the straight line. (Ryzhonkov *et al.* 2008 [1]. Reproduced with permission of BKL publishers.)

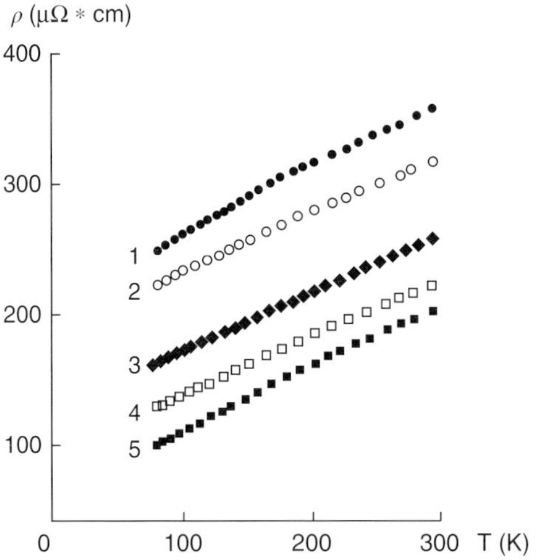

Figure 4.21 Temperature dependence of electrical resistance for Ni–P nanopowder with various particle sizes: 1 – 14 nm; 2 – 30 nm; 3 – 51 nm; 4 – 102 nm; 5 – large crystal specimen. (Ryzhonkov *et al.* 2008 [1]. Reproduced with permission of BKL publishers.)

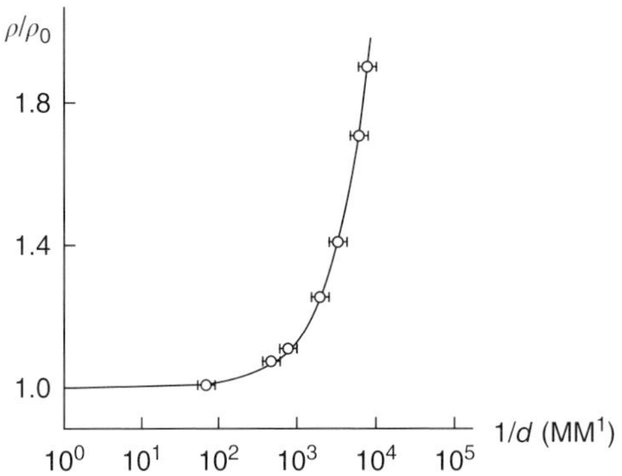

Figure 4.22 Dependence of relative specific electrical resistance of nanostructured Cu on average grain sizes. Straight line is indicating calculated curve; ρ_0 denotes specific electrical resistance for monocrystal copper. (Ryzhonkov *et al.* 2008 [1]. Reproduced with permission of BKL publishers.)

Experimental dependency changes in electrical resistance by an increase in temperature for Ni–P system with particle sizes from 14 to 102 nm are shown in Figure 4.21, which shows that when particle size increases, resistance of specimens decreases but still remains higher than that of large crystal material.

Dependence of electrical resistance for nanostructured copper, obtained by intensive plastic deformation method, on the reciprocal values of average grain size is presented in Figure 4.22. During the acquisition process, grains with a size of 100 nm formed in the material. Specimens were annealed to determine the dependence of electrical resistance on grain size. In the graph ρ is expressed in relative units, whereas for ρ_0 the value, to which the electrical resistance gravitate when approaching the melting point. As seen from the figure, obtained dependence exhibits a nonlinear pattern. When the grain size exceeds 10 μm, the electrical resistance does not change significantly. The growth of electrical resistance becomes clearer in the course of further grain size reduction, and sharp changes are observed at approximation to nanoregions.

Derived size dependence is valid for ceramic materials too. In Figure 4.23, the electrical resistance dependencies of TiB_2 films on their thickness and annealing temperature and the influence of grain size on electrical resistance are presented.

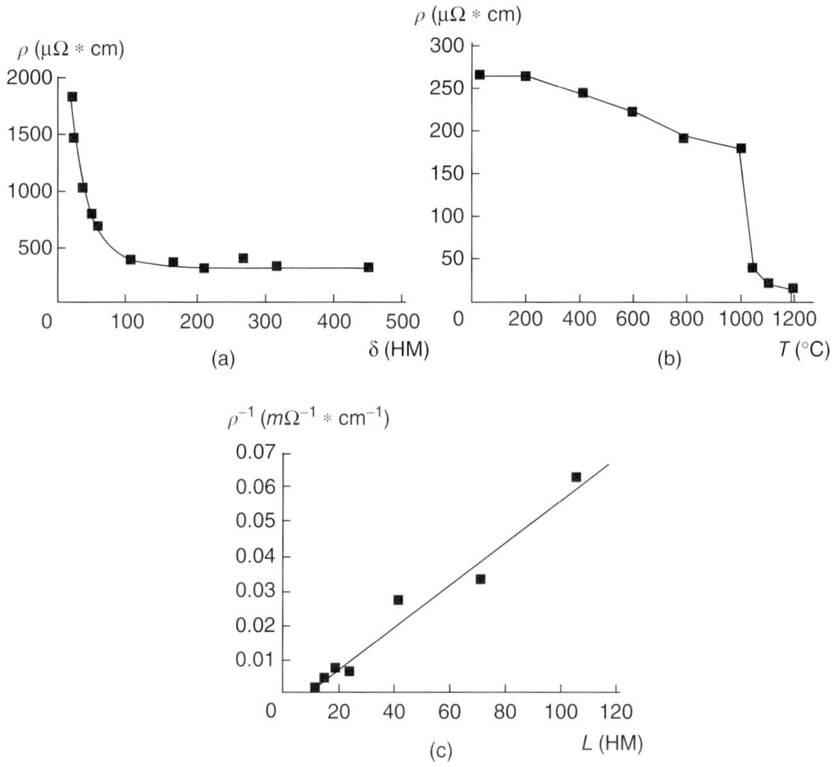

Figure 4.23 Influence of (a) thickness, (b) annealing temperature, and (c) grain size on electrical resistance (a, b) and conductivity (c) for TiB_2 films. (Ryzhonkov *et al.* 2008 [1]. Reproduced with permission of BKL publishers.)

4.4 Electron Work Function in Nanomediums

Size dependence of electron work function is important to understand contact phenomena and emission properties of nanoparticle system.

Work function is energy that needs to be spent for the removal of electrons from condensed medium to a place in vacuum where their kinetic energy will be equal to null. Theoretically, work function depends on Fermi energy E_F and potential barrier value, which is necessary to be overcome by electron for it to leave the particle. The main components of potential barrier are work against potential jump on the metal surface W_p and work against image forces W_{image}. In metal nanoparticles, both work function components can be changed.

The term *image force* can be derived through electrical fields' calculation method, which is based on the mental movement of any symmetrical object (e.g., electron) toward the border of substance. Electron will be equal to an object, which remains with a negative charge in object. As theoretical evaluations show, size dependence of work against image forces $W_{image}(R)$ on particle radius R can be expressed by the following equation:

$$W_{image}(R) = W_{image\ \infty} + 5.40/R \tag{4.13}$$

where $W_{image\ \infty}$ is work against imaging force in flat metal surface.

Hence, with a decrease in particle radius, $W_{\text{image}}(R)$ value increases.

Determination of work against potential jump is conducted through the half-empirical method for particles of model with FCC structure. This method is based on the identification of potential jump on the metal surface whose atoms have a negative electrical charge.

Based on calculations, with an decrease in diameter of faceted W, Pt, and Au particles up to ~10 nm, potential jump value does not change but then slowly decreases. Such decreasing for particles with a diameter of 2 nm is 0.8 eV for Pt and 0.32 eV for Au particles, respectively.

Moreover, one of the reasons for work function change in nanoparticles is a decrease in Fermi level. This effect becomes distinct at particle sizes less than 10 nm. As calculation showed, in spherical wolfram particles with a radius of 10 nm, E_F decreases until 5.77 eV, compared with 5.80 eV for large crystal metal. In spite of such insignificant changes in absolute values of the Fermi energy, this leads to a decrease in emission of W nanoparticles at 1000 K to 70% from appropriate value in bulk material.

In particular, during the calculation of size dependence of work function φ_R for spherical particle with a radius R as energy difference of non-ionized particle φ_∞ and after removal of electron, the following equation was obtained:

$$\varphi_R = \varphi_\infty \left(1 + \alpha/R + \beta/R^2\right) \tag{4.14}$$

where α, β are coefficients, $\alpha = 0.1$ nm, and $\beta = 0.001$ nm, wherein $R \geq 1.5$ nm.

In another model, the work function was determined as the difference between the energy used for the transfer of charge $+e$ to spherical particle and the energy used during the removal of $-e$ charge at distance x_0 from its surface to infinity. In this approximation, the following formula was obtained:

$$\varphi_R = \varphi_\infty \left(4\zeta + 2/\left(1 + \zeta^2\right)(2 + \zeta)\right) \tag{4.15}$$

where $\zeta = x_0/R$. R in both dependency cases is situated in the denominator, which should increase the work function with a decrease in particle radius.

Also, metal nanoparticles are characterized by quantum size effects, which have influence on changes in work function law. According to result from electron structure calculations, with a decrease in the number of atoms in the particle, the distance between vacuum and the highest completed electron level increases. This leads to an increase in work function, which, in large crystal silver and atomic particle, is 4.5 and 6.1 eV, respectively.

Calculated work function dependencies on the size and shapes of wolfram particles are presented in Figure 4.24. As can be seen in the graphs, the decrease in particle sizes for FCC lattice is 2–2.5 times more than that of BCC. Discontinuous change in work function with a small increase in diameter can be observed as a result of a large change in particle shape.

It is necessary to mention that calculation results should be treated with caution, despite being obtained in accordance with experiments that can always be done through free parameters. For example, concepts such as electronegativity, valence bond, and spatial localization of conducting electrons on metals seem highly debatable.

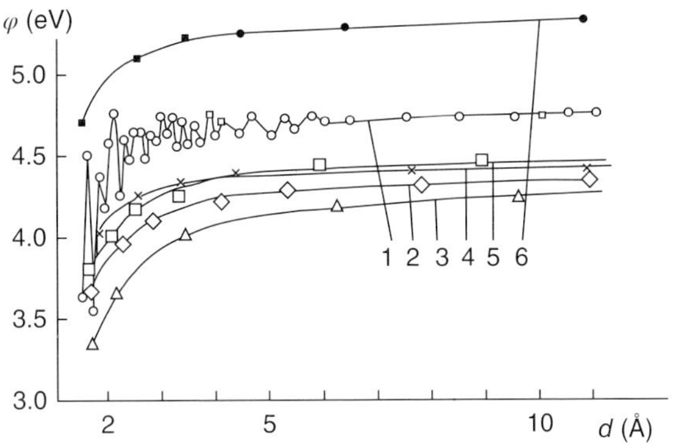

Figure 4.24 Calculated work function dependencies on the size of wolfram particles possessing different shapes: 1 – spherical, 2 – rhombododecahedral, 3 – cubic, 4 – cubic octahedral, 5 – truncated octahedral, 6 – octahedral. (Ryzhonkov *et al.* 2008 [1]. Reproduced with permission of BKL publishers.)

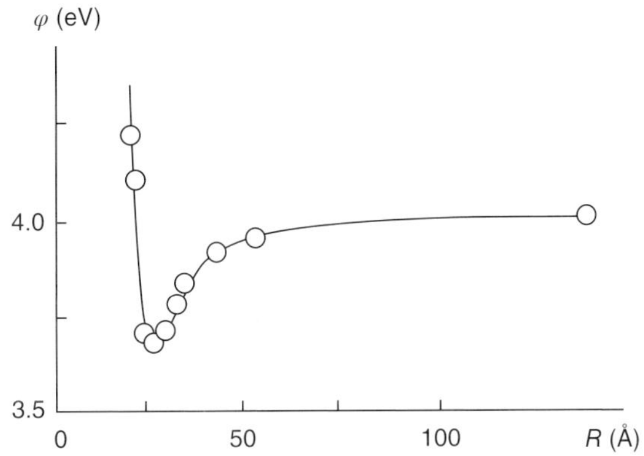

Figure 4.25 Experimental dependence of electron work function on Au particle size. (Ryzhonkov *et al.* 2008 [1]. Reproduced with permission of BKL publishers.)

Figure 4.25 shows the experimental dependence of work function on the size of insular gold films on quartz substrate. Determined law have minimum, with low work function at preceded particles size decrease. Analogous dependencies of work function changes on particle size were also obtained for Ag, Al, Fe, and Mg.

4.5 Superconductivity Phenomenon in Nanomaterials

Experimentally it was found that in some metals and alloys, specific electrical resistance at nearly definite temperature T_c, called the transition temperature, sharply drops to superconducting state. Limiting in the phonon spectrum caused by low frequencies will occur in nanoparticles, due to the lattice vibrations with larger wavelengths than the particle size. Hence, phonon spectrum from long wavelengths (or smaller frequencies) is clipped. Such change in phonon spectrum is termed tightening. On the other hand, in nanoparticles, strengthening of spectra of long wavelength phonon mode occurs because of surface vibrations, leading to a decrease in average phonon frequency and, in turn, growth of electron–phonon interaction parameter. This process is referred to as softening. Electron–phonon spectrum softening can also be caused by an increase in critical temperature T_c.

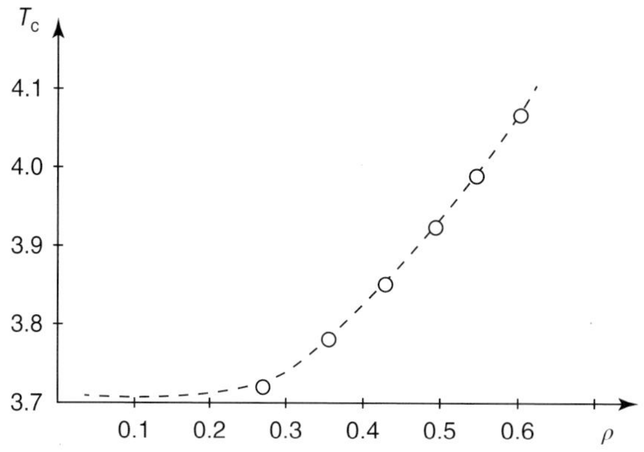

Figure 4.26 Dependence of transition temperature to superconducting state for Sn particle with a radius of 10 nm from its packed thickness. (Ryzhonkov *et al.* 2008 [1]. Reproduced with permission of BKL publishers.)

Tightening of phonon spectrum leads to an increase of transition temperature to superconducting state. To calculate phonon numbers in nanoparticle, it is necessary to multiply its spectral density to fill and integrate values from all frequencies. At this time, due to the cutting of long wavelength spectrum upon reaching the point, in which the phonon number for volume unit in the bulk metal and nanoparticle will be the same, it will be necessary to increase the temperature of the latter. From here it follows that T_c in nanoparticle must be larger than the temperature of superconducting transition for large crystal material.

In particle assembly, one reason of T_c growth exists: an increase in nanoparticle packaging thickness ρ, which is determined as the relation of specimen thickness to bulk material thickness. As shown in Figure 4.26, an increase in Sn particle packaging thickness with a radius of 10 nm leads to an increase in transition temperature to superconducting state.

Correlation of length or coherency length, with distance ξ between pairs of electrons, can be evaluated by the following equation:

$$\xi = hv_F/k_B T_c \tag{4.16}$$

where h is Planck constant, v_F is electron speed in Fermi level, k_B is Boltzmann constant, and T_c is transition temperature to superconducting state.

Estimation shows that $\xi \approx 10^{-6}$ m, which means that pair-forming electrons are located at a distance of 10^4 level crystal lattice periods from each other. In other words, all the electron system of superconductor represents a linked team, spreading to large atomic level distances.

Several methods for the evaluation of minimal particle size were developed, which can be transferred into superconducting state. One of the marks based on estimation of electron numbers n can form pairs according to the following relation:

$$n = k_B T_c N_e/E_F \tag{4.17}$$

where k_B is Boltzmann constant, N_e is number of free electrons, and E_F is electron energy in Fermi level. Calculations using this formula give value n of $10^{-3}N_e$ level. Hence, in a particle with $N_e \sim 10^{-3}$, the number of electrons for material transition to superconducting state will not be enough. The next method is bind with evaluation of value, calling as critical volume V of transition to superconducting state:

$$V = \lambda_F 2\xi_0 \tag{4.18}$$

where λ_F is electron wavelength in Fermi level and ξ_0 is coherency length at $T = 0$ for large crystal metal. For particles whose volumes are less than the calculated value using the formula, quantization of electron spectrum is also necessary to mention. Superconductivity becomes impossible when the distance between electron energy levels is comparable with energy of electron pair formation. Calculations showed that for Pb particle with a diameter of 2.2 nm containing 736 electrons, the superconducting state is unreachable and that for Sn particles, this value is equal to $\approx$ 5 nm.

Based on evaluation, the energy of electron pair formation, with a decrease in particle size, became comparable with the energy of heat fluctuations, which can transition it from the superconducting state to the usual state, and vice versa. For Al nanoparticles, for example, the critical volume is 5 nm^3 when the energy differences between superconducting and usual states are equal to $k_B T_c$.

It is necessary to give attention to T_c, which influences the size dependence of nanoparticles. As a rule, experiments were conducted on a large array of particles that interact with each other or surrounding medium. This will result in the degradation of transition to superconducting state, increasing with a decrease in particle sizes. This effect, often called fluctuation, becomes distinct when $\xi / k_B T_c \sim 0.001$. As soon as the fluctuation effects dominate in the particle, an increase in critical temperature will lead to their decrease, and then disappearance of superconductivity is observed.

In some metal nanopowders of pure metals, T_c increases with a decrease in particle size up to $\sim$ 5 nm. An increase in superconducting critical temperature with a decrease in particle size is observed in Al (Figure 4.27).

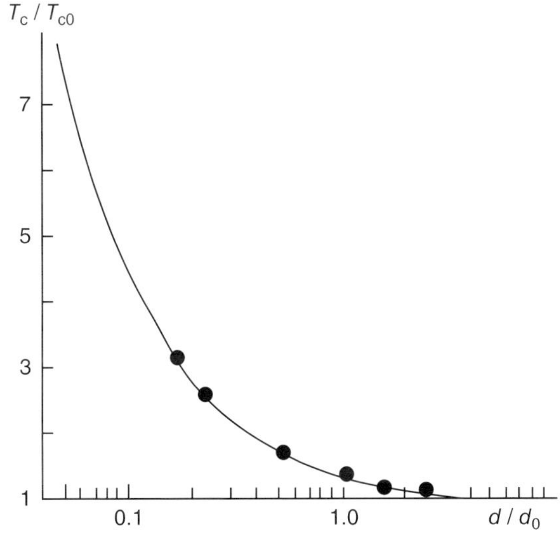

Figure 4.27 Dependence of relative superconductivity temperature T_c on relative diameter of Al particle: T_{c0} – superconducting transition temperature of bulk metal; d_0 – some diameter in which $T_c = T_{c0}$; straight line – calculation result. (Ryzhonkov *et al.* 2008 [1]. Reproduced with permission of BKL publishers.)

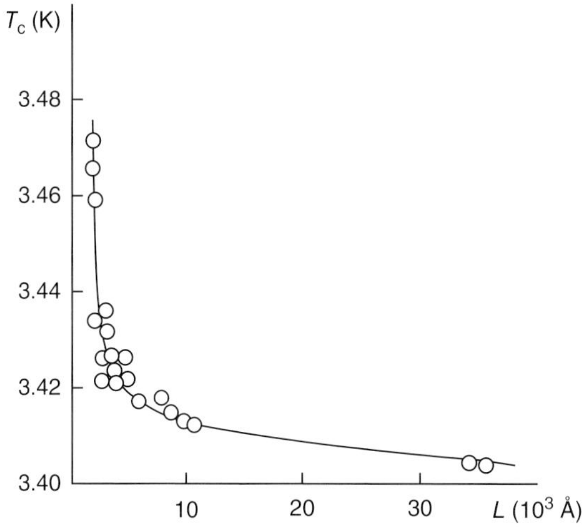

Figure 4.28 Dependence of T_c on thickness of the indium film. (Ryzhonkov *et al.* 2008 [1]. Reproduced with permission of BKL publishers.)

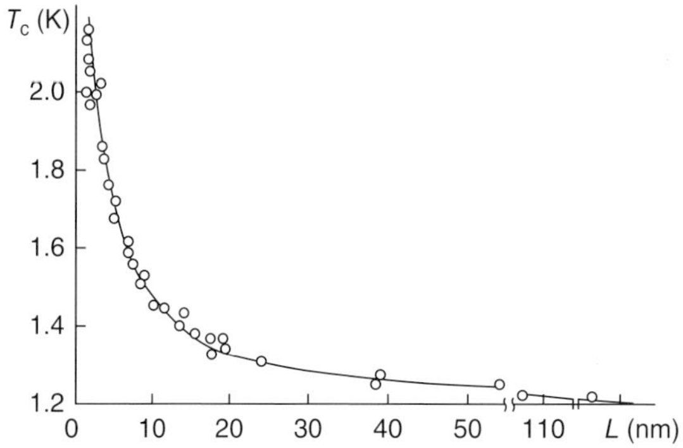

Figure 4.29 Dependence of T_c on thickness of the aluminum film. (Ryzhonkov *et al.* 2008 [1]. Reproduced with permission of BKL publishers.)

In metal film systems on foreign substrate, a significant increase in T_c by a decrease in crystallite size was observed. Temperature growth for transition into superconducting state for In (Figure 4.28), Al (Figure 4.29), and Sn, Mo, and Ga starts at film thickness around 100 nm.

However, several experimental results that indicate a decrease in temperature for transition to superconducting state exist. This was observed, for example, in Pb nanoparticles, in which T_c decreased during reduction in their size (Figure 4.30). Also, a decrease in temperature for transition to superconducting state was established for niobium nitride nanopowder $NbN_{0.9-1.05}$ with a size of 28–44 nm. Analogous results were observed for oxide superconductor Bi–Sr–Ca–Cu–O with a particle size $\approx$ 10 nm, obtained by crystallization from amorphous state.

In a number of systems, in particular Mo–SiO_2, Mo–Ge, Mo–Y, Al–Al_2O, In, Ti, and porous glass, initial increase in T_c and then its lowering are observed.

Thus, size dependence on temperature for transition to superconducting state is not established clearly. It follows from the earlier texts that as regards dependence on nature, shape, specimen preparation, and saving conditions, T_c might be not only higher but also lower than the temperature for transition to superconducting state for large crystal material [1].

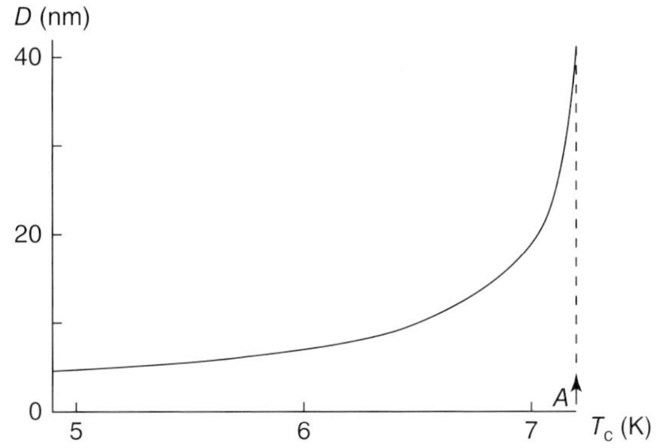

Figure 4.30 Size dependence of T_c for lead particles; *A* denotes T_c for bulk metal. (Ryzhonkov *et al.* 2008 [1]. Reproduced with permission of BKL publishers.)

Case Study 1: Surfactant Effects on Dispersion Characteristics of Copper-Based Nanomaterials

- Powder agglomeration and thermal conductivity in copper-based nanofluids were studied by Saterlie *et al.* [2]. Copper nanoparticle synthesis was achieved using various surfactants, such as polyvinylpyrrolidone, oleic acid, and cetyltrimethylammonium bromide. In this study, the use of surfactants during the synthesis of copper nanopowders has important consequences on the dispersion of the powders in a base fluid.
- The influence of solvents and surfactants on the preparation of copper nanoparticles by a chemical reduction method was studied by Dang *et al.* [3]. Based on this study, polyvinylpyrrolidone worked as both size controller and polymeric capping agent because it hindered the nuclei from aggregating through polar groups, which strongly absorb the copper particles on the surface with coordination bonds.

Case Study 2: Applications of Superconducting Nanomaterials

- BSCCO/$SrTiO_3$ one-dimensional superconducting photonic crystal (PC) was studied for many applications [4]. In this theoretical study, the transmittance properties of a one-dimensional superconducting dielectric PC were introduced based on the transfer matrix method (TMM). Focus was directed on the so-called cutoff frequency whose implementation can be useful when using PC as a good reflector besides its other applications. This study showed that cutoff frequency is very sensitive to temperature variation and that photonic band gap can be tuned by varying the system temperature, thus referring to wide applications of superconducting nanomaterials in transistor, magnetic, and electronic devices.

Control Questions

1) Describe the dispersion characteristics of nanomaterials.
2) Determine the specific surface area of nanomaterials.
3) Determine size distribution mechanisms in nanomaterials.
4) Discuss surface boundary and morphology features in nanosized materials.
5) Describe the role of grain boundaries in studying morphological characteristics of nanomaterials.
6) Describe the main morphologies in nanodisperse particles.
7) List and determine electrical properties of nanomaterials.
8) Describe changes in electron free path of nanomaterials and their effect on the electrical conductivity property of nanomaterials.
9) Discuss electrical conductivity characteristics of nanomaterials.
10) Determine electron work function in nanomediums.
11) Describe superconductivity phenomenon in nanomaterials.

References

1 Ryzhonkov, D.I., Levina, V.V., and Dzidziguri, E.L. (2008) *Nanomaterials, BINOM*, BKL Publishers, Moscow.

2 Saterlie, M.S. *et al* (2012) Surfactant effects on dispersion characteristics of copper-based nanofluids: a dynamic light scattering study. *Chem. Mater.*, **24** (17), 3299–3306.

3 Dang, T.M.D. *et al* (2011) Synthesis and optical properties of copper nanoparticles prepared by a chemical reduction method. *Adv. Nat. Sci.: Nanosci. Nanotechnol.*, **2**, 025004 (pp. 7).

4 Aly, A.H. *et al* (2015) BSCCO/$SrTiO_3$ one dimensional superconducting photonic crystal for many applications. *J. Supercond. Novel Magn.*, **28** (6), 1699–1703.

Further Reading

Alshehri, A.H., Jakubowska, M., Młożniak, A., Horaczek, M., Rudka, D., Free, F., and Carey, J.D. (2012) Enhanced electrical conductivity of silver nanoparticles for high frequency electronic applications. *ACS Appl. Mater. Interfaces*, **4** (12), 7007–7010.

Croitoru, M.D., Shanenko, A.A., and Peeters, F.M. (2009) Tuning the superconducting properties of nanomaterials, in *Complex Phenomena in Nanoscale Systems*, NATO Science for Peace and Security Series B: Physics and Biophysics (eds G. Casati and D. Matrasulov), Springer, Dordrecht, pp. 1–14.

Hanemann, T. and Szabó, D.V. (2010) Polymer-nanoparticle composites: from synthesis to modern applications. *Materials*, **3**, 3468–3517.

Huang, X. and El-Sayed, M.A. (2010) Gold nanoparticles: optical properties and implementations in cancer diagnosis and photothermal therapy. *J. Adv. Res.*, **1** (1), 13.

Lu, H., Liu, Z., Yan, X., Li, D., Parent, L., and Tian, H. (2016) Electron work function-a promising guiding parameter for material design. *Sci. Rep.*, **6**, 24366.

Parveen, S., Rana, S., and Fangueiro, R. (2013) A review on nanomaterial dispersion, microstructure, and mechanical properties of carbon nanotube and nanofiber reinforced cementitious composites. *J. Nanomater.*, **80**, Article ID 710175, 19 pp.

Pietrzak, T.K., Maciaszek, M., Nowiński, J.L., Ślubowska, W., Ferrari, S., Mustarelli, P., Wasiucionek, M., Wzorek, M., and Garbarczyk, J.E. (2012) Electrical properties of V_2O_5 nanomaterials prepared by twin rollers technique. *Solid State Ionics*, **225** (4), 658–662.

Su, H., Li, Y., Li, X.Y., and Wong, K.S. (2009) Optical and electrical properties of Au nanoparticles in two-dimensional networks: an effective cluster model. *Opt. Express*, **17** (24), 22223–22234.

Yurkov, G.Y., Fionov, A.S., Koshkarov, Y.A., Koleso, V.V., and Gubin, S.P. (2007) Electrical and magnetic properties of nanomaterials containing iron or cobalt nanoparticles. *Inorg. Mater.*, **43** (8), 834–844.

5

Physical Properties of Nanomaterials: Graphene

Translated materials from the original work of Ryzhonkov, D.I., Levina, V.V. and Dzidziguri, E.L. were used in this chapter.

> *"One thing I have learned in a long life: that all our science, measured against reality, is primitive and childlike – and yet it is the most precious thing we have."*
>
> Albert Einstein

5.1 Ferromagnetic Characteristics of Nanomaterials

Nanomaterials are very diverse, unusual, and often unique magnetic properties, and hence, researchers' attention has been drawn toward great perspectives for the creation of new highly effective magnetic materials.

5.1.1 Substance in Single-Domain Condition

The single-domain structure determines the specific magnetic properties of ferromagnetic materials. Upon decrease in size of these materials, single-domain structure might be energetically advantageous in such condition than multi-domain structure of bulk ferromagnetic materials.

The formation of multi-domain structure is based on the intention of ferromagnetic material to have minimal free energy, which is, in this case, fulfilled with components such as exchange, magnetostatic and magnetostrictive energy, and crystallographic anisotropy energy. A decrease in ferromagnetic energy is achieved by parallel lining up of electron spins with minimal crystallographic anisotropy energy and with dominating direction to axis of "easy" magnetization. To close the formed magnetic flow by electrons, a large number of spontaneous regions (*domains*) magnetized until saturation will form in bulk materials. During this process, the quantity of magnetic poles decreases, leading to a decrease in magnetostatic energy.

During reduction of ferromagnetic sizes or their splitting into tiny powders, particle diameter gradually becomes commensurable with equilibrium domain sizes. In such a way, as a result of the crushing of the material, moment occurs when all the volume of particle is taken by one domain; that is,

Nano- and Biomaterials: Compounds, Properties, Characterization, and Applications,
First Edition. Zhypargul Abdullaeva.

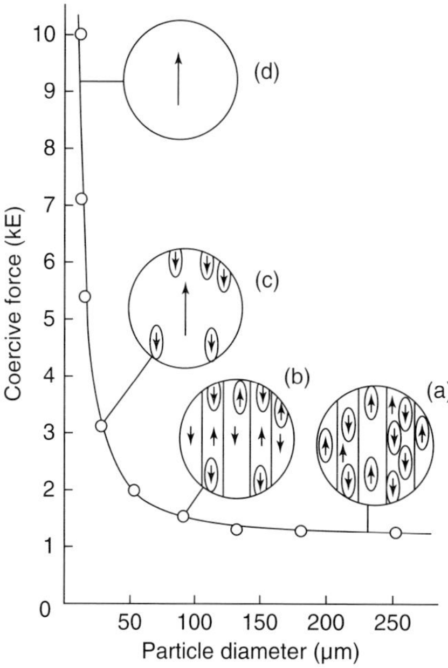

Figure 5.1 Binding of Mn–Bi alloy particle diameter with coercive force and schematics of domain structures: (a) multi-domain structure; (b) multi-domain structure without surface-connecting regions; (c) transition form; and (d) single-domain structure. (Reproduced with permission of BKL Publishers.)

single-domain condition occurs. The transition from multi-domain (Figure 5.1a) to single-domain (Figure 5.1d) state will happen under several intermediate conditions.

First of all, the multi-domain structure will lose surface-connecting regions (Figure 5.1b). After that, condition with transition magnetic structure will form when there is only one basic domain in particle, and near the surface, not just large-connecting regions will remain (Figure 5.1c).

Domain sizes d in rectangular crystal with thickness l, starting from minimal magnetic energy, can be evaluated by the following relation:

$$d = 3.04 \times 10^{-3} \cdot \sqrt{\gamma l / I_s} \tag{5.1}$$

where I_s is the saturation magnetization in tesla and γ is the domain energy wall, fitting with square unit, in Joule per square meter.

According to the last equation, the width of the domains is proportional to $\sqrt{l}$. This means that during dispersion, width decreases more slowly than particle size. Finally, d becomes greater than nanoparticle diameter, and single-domain structure without domain walls will appear. In Figure 5.2, the magnetization distribution in cobalt particle is obtained by interference electron microscopy: magnetization lines are not connected and magnetic flow goes beyond the particle.

Change in particle ferromagnetic properties is determined by three characteristic sizes. The first is the critical radius of single-domain R_0. In the absence of outer magnetic field, homogeneous magnetization lower than the given size causes less free energy than any other condition with magnetization distribution on particle volume.

Let us evaluate the critical radius for single-domain R_0. For certainty let us assume that nanoparticles are spherical. If it is separated into domains with width

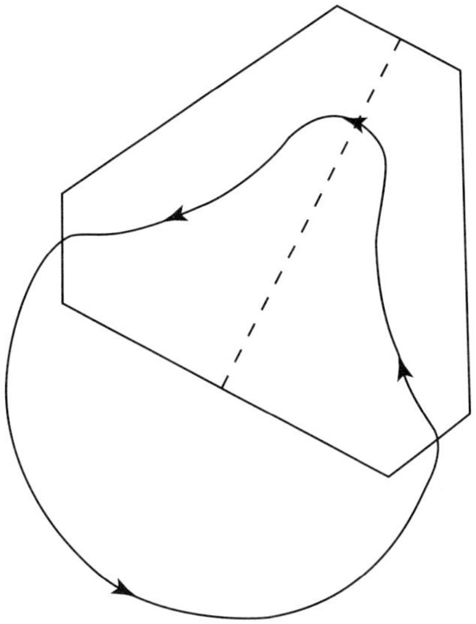

Figure 5.2 Magnetization distribution in the cobalt particle. (Reproduced with permission of BKL Publishers.)

d, then the equation can be roughly written as

$$d = \sqrt{18\gamma \mu_0 R / I_s} \tag{5.2}$$

where I_s is the saturation magnetization in tesla; γ is the domain energy wall, fitting with square unit, in joule per square meter; μ_0 is the magnetic sensitivity, and R is the particle radius in meter.

If the single-domain condition will be realized, then $d = 2R_0$. Hence, it can be written as

$$2R_0 = \sqrt{18\gamma \mu_0 R / I_s} \tag{5.3}$$

and, after bringing to the square,

$$R_0^2 = 9\gamma \mu_0 R / (2I_s^2) \tag{5.4}$$

For iron $I_s = 2.15\,\text{T}$ and $\gamma = 1.6 \times 10^{-3}\,\text{J}\,\text{m}^{-2}$, in accordance with the last equation $R_0 = 2\,\text{nm}$.

More strict calculations are made for isolated Co, Ni, and Fe spherical particles, which show that single-domain critical sizes are equal to 8–18, 7.5–17, and 21–40 nm, respectively.

When considering any set of nanoparticles, the critical size for single domain will be determined by their concentrations. The tendency is that in assembly of ferromagnetic particles, the critical size of single domain will increase.

The radius of absolute single-domain R_0' ($R_0' < R_0$) is the second size characteristic of ferromagnetic nanoparticles. Lower than this value, condition with homogeneous magnetization cannot be eliminated by outer magnetic field during magnetic reversal process.

5.1.2 Superparamagnetism in Nanoparticles

Finally, the third size characteristic is the critical radius of superparamagnetic behavior of a_0^* particle.

Superparamagnetism is a special condition appearing in small ferromagnetic particles when their sizes decrease significantly lower than critical. This phenomenon is realized in assembly with ferromagnetic single-domain particles where, as a result of heat fluctuations, chaotic rotations by magnetic moment vectors will occur. As a result, the system will behave as paramagnetic, with only the difference in magnetic moment of ferromagnetic particles being larger up to 10^5 times.

Thus, superparamagnetism is a quasi-paramagnetic behavior of systems containing complex, very tiny ferro- and ferrimagnetic particles.

The appearance of superparamagnetism in nanomaterials is realized when in large particles, the magnetic moment vector of particle M is oriented along the direction of lighter magnetization, determined by the sum of magnetic anisotropy and magnetic moment vector. From this direction, it is necessary to overcome the energy barrier, which is proportional to anisotropy energy $K_{\text{eff}}V$, where K_{eff} is constant for total anisotropy and V is the particle volume. When an average heat energy $k_B T$ becomes commensurable with or larger than anisotropy energy ($k_B T \geq K_{\text{eff}}V$), the turn of magnetic moment by heat fluctuations will be probable. For example, in typical ferro- and ferrimagnetic substances, $K_{\text{eff}} \approx 10^{-2} - 10^{-6}\,\text{J}\,\text{m}^{-3}$; thus, at $T \approx 100\,\text{K}$ heat fluctuations become visible in particles, the volume of which is less than $10^{-24} - 10^{-27}\,\text{m}^3$, which agrees with linear sizes 1–10 nm. In other words, the behavior of a set of nanoparticles in relation to temperature influence is similar to that of gas of paramagnetic molecules. Only in gas, as a result of heat fluctuations, will orientations of molecules with magnetic moments undergo change and self-titled particles remain inert. Also their magnetic moment will undergo changes. But qualitative influence of temperature is the same for both cases.

From above it becomes clear that particle assembly loses ferromagnetic properties as it transitions to superparamagnetic state. Hysteresis loop degenerates as magnetization curve, that is, equality of coercive force and remnant magnetization.

Superparamagnetism was experimentally observed in particle systems of Fe, Co, and Ni. The Mössbauer effect is very sensitive to this transition. Figure 5.3 presents the Mössbauer spectra of Fe nanopowder obtained by chemical dispersion method. During the transition from ferromagnetic to superparamagnetic state, sextet of lines (i) degenerates into one central line (ii). As spectra contain sextet and central line both at the same time, there are ferromagnetic and superparamagnetic components in a given specimen.

The square unit of appropriate peaks is proportional to the quantitative composition of each component. In specimen, the spectra of which are presented in Figure 5.3, approximately 15% of substance exists in superparamagnetic state. As sizes of superparamagnetic material are strictly determined, then it can be assumed that 15% of particles have a size of 10 nm. By this way, the Mössbauer study gives a possibility for evaluation of size characteristics of nanopowder.

5.1.3 Size Dependence on Coercive Force

Size dependence on coercive force H_c can be presented schematically as follows. First, with a decrease in particle diameter, H_c grows (Figure 5.4) and reaches a maximum at nanomaterial size of around 10 nm. After that, a sharp decrease in H_c is observed, which becomes null at the region of superparamagnetic state.

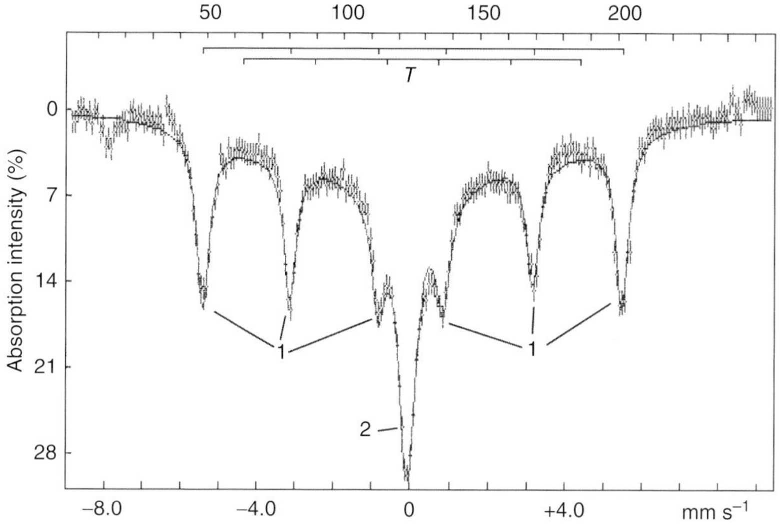

Figure 5.3 Mössbauer spectra for iron nanopowder. (Reproduced with permission of BKL Publishers.)

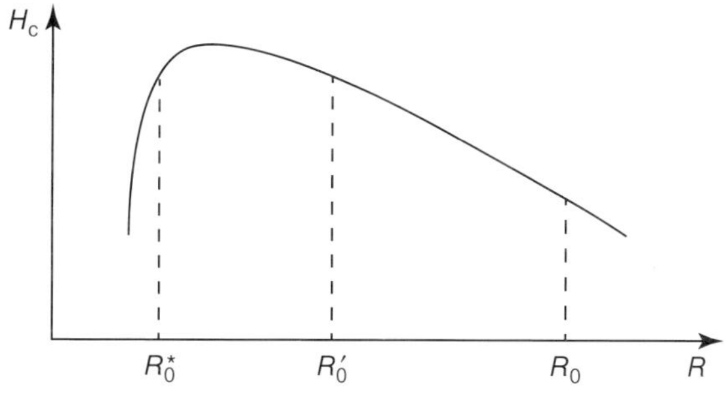

Figure 5.4 Qualitative dependence of coercive force on particle radius: R_0 is the single-domain critical size; R_0' is the absolute single-domain radius; R_0^* is the critical radius of superparamagnetism. (Reproduced with permission of BKL Publishers.)

Extremal character of size dependence on coercive force is explained by different domain structures of particles during change in their diameter.

The size dependence on coercive force for the assembly of iron and cobalt nanoparticles at temperatures of 4.2 and 300 K is presented in Figure 5.5. Samples were obtained by metal steam condensation method in the inert gas medium at paraffin matrix. Critical single-domain sizes, determined by maximum of size dependence states H_c, are 24 and 28 nm for Fe and Co, respectively, which well agrees with theoretical evaluations.

Nanopowders of Fe, Ni, and alloy $Fe_{0.91}Si_{0.09}$ with minimal particle size of 8, 12, and 6 nm, respectively, were obtained by ball milling. The conducted measurements showed that a decrease in Fe nanoparticle size from 80 to 8–10 nm is accompanied by a nearly three times H_c increase. Maximum is observed on size dependence of Ni nanopowders on coercive force, in accordance with a diameter of 15–35 nm. However, during a particle size decrease up to 12 nm, H_c value sharply decreases up to five times. A decrease in nanoparticle size for $Fe_{0.91}Si_{0.09}$ alloy from 40 to 6 nm leads to a fivefold H_c growth.

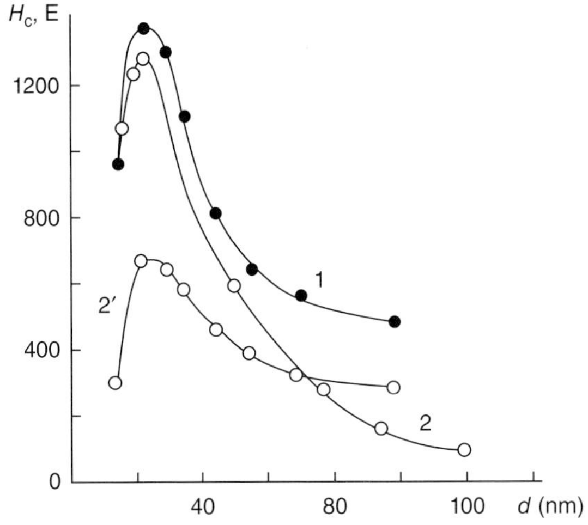

Figure 5.5 Dependence of coercive force on particle size: 1 – Fe at 4.2 K; 2 and 2′ – Co at 4.2 and 300 K, respectively. (Reproduced with permission of BKL Publishers.)

5.1.4 Size Dependence on Saturation Magnetization

Figure 5.6 presents typical size dependence on saturation magnetization of I_s. In the graph, saturation magnetization of Ni nanopowder experiences a nearly two times reduction upon decrease of particle size from 140 to 20 nm.

I_s of cobalt nanopowder is analogous. The saturation magnetization of spherical iron particles is less than that of large-crystal material, even at a size around 100 nm. With a decrease in diameter of particles, saturation magnetization initially decreases, and then starting from 35 nm, it remains stable.

A study of nanostructured Ni with an average grain size of 70–100 nm showed that its saturation magnetization is less than approximately 10% compared with that of large-grained Ni. The same result was observed in submicrocrystal nickel obtained by deformation–thermal processing. Currently, there is no single opinion regarding reasons for saturation magnetization changes in nanomaterials.

One possible explanation can be assumed. With a decrease in particle size, more significant part of atom spins lying at the surface has a stable direction, which does not fit with particle size. As a result, in ferromagnetic nanopowders, two spin subsystems form. One of them is collinear in volume and the second is

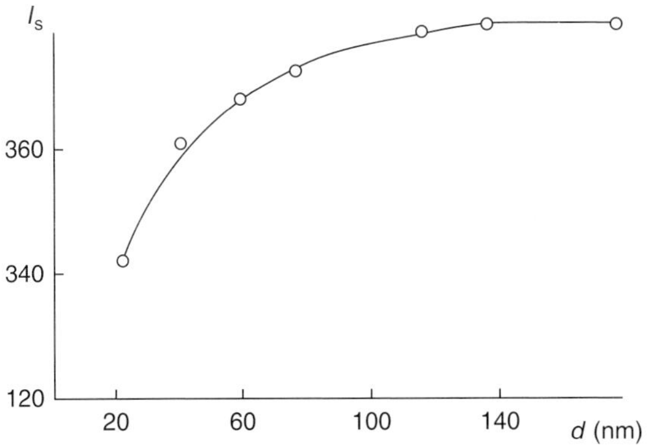

Figure 5.6 Size dependence of saturation magnetization for Ni at 4.2 K. (Reproduced with permission of BKL Publishers.)

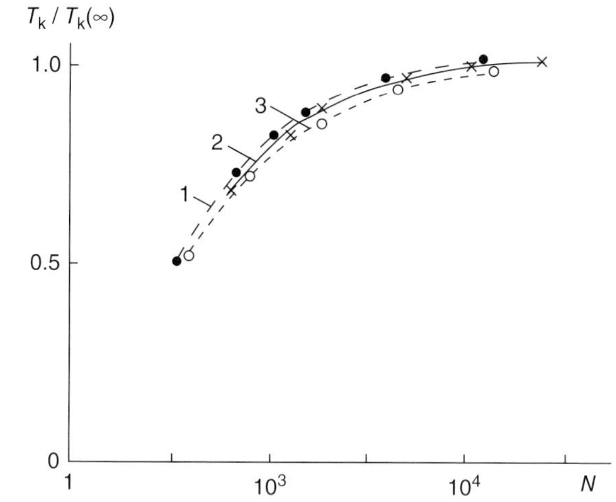

Figure 5.7 Size dependences of Curie temperature, calculated by layered model for cubic octahedron (1), octahedron (2), and cube (3) with FCC lattice. (Reproduced with permission of BKL Publishers.)

in subsurface layer, which have constituent of magnetization, perpendicular to the first one.

With the interaction of parallel-located particles one more possible explanation of size dependence on saturation magnetization is binding. Interaction of closely located particles results in ferromagnetic property if their magnetic moments are lined to one side. Antiferromagnetic condition when the magnetic moments of particles are lined faced to each other is more energetically advantageous. Such pairs cannot contribute to the magnetization of specimen. To break them apart, larger fields are necessary.

5.1.5 Size Dependence on Curie Temperature

With a decrease in particle size, the Curie temperature will also undergo changes. *Curie temperature* is the temperature above which self-magnetization does not occur. Calculations of size dependence on the Curie temperature for atomic numbers N composing the nanoparticle were carried out. Obtained graphs in relative units for various shape nanoparticles are presented in Figure 5.7. Calculation results show that a decrease in Curie temperature is not large and reaches 10% for particles with a size of 2 nm.

In experiments, it was revealed that changes in the Curie temperature for ferromagnetic nanoparticles have similar obtained values. For example, T_K for bulk Ni is equal to 631 K, and for particles with a size of 3 nm, it is equal to 565 K (Figure 5.8).

5.2 Thermal Property Features in Nanomaterials

Similar to other physical properties, heat is characterized by size dependence, as well as a decrease in linear value of material extension. Characteristics of material, such as specific heat value, heat conductivity, and Debye temperature, depend on lattice dynamic, which will be presented later, and change due to a number of

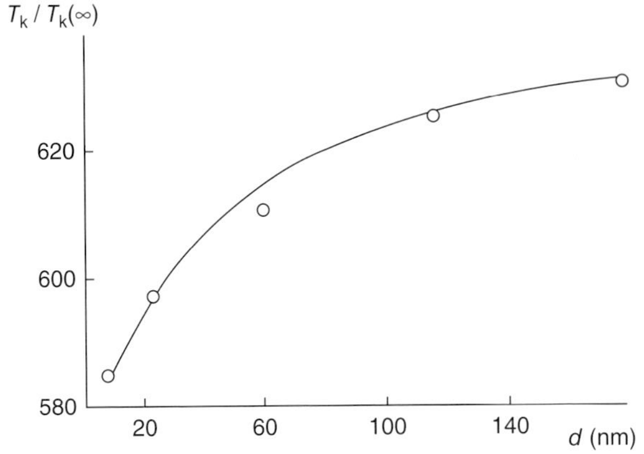

Figure 5.8 Size dependence of Curie temperature for nickel. (Reproduced with permission of BKL Publishers.)

nanostate features. This happens firstly due to the existence of a number of atoms near the surface of nanomaterials.

5.2.1 Size Dependence on Heat Conductivity

As it is known, heat movement of atom lattice is based on its fluctuations around some equilibrium state. The number of crystal fluctuation types, according to the Debye theory, is equal to atomic numbers N, and the total number of fluctuations in bulk material is equal to $3N$, with three levels of freedom to each fluctuation. According to this, the following equation is derived [1]:

$$\int_0^{\nu_{max}} g(\nu)d\nu = 3N \tag{5.5}$$

where ν is the fluctuation frequency, $g(\nu)$ is the thickness of fluctuation states, $g(\nu)d\nu$ is the number of fluctuations with frequency from ν to $\nu + d\nu$, and ν_{max} is the maximum frequency of fluctuation for crystal lattice determined from the full number of fluctuations to the value of free lattice fluctuation levels.

In size-limited crystals, their wavelengths do not exceed twice the diameter of particle d. As a result, the fluctuation spectra of nanomaterials at low-frequency states differ from those of large-crystal materials and are limited by some minimal value $\nu_{min} \sim c/2d$, where c is light speed. Hence, the total number of fluctuations for particle containing N atoms can be determined as

$$\int_{\nu_{min}}^{\nu_{max}} g(\nu)d\nu = 3N \tag{5.6}$$

The value of ν_{min} generally depends on substance nature, shape, and size of particle.

As theoretical studies showed, the frequency distribution function $g(\nu)$ of rectangular nanoparticle is determined by the following formula:

$$g(\nu) = a_1 V\nu^2 + a_2 S\nu + a_3 L \tag{5.7}$$

where V, S, L are the volume, square area, and total length of nanoparticle ribs, respectively, and a_1, a_2, a_3 are the coefficients.

On the other hand, according to the Debye theory, heat conductivity C_υ for large-crystal solid material at absolute low temperatures T, which correspond to the condition $h\nu < k_B T$, is determined by equation

$$C_\upsilon = bVT^3 \tag{5.8}$$

where V is the material volume and b is the coefficient.

Taking into account Eq. (5.7), then the heat conductivity for nanoparticles can be obtained by the following equation:

$$C_\upsilon(r) = b_1 VT^3 + b_2 ST^2 + b_3 LT \tag{5.9}$$

where b_1, b_2, b_3 are the coefficients.

Let us assume that ν_{max} in nanomaterials fits with maximum frequency fluctuation of the lattice of bulk crystals. Then, the first member shown in Eq. (5.9) appears as contributor to heat conductivity of large-crystal solid material according to Eq. (5.8). However, in the case of nanosubstance, in the expression for heat conductivity, contributors caused by large surface of the second and third summands are present. Hence, at $h\nu_{max} < k_B T$, the heat conductivity of nanomaterial $C_\upsilon(r)$ is always higher than heat conductivity of large-crystal material C_υ.

Similar results during the determination of size dependence on heat conductivity are also obtained by quantum approach. Truly, the temperature interval in which lattice fluctuation can be observed based on quantum representations is very narrow. It is determined by the so-called degeneration temperature T_{D}, at which quantum effects in ideal gas will start to appear:

$$T_{\text{D}} = (h^2/mk)(N/V)^{2/3} \tag{5.10}$$

where m is the mass, N is the number of atoms, and V is the system volume.

By substitution of appropriate number values into given equation, degeneration temperature value is determined by 10 K at level. Hence, the quantum mechanical study of lattice fluctuations is possible at $T < 10\,\text{K}$. At higher temperatures, the heat movement of crystal should be observed at classical positions.

According to quantum approximation, the total number of fluctuations for spherical particle with radius r containing N atoms is determined by the following formula:

$$\nu(N) = (2/9\pi)r^3 k_{\text{D}}^3 + (1/4)r^2 k_{\text{D}}^2 + (2/3\pi)r k_{\text{D}} \tag{5.11}$$

where k_{D} wave vector corresponding to the maximum of frequency of fluctuations $\nu_{\text{max}} = k_{\text{D}} c/2\pi$.

Wave vector is a vector determining the distribution direction and spatial period of flat monochromatic wave. The module of wave vector is called wave number k, which determines spatial period for wave or wavelength λ: $k = 2\pi/\lambda$.

As in Eq. (5.9), summands in the right side of Eq. (5.11) corresponding to volume, surface, and linear contributions are highlighted.

By highlighting volume contribution, expression for heat conductivity of crystal with radius r in the temperature regions $h\nu_{\text{max}} < k_{\text{B}} T$ will be

$$C_\upsilon(r) = C_\upsilon + k_1 T^2/r + k_2 T/r^2 \tag{5.12}$$

where C_υ is the heat conductivity of large-crystal material and k_1, k_2 are coefficients.

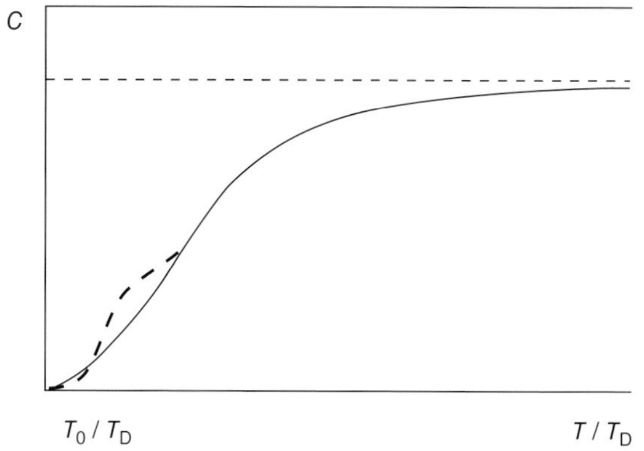

Figure 5.9 Size dependence of heat conductivity C: straight line – Debye theory; horizontal dotted line – limit of the Dulong–Petit law; dotted curve line – binding with quantum effect deviation from the Debye theory. (Reproduced with permission of BKL Publishers.)

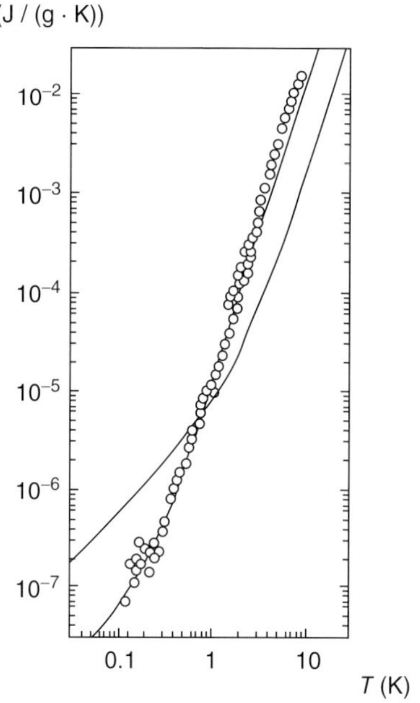

Figure 5.10 Specific heat conductivity C for silver nanoparticles with a diameter of 10 nm at $T \leq 10$ K; straight line – heat conductivity for bulk silver. (Reproduced with permission of BKL Publishers.)

Theoretical evaluations showed that in low-temperature regions at $T \to 0$, heat conductivity $C_\upsilon(r)$ decreases faster than heat conductivity of large-crystal material C_υ: $\Delta C = C_\upsilon(r) - C_\upsilon < 0$, suggesting that below temperature T_0, $\Delta C < 0$. Temperature dependence on heat conductivity is schematically presented in Figure 5.9. At $T > T_0$, the difference becomes larger than null. At higher temperatures, heat conductivity tends to be extremal corresponding to the Dulong–Petit law: $C_\upsilon \to 3R$.

Experimental data from theoretical studies determined the quantum size effect for heat conductivity of silver nanoparticles: at $T < 1$ K, heat conductivity of particle was less, but at $T > 1$ K, heat conductivity was higher for large-crystal silver nanoparticles (Figure 5.10).

Also, studies on the heat conductivity of lead nanoparticles with sizes of 2.2, 3.7, and 6.6 nm and of indium nanoparticle with a diameter of 2.2 nm showed that at

Table 5.1 Polynomial for heat conductivity coefficients $C(T) = aT + bT^2 + cT^3$ [1].

Specimen	a (mJ (K^2 mol)$^{-1}$)	b (mJ (K^3 mol)$^{-1}$)	c (mJ (K^4 mol)$^{-1}$)
Cu, large crystal	0.68	0.01	0.051
Cu, $d = 50$ nm	1.03	0.32	0.066
CuO, $d = 50$ nm	0	0	0.410

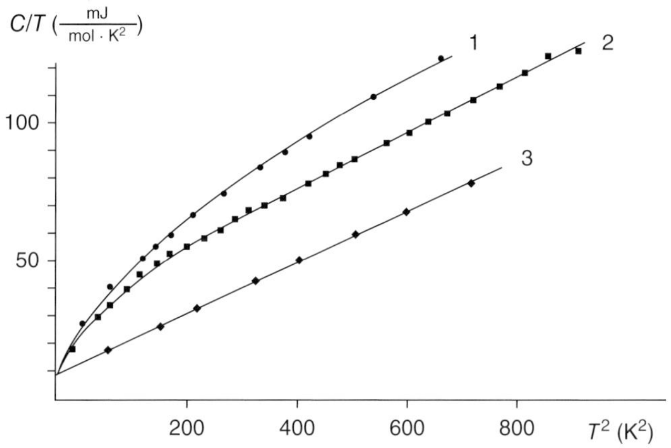

Figure 5.11 Temperature dependence of heat conductivity for Pd nanoparticles with a diameter of 3.0 nm (1) and 6.6 nm (2) and bulk palladium (3). (Reproduced with permission of BKL Publishers.)

$T < 10$ K, heat conductivity $C_v(r)$ for nanopowders was 25–27% more than heat conductivity C_v for appropriate large-crystal metals.

At temperature intervals from 1 to 20 K and 300 to 800 K, heat conductivities of large-crystal copper nanoparticles and copper nanopowders with a particle size of 50 nm were also studied. For temperature dependence at $T \leq 20$ K, the polynomial $C(T) = aT + bT^2 + cT^3$ was applied. Obtained polynomial coefficient values a, b, and c are given in Table 5.1 (Figure 5.11).

Based on results, quadratic term (bT^2) exists only in the temperature dependence of copper nanoparticles on heat conductivity. Coefficients of copper nanopowders at linear and cubic terms are more than the appropriate values for large-crystal specimen. Bulk copper at all studied temperatures had the smallest heat conductivity, which was 1.2–2.0 times lower than the appropriate values for copper nanoparticles at temperatures up to 450 K. Further increase in temperature leads to an intensive growth of nanopowder, which causes a decrease in heat conductivity until values correspond to the bulk copper.

Similar results were obtained for Ni nanoparticles with a diameter of 22 nm; their heat conductivity is approximately two times more than the values for bulk nickel at 300–800 K. Growth in $C_v(r)$ of In, Ga, and V nanoparticles was also proven experimentally. As an example, heat conductivity values for amorphous bulk materials, nanomaterials, and large-crystal materials are presented in Table 5.2. Significant differences in heat conductivity are observed in samples,

Table 5.2 Heat conductivity for amorphous material, nanomaterial, and large-crystal material.

Material	C_p for amorphous material (J (K mol)$^{-1}$)	C_p for nanomaterial (J (K mol)$^{-1}$)	Grain size of nanomaterial (nm)	C_p for large-crystal material (J (K mol)$^{-1}$)
Pd	27	37	6	25
Ru	—	28	15	23
$Ni_{80}P_{20}$	23.4	23.4	6	23.2
Sc	24.7	24.5	10	24.1

Source: Reproduced with permission from the BKL Publishers.

which are related to deformation, which in turn has an influence on $C_v(r)$ due to significant structure distortions.

5.2.2 Heat Conductivity of Crystal Lattice in Nanomaterials

According to definition, heat conductivity of lattice is caused by a transfer of heat through crystal lattice fluctuations (phonons) under the influence of applied temperature gradient. In a given model, fluctuations of atoms in the lattice are collective, which can be likened to "phonon gas," wherein each phonon spreads freely in volume within material. In such way, the concept of phonons appears as a result of quantum description of lattice fluctuation.

For large-crystal materials under low-temperature conditions, the following equation for temperature dependence on lattice heat conductivity λ_{lattice} was analytically obtained:

$$1/\lambda_{\text{lattice}} = A\Big/\left[T^3 e^{\frac{\theta_D}{\alpha T}}\right] + B/T^3 + C/T^2 + D/T \tag{5.13}$$

where $A, B, C, D,$ and α are coefficients and θ_D is the Debye temperature.

In Eq. (5.13), the first summand results from the scattering of phonons, whereas the second summand describes phonon scattering on grain boundaries. The contribution to heat conductivity dislocations and point defects is described by summands proportional to T^{-2} and T^{-1}.

The contribution of various factors to heat conductivity differs for nanomaterials and large-crystal analogs, which is caused, in particular, by nanostructure features. For example, in equilibrium state, dislocations in nanomaterials are almost absent and hence phonon scattering will not happen. Impurity atoms will enrich the surface of nanoparticles if the surface energy decreases and vice versa and are not distributed homogeneously in nanoparticle volume; thus, the scattering of phonons on them cannot be determined. Thus, it can be concluded that in nanomaterials, scattering on phonons, as well as on the borders of grain structures, should dominate. Accordingly, the equation for lattice conductivity will change.

Taking into account the contribution changes for various factors in λ_{lattice} in nanomaterials, we come to the following equation:

$$\lambda_{\text{lattice}} = A_{\text{spec}}T^3 + B_{\text{spec}}T^2 S/V + C_{\text{spec}}TL/V \tag{5.14}$$

where $A_{\text{spec}}, B_{\text{spec}}, C_{\text{spec}}$ are coefficients and V, S, L pertain to volume, surface area, and total length of nanoparticle ribs, respectively.

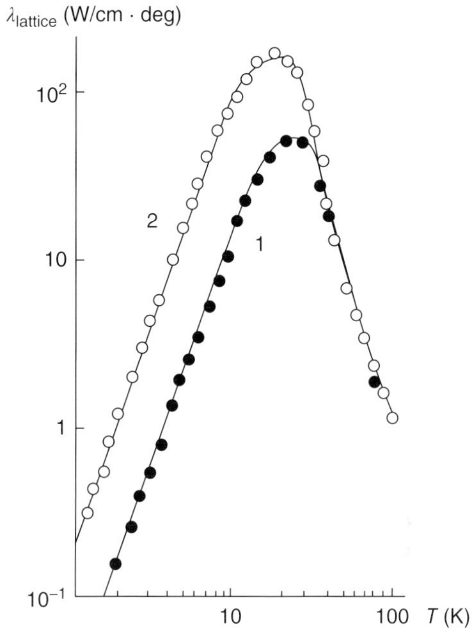

Figure 5.12 Experimental temperature dependences of lattice conductivity for LiF monocrystals, with cross-section: curve 1 – 0.123 × 0.091 cm^2; curve 2 – 0.755 × 0.697 cm^2. (Reproduced with permission from the BKL Publishers.)

Following Eq. (5.14), at low absolute temperatures, contribution by second and third summands will increase with a decrease in particle size and hence, the lattice conductivity should increase. A decrease in temperature should bring the same effect, insofar as this average length for phonon free path is increasing. As soon as the length of phonon free path exceeds linear sizes of a crystal, the dominating mechanism will be phonon scattering on boundaries. In this case, summands in Eq. (5.14) become proportional to the particle radius. As scattering and particle size decrease, conductivity should also drop.

Let us look at some experimental results. Experimental dependences of lattice conductivity for lithium fluoride on temperature are given in Figure 5.12.

5.2.3 Debye Temperature in Nanomaterials

Debye temperature and other heat properties are expected to change in nanomaterials, compared with bulk materials. *Debye temperature* is a characteristic temperature of hard materials. Above this temperature, all crystal lattice fluctuations are excited, but below it, some fluctuation conditions start to "freeze solid." Debye temperature θ_D is determined by the following relation [1]:

$$\hbar\theta_D = h\nu_{max} \tag{5.15}$$

As experimental data show, Debye temperature decreases more in nanomaterials than in large-crystal materials because of the change in view and boundaries of phonon spectra for small crystal. For larged-size specimen, in Eq. (5.9), summands such as S and L can be ignored. Then for bulk materials with wave vectors $\hbar$, dependency (5.10) will become

$$N = (2/9\pi)r^3\hbar \tag{5.16}$$

Table 5.3 Change in the relative Debye temperature $\theta_D(r)/\theta_D$ depending on nanoparticle size. (Reproduced with permission from the BKL Publishers.)

Metal	Particle diameter (nm)	$\theta_D(r)/\theta_D$
Ag	10–20	0.75–0.83
Al	15–20	0.50–0.67
	1.0	0.69
Al	2.0	0.92
	10.0	0.995
In	2.2	0.80
Pb	2.2	0.87
	3.7	0.90
	6.0	0.92
	20.0	0.94
Pd	3.0	0.83
	6.6	0.89
V	3.8	0.83
	6.5	24.5

According to theory $\theta_D = (h\hbar_D c)/(2\pi\hbar_B)$, after a number of transformations, the following equation can be obtained, which binds the Debye temperature in nanomaterial and large-crystal material:

$$\theta_D(r)/\theta_D \approx 1\text{-}3\pi/(8r\hbar) \tag{5.17}$$

Hence, the lower the radius of nanoparticle, the more its Debye temperature will differ from the value characterized for bulk crystal.

Related to particle size decrease, lowering in the Debye temperature was observed in most researches, the results of which are given in Table 5.3.

5.3 Optical Characteristics of Nanomediums

Optical properties are determined by interaction of materials with electromagnetic radiation at various wavelengths and are different for bulk materials, micron-size materials, and particles with diameters less than their wavelength for incident radiation, as experiment had showed. Moreover, interaction of light wavelengths with solid materials, depending on their sizes, is described by various theories. Classical theory on the optical characteristics of bulk materials was developed by G. A. Lorentz at the beginning of the twentieth century. In the given approximation, material electrons and ions are simple harmonic oscillations, on which electrical forces by incident light are acting. Experimental studies had compared the number of optical properties of small particles and macroscopic solid material. In particular, M. Faraday drew attention on the color similarity of colloidal solution and gold film and, based on that, expressed his assumption about the dispersion structure of colloidal solution. Strict theory for light scattering on small spherical particles was developed in 1908 by G. Mie.

Recently, a number of new materials possessing specific optical properties have been obtained, such as nanoparticle suspensions in matrix, granulated films, cermets, and composite materials. These specific materials have linear sizes that are less than light radiation wavelength.

Wavelength of visible light λ lies in the interval of $(3.8 - 7.6) \times 10^{-7}$ m, which is larger than nanoparticle sizes. Optical characteristics of nanomediums have been described by a number of theories. It should be mentioned, that among them any or that allowance can be applied. For example, the classical model of Drudge should be applied with a length limit condition for electron free path by particle sizes. The Maxwell–Garnett theory is usually used to describe properties of particles with sizes less than light wavelength. The Mie theory refers to optical properties of non-interacting nanoparticle system. The quantum mechanical theory of Gor'kov–Eliashberg describes optical properties from a quantum size point of view.

5.3.1 Light Scattering Features of Tiny Particles

Let us refer to a model experiment where particle is located in a homogeneous medium and placed in the beam path of electromagnetic radiation with initial intensity of I_i (Figure 5.13). The medium is considered homogeneous when heterogeneity at atomic or molecular scale is less than the incident light wavelength. The radiation with intensity of I_t falls onto the collector, located behind the particle. If the particle is removed, then the intensity accepted by the collector will be equal to initial I_i, wherein $I_i > I_t$. Hence, the presence of the particle leads to damping or beam extinction.

Extinction is the attenuation of electromagnetic wave during its passage through the medium caused by scattering and absorption.

Scattering of electromagnetic waves by any system is related to their heterogeneity. The physical principles of scattering remain similar in all systems regardless of their heterogeneity type.

Electromagnetic wave falling on any barrier, which might be an individual electron, atom, molecule, or particle of solid or liquid material, excites fluctuation movements in electrical charge carriers in materials. During the opposite transition of material into stationary state, electromagnetic energy is radiated in all directions. Secondary waves are radiation especially scattered by barrier.

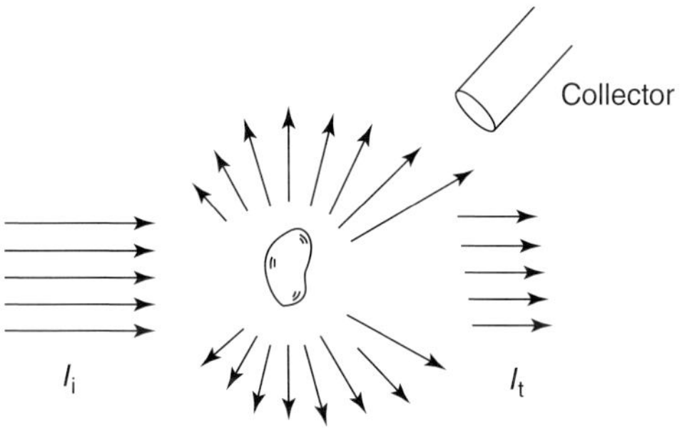

Figure 5.13 Light scattering by a random particle. (Reproduced with permission from the BKL Publishers.)

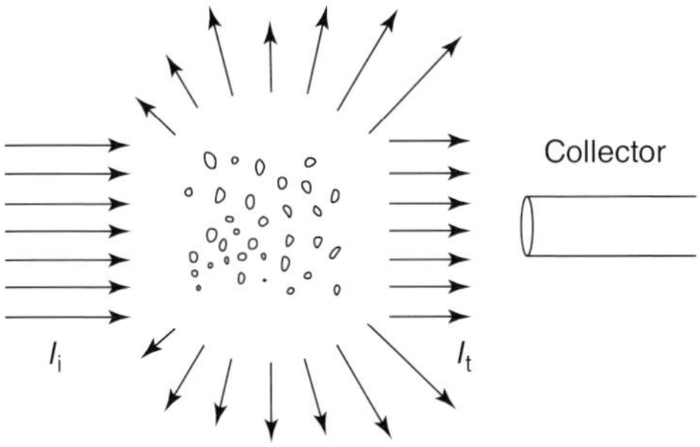

Figure 5.14 Light scattering by particle conglomeration. (Reproduced with permission from the BKL Publishers.)

Except during reradiation, excited carriers of elementary charges can convert part of their falling electromagnetic energy into other forms, for example, heat energy. Such process is called absorption. In general, scattering and absorption are not mutually independent processes. The complex of measured values I_t/I_i in some diapason of wavelengths for homogeneous layer of material is called transmission range, absorption of extinction.

In the case wherein the medium in which the material is included is not absorptive, the difference $I_i - I_t$ is determined by absorption and scattering only in the particle. Extinction generally depends on the chemical composition of material, its size and shape, orientation due to incident light, surrounding equilibrium, frequency, and polarization of incident light. Under real conditions, it usually has to interact with electromagnetic radiation with a large number of particles (Figure 5.14).

According to practice, if the particles are crushed into small pieces after measuring its transmission spectra, then the discrete medium transmission spectra will be different with initial ones. It is emphasized that the chemical composition of a substance in both cases remain the same and only dispersity will change. However, this will lead to macroscopic optical properties; for example, distance and absorption significantly differ depending on which disperse condition the given material is.

Absorption, as a rule, is one of damping of incident light in bulk homogeneous materials. However, in the case of particles with small linear sizes, extinction might be caused by both absorption and scattering. Demonstration of these two limited conditions, by which extinction can result, is possible in the following simple experiment: As shown in Figure 5.15, two transparent vessels are filled with water and installed on the demonstration table for projection of their image on the screen. In one of the vessels, some drops of milk were added, and in another, black ink. The increase in the amount of added substance changes the tone of screen image from transparent to reddish and black in the case of milk and ink, respectively. However, during definite concentrations of solutions, both emulsion images on the screen become black.

Differentiation of each vessel by the amount of light reaching the screen is not possible, and the outer view of vessels is completely different: the vessel containing milk is white, whereas that containing ink is black. Given this difference, extinction in both cases was nearly the same, but was caused by different reasons. Milk is an emulsion consisting of very poorly absorbing particles

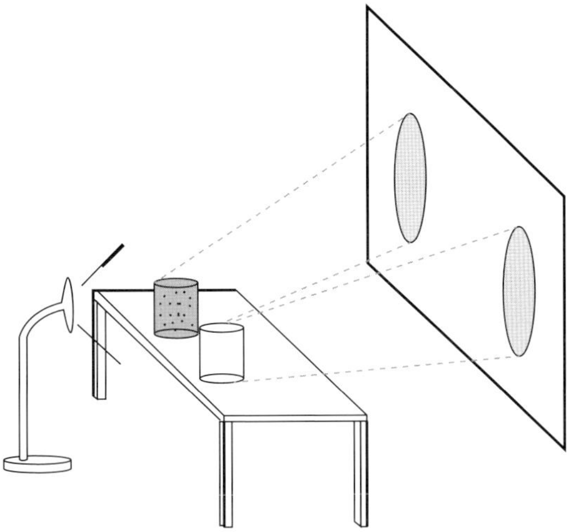

Figure 5.15 Experiment based on demonstration of scattering and absorption influence on extinction. (Reproduced with permission from the BKL Publishers.)

whose attenuation can be determined by scattering, whereas black ink is an emulsion composed of very tiny carbon particles whose intensity is changed by light, mainly caused by absorption. This experiment is qualitative, and its strict quantitative interpretation is complicated by the influence of multiple scattering. But this experiment clearly shows the difference between extinction caused by scattering and extinction caused by absorption. Relative contributions for absorption and scattering to extinction cannot be determined by observing only one passed light. For such determination, additional independent experiments will be necessary.

5.3.2 Extinction by Dielectric Nanoparticles

Differences and similarities exist between extinction spectra of disperse particles of different sizes and absorption spectra of bulk materials. Let us consider this on extinction curves, calculated for three different radii of water drops in air medium. Extinction dependences Q_{ext} from the reverse wavelength $1/\lambda$ for particles with various diameters are given in Figure 5.16.

It is seen from the figure that all curves have series of broad and narrow peaks. For particles with sizes of 1 μm and 200 nm, oscillations converge to a certain value, and further extinction will not change. If the particle diameter become equal to 50 nm, which is larger than the incident light wavelength, then extinction in spite of oscillation, having tendency to increase and will not reach the limited values.

In these spectra, peaks will remain to exist in the range of volume absorption. In particular, extinction peak near a value of 6 μm^{-1} for drop with a diameter of 50 nm is the same as absorption peak for bulk material, showing that for nanoparticles where absorption prevails over scattering, a significant absorption of wavelengths can be observed too. Extinction spectra of radiation energy for spherical MgO particles with different average sizes are given in Figure 5.17.

Scales along both axes are logarithmic. For comparing of bulk properties and nanoparticle properties of the same material in Figure 5.18b, absorption

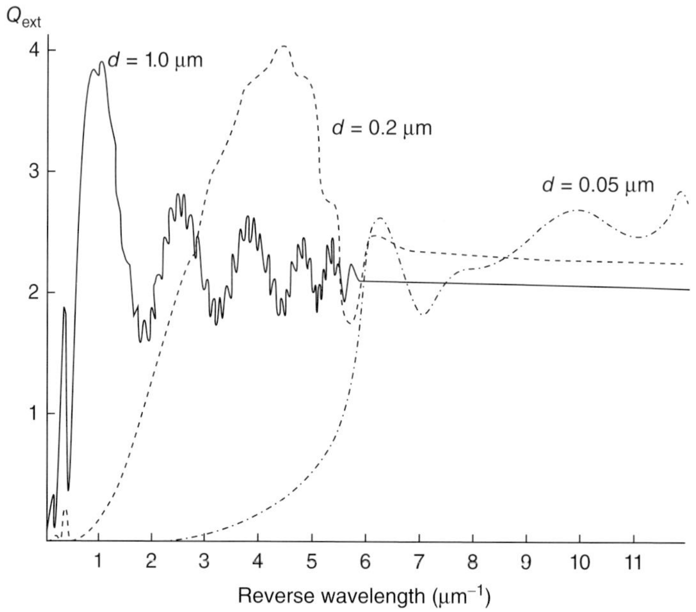

Figure 5.16 Extinction of water drops with various sizes in air. (Reproduced with permission from the BKL Publishers.)

coefficient graph for bulk material was presented. From the above presented dependences, it is seen that attenuation radiation in dispersion layer of MgO, significantly differs from the attenuation in bulk material. In particular, for visible light diapason and near it, bulk MgO samples are highly transparent (Figure 5.17b). However, in disperse layer of bulk MgO, extinction on this area is high enough; moreover it is growing linearly with increase in scattering energy (see Figure 5.17a). From the given comparison, it can be concluded that extinction in MgO nanoparticle layer in the visible diapason is determined by scattering.

Theoretically, in small particles, scattering is proportional to the quarter level of photon energy, compared to wavelengths. On a graph with logarithmic scales, extinction dependence on radiation energy is presented as linear function. Straight regions, as it is seen in the Figure 5.17a, exist in all calculated curves, and the longest straight line is observed for particles with sizes of 10 and 50 nm. At a diameter of 200 nm, straight region shortens, and in particles with a diameter of 1 μm, it is quite small.

Extinction is caused by scattering and almost does not depend on photon energy when particle sizes are greater than wavelength. It is presented as a horizontal line graphically. A wide region exists for incident light wavelengths, where extinction for particles with an average size of 1 μm is almost constant. Horizontal regions are also observed less extensively on the extinction graphs for particles with a diameter of 200 and 50 nm.

Extinction for particles with a diameter of 10 nm at a radiation energy of ~ 7 eV is almost growing vertically. At the same time, this region corresponds to the edge of absorption band of bulk MgO. Extinction in MgO nanoparticles at infrared wavelength diapason is determined mainly by absorption.

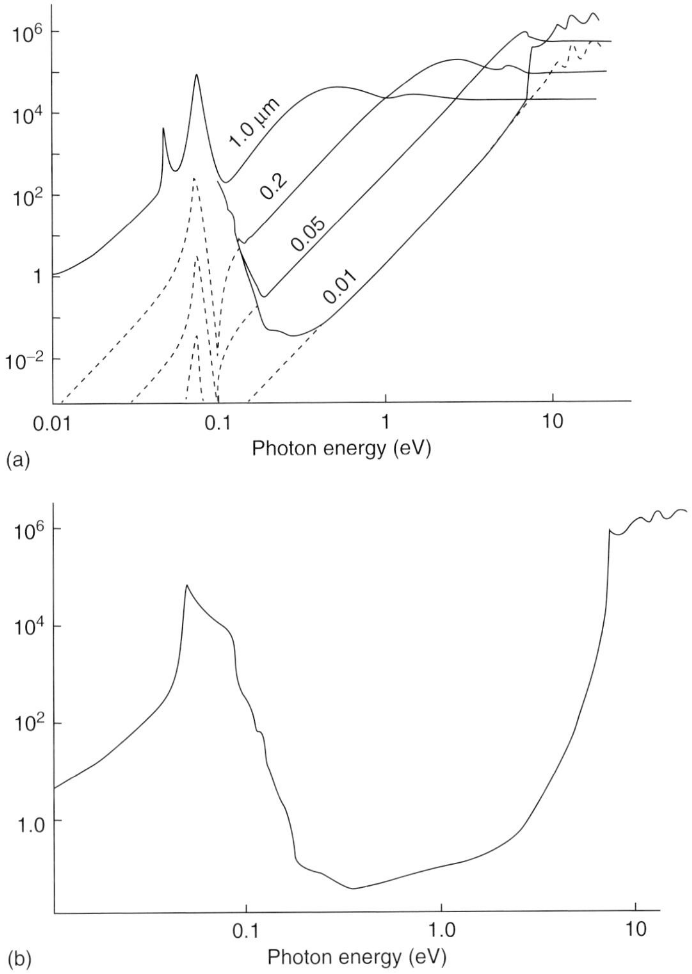

Figure 5.17 (a) Calculated extinction spectra for MgO nanoparticles with various diameters and (b) absorption spectra of bulk MgO. (Reproduced with permission from the BKL Publishers.)

According to calculations, maximum falls on 0.075 eV, while in bulk material, absorption maximum falls on energies around 0.05 eV. This difference is explained by the appearance of surface fluctuations in nanoparticles due to collective ionic lattice excitements.

At the infrared diapason, scattering is present during extinction of MgO nanoparticles, though their absolute values are significantly less (illustrated in Figure 5.17 as dotted line). Maximum of scattering is also observed around 0.075 eV but then sharply decreases to a radiation energy around 0.1 eV, which is illustrated on graphs by a deep minimum. Through this way, passage of light with definite frequency through nanoparticle conglomerates is maximal, though scattering always disappears. Hence, nanoparticle surface can work as a selective filter of infrared radiation by passing the definite wavelength and by strongly scattering the neighboring frequencies.

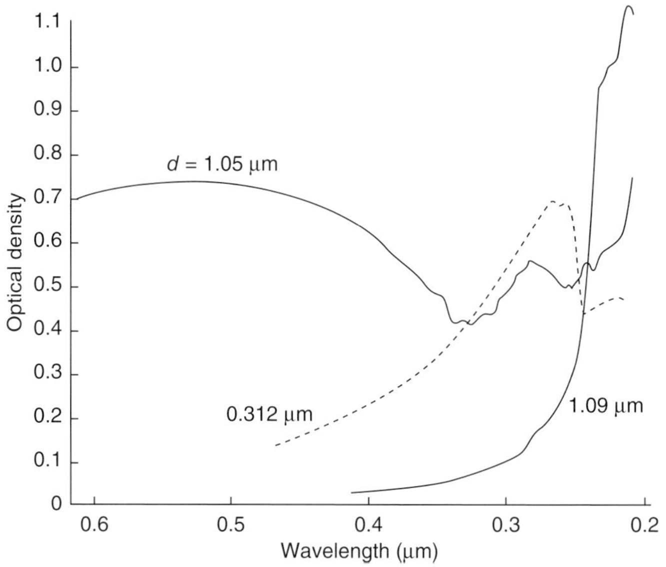

Figure 5.18 Experimental extinction spectra for polystyrene sphere emulsions with various sizes in water. (Reproduced with permission from the BKL Publishers.)

Experimental extinction spectra for polystyrene sphere emulsions in water are shown in Figure 5.18. As water is transparent at wavelengths of 0.2–1.3 μm, then measurements will also be limited by diapason. Graphs are illustrated in such form depending on equipment they are created.

From the obtained results, with a decrease in average particle sizes, the extinction region shortens: material turns transparent at large wavelength intervals.

5.3.3 Extinction in Metallic Nanoparticles

In metallic nanoparticles, extinction spectral characteristics have a number of features and largely differ from dielectric material spectral characteristics. As in metals, contribution of free electrons to absorption will dominate above all other mechanisms and then dominates in the frequency line from the radio diapason to the far-ultraviolet region.

Estimated extinction spectra in polydisperse system of spherical aluminum particles with an average diameter of 10 nm are shown in Figure 5.19a. Scales along both axes are logarithmic. In Figure 5.19b, absorption spectra of bulk Al are shown for comparison.

In contrast to bulk material, Al nanoparticles at visible region of the extinction spectra have an absorption peak appearing at energy of about 8 eV. As it is seen in Figure 5.20, maximum fits with the region where the absorption of bulk material is monotonically decreasing, which can be explained by resonance appearing during the collective movement of free electrons in fluctuation restriction by nanovolume.

Based on estimations, an increase in particle size leads to a shift in absorption maximum to the region of small energies, broadening, and, at a diameter

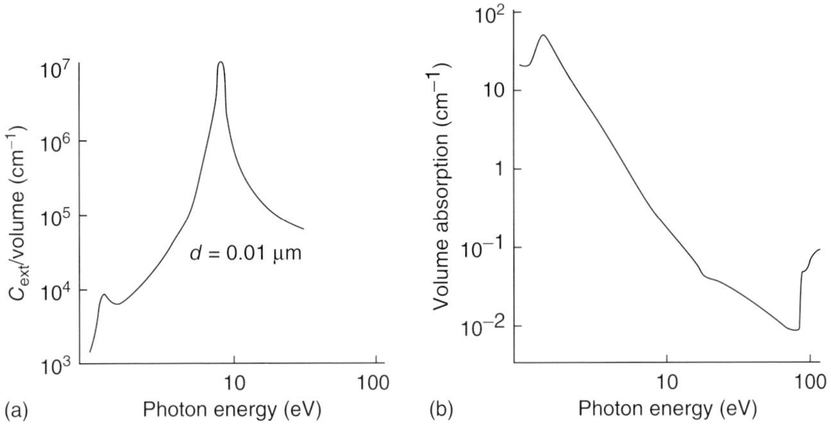

Figure 5.19 (a) Estimated extinction spectra for spherical aluminum nanoparticles and (b) absorption spectra of bulk aluminum. (Reproduced with permission from the BKL Publishers.)

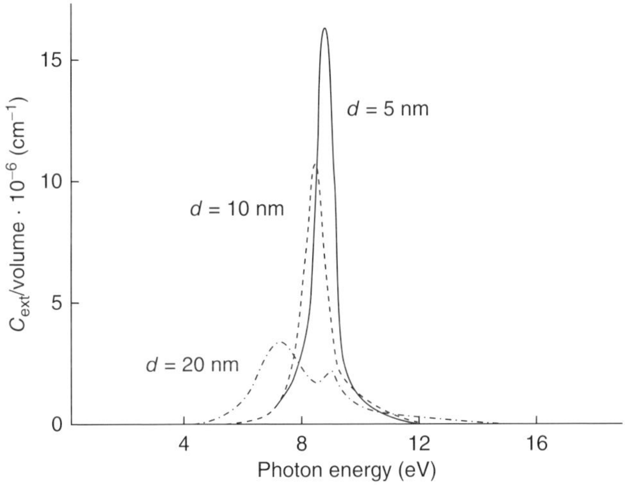

Figure 5.20 Estimated extinction to the volume unit for spherical Al nanoparticles with various diameters. (Reproduced with permission from the BKL Publishers.)

of 20 nm, bifurcation (Figure 5.20). Conducted estimations have an experimental proof. In particular, granulated Au films with size structure components of 4 nm at region $\lambda = 500 - 600$ nm have clear absorption maximum. Also, absorption maximums were observed in visible diapason for Ag, Cu, Au, Li, In, Na, K, and Ca nanoparticles. Estimation results for isolated Ag, Au, and Cu nanoparticles with a size of 10 nm are shown in Figure 5.21.

In metallic nanoparticles it is also necessary to mention effects related to average length restriction for electron free path. Estimation extinction results of spherical Al nanoparticles, with a change in average length for electron free path, depending on material size, are presented in Figure 5.22. A decrease in particle

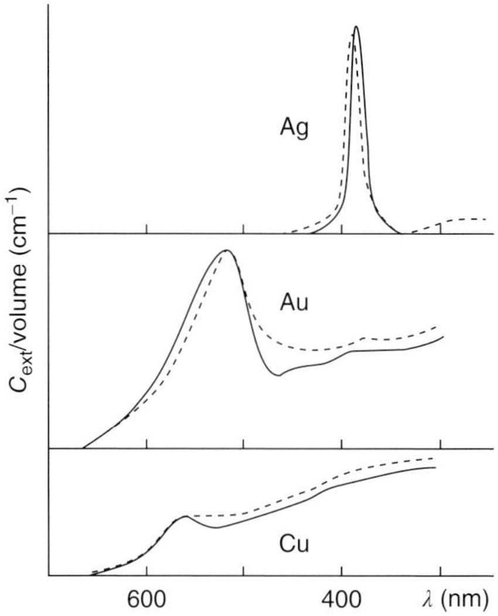

Figure 5.21 Absorption spectra of Ag, Au, and Cu nanoparticles. (Reproduced with permission from the BKL Publishers.)

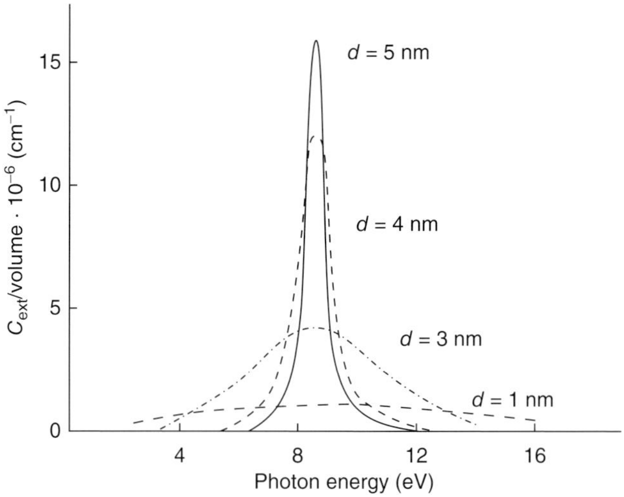

Figure 5.22 Extinction spectra of Al nanoparticles with various diameters. (Reproduced with permission from the BKL Publishers.)

diameter leads to a widening of absorption peak and a reduction of height, but the maximum remains unaltered.

Experimental extinction dependences on particle sizes in the colloidal gold solution are presented in Figure 5.23. Obtained curves illustrate optical effects by metallic nanoparticles due to restriction of collective fluctuation volumes and decrease in average length of electron free path. Dependences for radii less than 2.6 nm (dotted lines in figure) correspond to a constant number of particles, and for large radii, they correspond to constant mass. In the figure, extinction by nanoparticles with a diameter of 2.6–10 nm does not have a maximum near the wavelength region $\lambda_F \approx 520$ nm, the state of which weakly depends on particle size. Broadening and decreasing of extinction maximum can be explained by

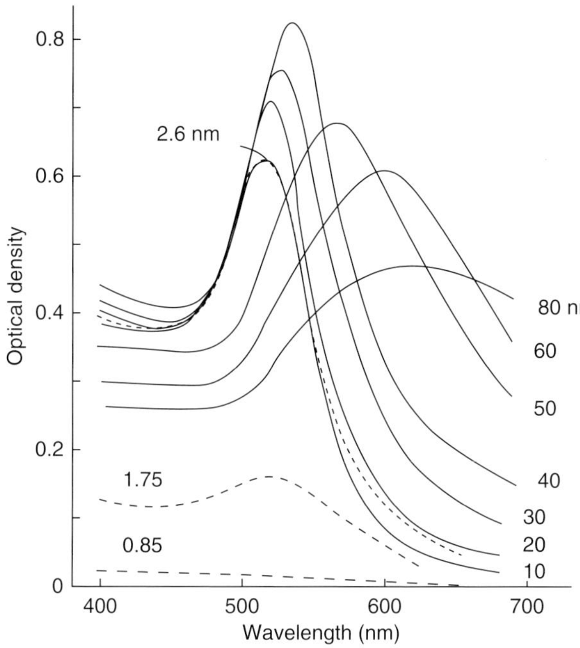

Figure 5.23 Absorption spectra of Al nanoparticles with various diameters. (Reproduced with permission from the BKL Publishers.)

decrease in average wavelength of free conductivity electron free path. On large wavelengths, absorption in material strongly falls, which leads to a ruby-red color, obtained during passage of white color through the liquid gold colloidal solutions.

Extinction maximum in particles with sizes larger than 10 nm is widening and shifting to the region of large wavelengths. Simultaneously change in solution color from ruby red to purple is observed, later to violet and then to pale blue for very large particles with a size of 80 nm.

5.3.4 Influence of Morphology and Polydispersity on Optical Properties of Nanomaterials

It is often considered that, if particle is smaller than a falling radiation wavelength, then electromagnetic wave does not sense particle structure details, and hence, the shape of particle has no influence on the absorption spectra. However, one of the interesting features of nanoparticles is that they can exhibit such optical properties, which are almost fully determined by their shape, and less fits with bulk material properties. Meanwhile, in polydisperse system, depending on particle size, extinction features are significantly smoothened until full disappearance.

Estimated graphs for polydisperse water drops are given in Figure 5.24. Obtained dependences show how gradually increasing size variation in nanomaterials influences extinction. Polydispersity assumes the well-known Gaussian distribution. In the figure, it is seen that with an increase in dispersity, ripple disappears first. A *ripple* is a sharp, nonregularly located splash of extinction curve for weakly absorbing spheres. By further gradual broadening in distribution, the

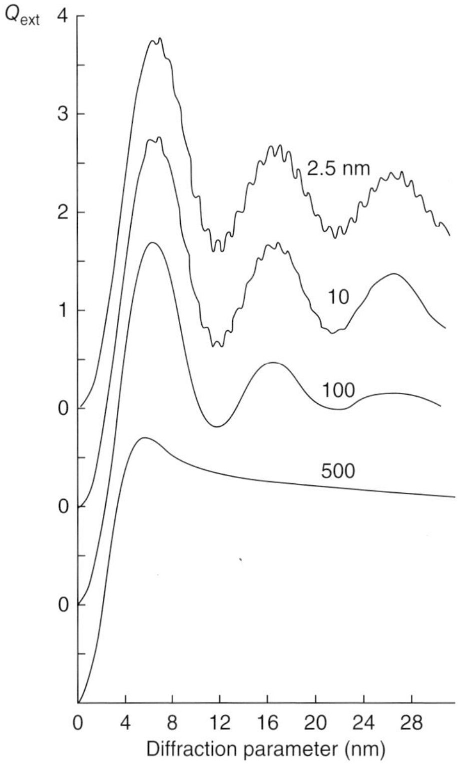

Figure 5.24 Influence of size distribution on visible light extinction in water droplets. Standard deviation values for Gaussian size distributions are given near curves. (Reproduced with permission from the BKL Publishers.)

interference structure clears. In the particle system with the widest distribution, only the maximum in the region with small values $1/\lambda$ remains, which corresponds to redness of passed light and asymptomatic approximation to limit value in the region of large $1/\lambda$.

In experiments with silver, more convincing results related to the influence of morphology on absorption spectra of small particles were obtained. In Figure 5.25, absorption spectra of three silver specimens with various

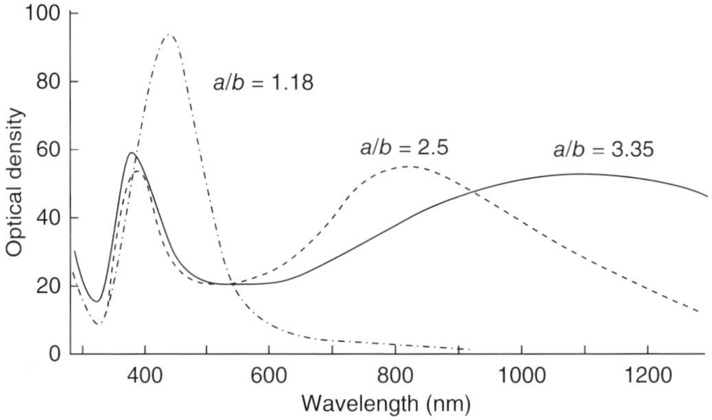

Figure 5.25 Absorption spectra for silver colloidal solutions. Particles shape is described by average half-axis ratio a/b. (Reproduced with permission from the BKL Publishers.)

average half-axis ratios (a/b) were illustrated. In almost all spherical particles ($a/b = 1.18$), only one absorption line near the wavelength of 420 nm was observed. On the spectra of more elongated particles ($a/b = 2.5$ and 3.35), a cleavage appears: one of the lines will move to the region of large wavelengths and another to the region of small wavelengths. The divergence of absorption lines increases with a growth in a/b ratio.

5.4 Diffusion in Nanomaterials

Most physical processes related to the reconstruction of material structure are caused by diffusion, such as creeping, annealing, recrystallization, diffusion–inductive migration of borders, and eutectoid decomposition. As a rule, different chemical reactions in solid state are controlled by diffusion processes.

Diffusion is a nonequilibrium process caused by molecular heat movement and establishment of equilibrium distribution of interphase concentrations. As a result of diffusion, alignment of chemical potentials in component mixture occurs.

Adequate experimental results show that diffusion processes play a significant role during the realization of unique properties in nanomaterials, such as plasticity, superplasticity, destruction, and structure reduction processes. During this time, as studies showed, diffusion parameters in nanomaterials are particularly greatly different from appropriate values in large-crystal materials. In other words, size effects can have an influence on diffusion processes in such objects.

5.4.1 Diffusion in Nanopowders

Studying size effects on diffusion process in small objects is experimentally very complex, hence the various model cases approved. For example, estimation of diffusion in spherical particles with radius R for two border conditions, namely, (1) presence of infinity source on the particle surface and (2) ultimate power, was done. The first case is rare in practice, but the second is close to many real situations, implemented particularly during annealing of various mixture powders. Also, in the model, it is accepted that diffusion coefficient is equal to equilibrium and will not change in the course of the process.

During problem-solving with the use of infinity source power, it is convenient to present results graphically (Figure 5.26), in coordinates c/c_0 and $1 - r/R$ at different values of dimensionless time $\tau = Dt/R^2$ where c_0 and c are the initial and final concentrations, respectively; r is the current concentration of radius, while spherical center corresponds to $r/R = 0$; t is the time; and D is the diffusion coefficient. In the figure, for comparison, estimated concentration curves are drawn for diffusion in plane parallel to plate with a width of $2R$.

Estimated dependences show that with a growth in τ, the difference in concentrations of diffusing substance in spherical and plane materials increases. The transfer of concentration front in sphere is faster than in plane specimen. This effect is caused by a geometrical factor.

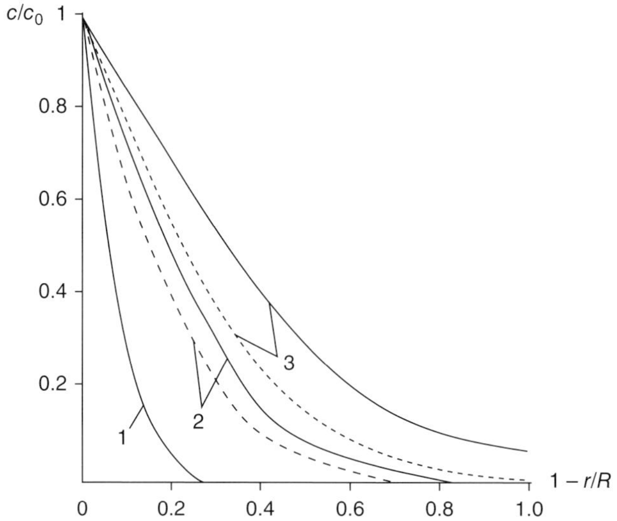

Figure 5.26 Concentration profiles in plane (dotted lines) and spherical (straight lines) specimen at different values of dimensionless time $\tau = Dt/R^2$: 1 – 0.005; 2 – 0.03; 3 – 0.08. (Reproduced with permission from the BKL Publishers.)

During problem-solving using the second border condition, it is accepted that on the surface of spherical particle, a concentration source c_0 of final force exists, which was focused in the layer with thickness of $\lambda \ll R$. During the course of diffusive annealing, concentration c in the layer will reduce. After completion of homogenization, uniform solution with concentration c_{cp} will form in the particle. In Figure 5.27, estimation results are presented as dependences c/c_{cp} from r/R at different values of dimensionless time $\tau = Dt/R^2$.

As followed from the given graphs, formation of homogeneous solution outside of sphere is practically over at time $t \approx 0.3R^2/D$. Evaluative estimation for particle

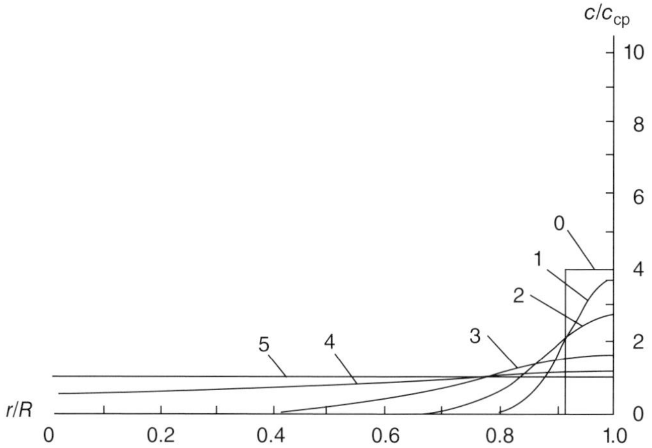

Figure 5.27 Concentration profiles in spherical samples for c_0/c_{cp} at different values of dimensionless time τ: 1 – 0.00128; 2 – 0.00582; 3 – 0.02048; 4 – 0.06192; 5 – 0.32768. (Reproduced with permission from the BKL Publishers.)

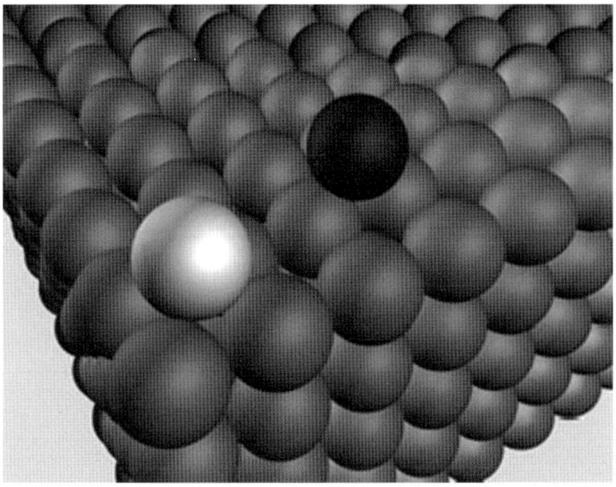

Figure 5.28 Schematic of location of adsorbed atoms on the crystal surface. (Reproduced with permission from the BKL Publishers.)

with a radius of 10 nm at coefficient of volume diffusion $0.3 \times 10^{-15}\,m^2\,s^{-1}$ shows that homogenization should end at 0.1 s.

Also a study of diffusion processes in nanopowders presents interest in relation to practical absence of vacancies and dislocations in their volume. These structural features of nanoparticles result in their small diameter values and size effects. Reduced values of volume diffusion in nanopowders should cause an absence of structural defects. Experiments show that with a decrease in linear size of particles, the relative transfer of substance by surface diffusion mechanism increases (Figure 5.28).

Surface diffusion is process, related to transfer of particles, as a rule by random movement of atoms or molecules, appearing on the surface of condensed material within the first surface layer above it.

Let us look at surface diffusion mechanisms. At temperatures different from absolute null, on the surface of any crystal, there are adsorbed atoms (Figure 5.29), the thickness of which is determined by

$$n_a = n_0 \exp(-E_a/k_B T) \qquad (5.18)$$

where E_a is the adsorbed atom formation energy, which is necessary for atom transfer from the edge stage position to adsorption on the smooth-atomic region surface, and n_0 is the surface thickness of atoms.

Figure 5.29 Schematic of contact isthmus profile. (Reproduced with permission from the BKL Publishers.)

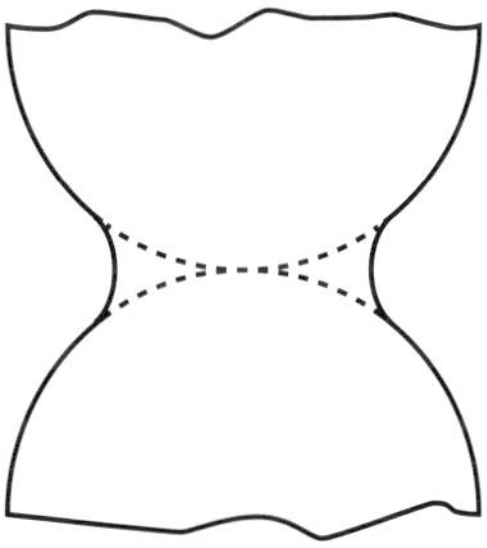

As estimations show, on the crystal surface with FCC structure, the plane (111) energy for absorbed atom $U_a \approx \varepsilon/3 \approx H_s/20$, where H_s is the sublimation temperature. Hence, absorbed atoms on the surface are very mobile and resemble spheres that seem rolling on the surface and transferring to act at multiple interatomic distances. This manner of movement is called "tumbleweed."

In the case of surface *heterodiffusion*, when impurity atoms, rather than surface atoms, are migrating on the crystal surface, two variants are possible. When the interaction energy for heterogeneous and homogeneous atoms is comparable, the transfer mechanism remains as before. When the infraction energy between impurity and surface atoms is large, the transfer of heterogeneous particles by "tumbleweed" mechanism is complicated. In this case, diffusion will occur by surface spreading of impurities, which is called "unrolling carpet" mechanism. When impurity atoms cover the surface by monoatomic layer, the process ends.

The path passed by atoms on the surface for t_a can be evaluated by the following equation:

$$l_a \approx (D_a t_a)^{1/2} \tag{5.19}$$

where D_a is the diffusion coefficient for adsorbed atoms.

It is necessary to mention one more phenomenon which is characteristic of nanomaterials. As it is known, in any system, simultaneous processes caused by aspiration to lower the free energy will occur. In nanopowders particularly, this energy is related to the presence of a developed surface. During the course of these processes, the contact isthmus between particles will form (Figure 5.29). Thermodynamic expediency of substance transfer to the region of contact isthmus will occur when free surface, and hence the surface energy of the whole system, will reduce.

Self-diffusion is a local case of diffusion in pure substances or solutions with constant composition, in which substance particles diffuse. The diffusive particle transfer of solid material can lead to a change in shape if surface tension, gravity, elastic, or electrical forces will act for a long time on the material surface [1].

5.5 Graphene

Graphene can be divided into several categories based on its properties and the possible applications: (i) graphene or reduced graphene oxide flakes for composite materials, conductive paints; (ii) planar graphene for low performance active and non-active devices; (iii) planar graphene for high-performance electronic devices [2]. Special characteristics of graphene such as thrombogenicity, biotoxicity and biocompatibility, antibacterial effects are highlighting its biomedical applications [3].

5.5.1 Structure of Graphene

Structure of graphene is composed of monolayer hexagonal lattice build of carbon atoms, where individual carbon atoms were connected by sp^2 bonds, similar to those of carbon nanotubes and fullerenes [4]. Zigzag edges in graphene structure possess high density of electronic states at the Fermi level, furthermore, the zigzag and armchair edges of graphene can be reconstructed and inter-converted under transmission electron microscopy [5]. Visual transparency of graphene was defined by fine structure constant, according to the Hall effect, conductance fluctuations, and the magnetic flux quantum, $h/2e$ [6]. Carbon nanotubes are obtained by rolling graphene along a given direction and reconnecting the carbon bonds. Hence carbon nanotubes have only hexagons and can be thought of as one-dimensional (1D) objects. Graphite, a three-dimensional (3D) allotrope of carbon, became widely known after the invention of the pencil in 1564, and its usefulness as an instrument for writing comes from the fact that graphite is made out of stacks of graphene layers that are weakly coupled by van der Waals forces. Hence, when one presses a pencil against a sheet of paper, one is actually producing graphene stacks and, somewhere among them, there could be individual graphene layers. Although graphene is the mother for all these different allotropes and has been presumably produced every time someone writes with a pencil, it was only isolated 440 years after its invention.

The structural flexibility of graphene is reflected in its electronic properties. The sp^2 hybridization between one s orbital and two p orbitals leads to a trigonal planar structure with a formation of a σ bond between carbon atoms that are separated by 1.42 Å. The σ band is responsible for the robustness of the lattice structure in all allotropes. Due to the Pauli principle, these bands have a filled shell and, hence, form a deep valence band. The unaffected p orbital, which is perpendicular to the planar structure, can bind covalently with neighboring carbon atoms, leading to the formation of a π band. Since each p orbital has one extra electron, the π band is half filled. Because of its unusual structural and electronic flexibility, graphene can be tailored chemically and/or structurally in many different ways: deposition of metal atoms or molecules on top; intercalation [as done in graphite intercalated compounds]; incorporation of nitrogen and/or boron in its structure; [in analogy with what has been done in nanotubes]; and using different substrates that modify the electronic structure. The control of graphene properties can be extended in new directions allowing for the creation of graphene-based systems with magnetic and superconducting properties that are unique in their 2D properties. Although the graphene field is still in its infancy, the scientific and technological possibilities of this new material seem to be unlimited. The understanding and control of this material's properties can open doors for a new frontier in electronics.

5.5.2 Electronic Properties of Graphene

Electronic band structure of graphene was studied where the energy variations for graphene hexagonal lattice were determined by the following set of equations [7]:

$$\vec{a}_1 = a\left(\frac{\sqrt{3}}{2}, \frac{1}{2}\right) \tag{5.20}$$

with

$$\vec{a}_2 = a\left(\frac{\sqrt{3}}{2}, -\frac{1}{2}\right) \tag{5.21}$$

and

$$\vec{b}_1 = \left(\frac{2\pi}{\sqrt{3}a}, \frac{2\pi}{a}\right) \tag{5.22}$$

with

$$\vec{b}_2 = \left(\frac{2\pi}{\sqrt{3}a}, -\frac{2\pi}{a}\right) \tag{5.23}$$

where $\vec{a}_1$and $\vec{a}_2$ – are the unit vectors of the graphene lattice, $a = 2.46$ Å is the lattice constant of graphene, $\vec{b}_1$and $\vec{b}_2$ – are the unit vectors of the reciprocal lattice of graphene, respectively, as depicted in Figures 5.30 and 5.31.

5.5.3 Topology of Hexagonal Lattice

The use of the term *topology* is related to a study of geometric properties and spatial (dimensional) relations unaffected by the continuous change of shape or size of figures. In terms of graphene structure, topology of hexagonal lattice is considered an arrangement of numbered carbon atoms in the lattice. For better understanding of structure, symmetry, and edge location definitions, more

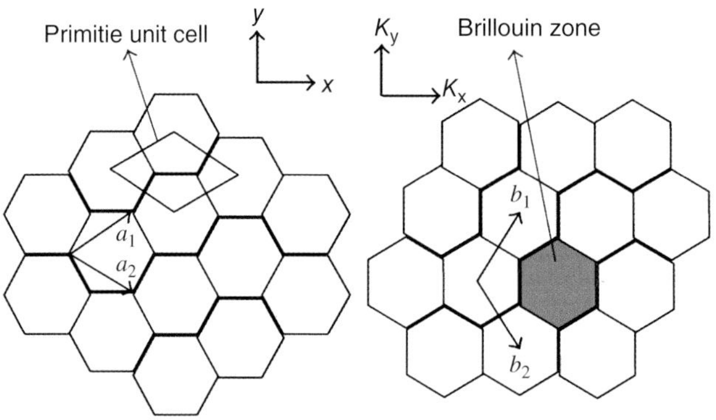

Figure 5.30 Primitive unit cell and the Brillion zone in graphene [7], https://creativecommons.org/licenses/by/3.0/.

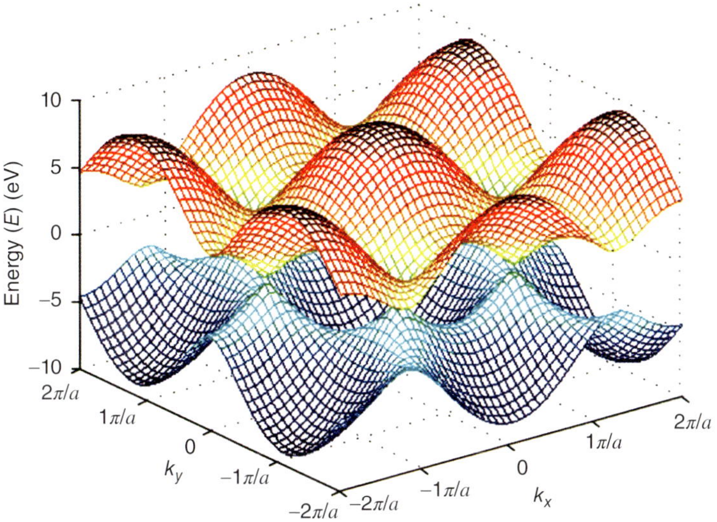

Figure 5.31 The energy dispersion variations in graphene [7]. https://creativecommons.org/licenses/by/3.0/.

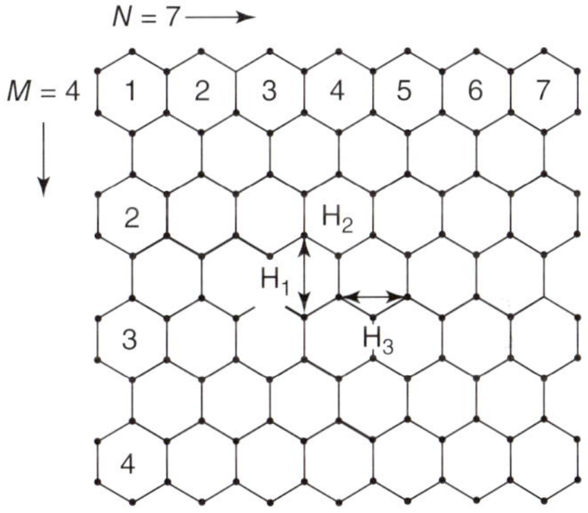

Figure 5.32 Graphene: topology of hexagonal lattice. (Reproduced with permission of Glukhova O.E.)

detailed study using mathematical calculation methods is necessary. General conclusions and notions were made through analysis software, and calculation programs are available regarding this issue. The topology of hexagonal lattice permits us to exactly define and show the graphene edges (zigzag and armchair) in its structure. Horizontal direction of $\boldsymbol{N}$, starting from numbers 1 to 7, determines the zigzag edge in the hexagon unit lattice. In Figure 5.32, the vertical $\boldsymbol{M}$ direction starts from top to bottom, numbered from 1 to 4, and determines the armchair edge in graphene lattice.

5.5.4 Physical Properties and Ionization Potential of Graphene

Physical properties of graphene include its bond length, atom energy, and semiconducting bandgap energy, and ionization potential (IP) is described in this section. IP is the amount of energy required to successively withdraw the 1st,

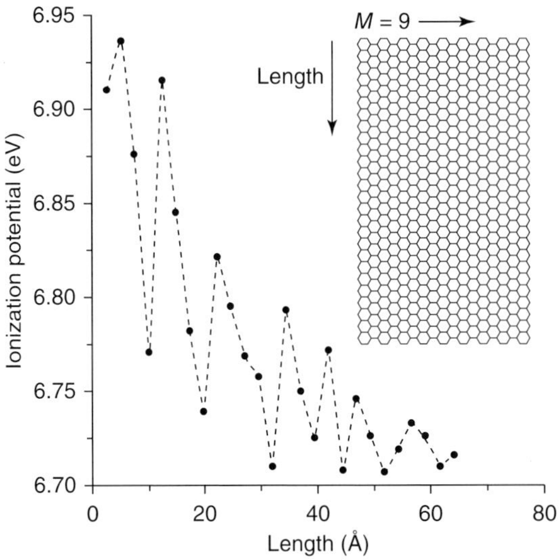

Figure 5.33 Ionization potential for graphene at $M = 9$. (Reproduced with permission of Glukhova O.E.)

Table 5.4 Physical parameters and ionization potential for graphene at $M = 9$.

$N \times M$	LN (Å)	LM (Å)	E_{atom} (eV atom^{-1})	E_g (eV)	IP (eV)
1 × 9	2.32	37.42	−42.10	0.43	6.91
2 × 9	4.77	37.00	−42.47	0.27	6.94
3 × 9	7.25	36.83	−42.65	0.05	6.88
4 × 9	9.72	36.85	−42.76	0.02	6.77
5 × 9	12.15	36.86	−42.83	0.22	6.92
6 × 9	14.64	36.94	−42.88	0.20	6.85
7 × 9	17.15	36.85	−42.92	0.08	6.78
8 × 9	19.6	36.85	−42.95	0.06	6.74
9 × 9	22.05	36.93	−42.97	0.12	6.82
10 × 9	24.50	36.93	−42.99	0.11	6.80
11 × 9	26.95	36.93	−43.00	0.02	6.77
23 × 9	56.58	37.01	−43.09	0.02	6.73
24 × 9	59.04	37.01	−43.09	0.05	6.73
25 × 9	61.50	37.01	−43.09	0.06	6.71
26 × 9	63.96	37.01	−43.10	0.02	6.72

Source: Reproduced with permission of Glukhova O.E.

2nd, or 3rd electron from an atom in the gaseous state [8]. For $M = 9$, indicating *armchair edges* in inset, as shown in Figure 5.33, an increase of length in the vertical direction during geometrical progression causes a decrease in atom energy and a decrease in semiconducting bandgap energy (Table 5.4). The value of IP decreases when length increases in the vertical direction of N zigzag edges (Figure 5.34).

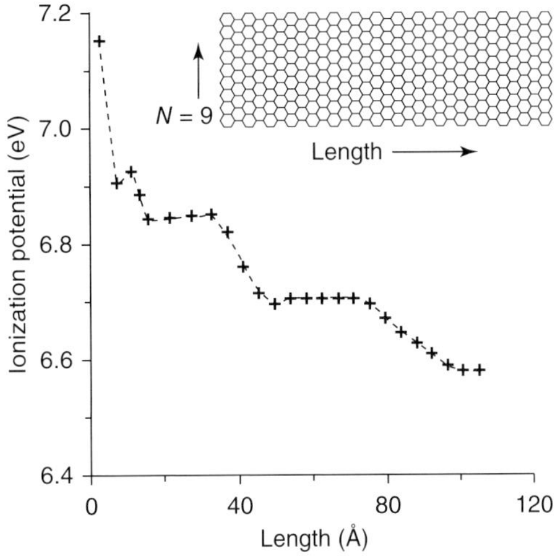

Figure 5.34 Ionization potential for graphene at $N = 9$. (Reproduced with permission of Glukhova O.E.)

Table 5.5 Physical parameters and ionization potential for graphene at $N = 9$.

$N \times M$	LN (Å)	LM (Å)	E_{atom} (eV atom^{-1})	E_g (eV)	IP (eV)
9 × 1	22.05	2.57	−41.886	0.17	7.15
9 × 2	22.05	7.04	−42.464	0.02	6.91
9 × 3	22.05	11.31	−42.681	0.08	6.93
9 × 4	22.04	15.58	−42.79	0.00	6.84
9 × 5	22.05	19.84	−42.85	0.00	6.84
9 × 6	22.05	24.15	−42.90	0.15	6.85
9 × 7	22.05	28.41	−42.93	0.11	6.85
9 × 8	22.04	32.66	−42.95	0.15	6.85
9 × 9	22.05	36.93	−42.97	0.12	6.82
9 × 10	22.05	41.19	−42.98	0.07	6.76
9 × 11	22.05	45.45	−43.00	0.02	6.71
9 × 12	22.05	49.71	−43.01	0.02	6.69
9 × 22	22.05	92.53	−43.06	0.03	6.61
9 × 23	22.05	96.8	−43.06	0.01	6.59
9 × 24	22.05	101.07	−43.06	0.00	6.58

Source: Reproduced with permission of Glukhova O.E.

In the case of $N = 9$, indicating *zigzag edges* in inset, with an increase of length in the horizontal direction, atom energy increases and semiconducting bandgap energies decrease (Table 5.5). The IP decreases with an increase in length M armchair edges (Figure 5.34).

5.5.5 Approaches in Graphene Synthesis

The synthesis of graphene can be accomplished in several ways and methods, which mainly can be classified into two large groups, namely, top-down

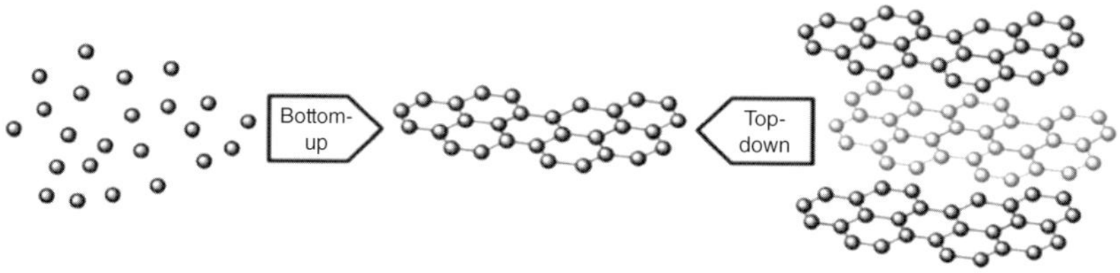

Figure 5.35 Schematic of "bottom-up" and "top-down" graphene synthesis. (Edwards *et al.* 2012. Reproduced with permission of Royal Society of Chemistry.)

and bottom-up methods (Figure 5.35). *Bottom-up methods* are based on the synthesis or formation of graphene from initial precursors and from carbon sources, including epitaxial growth on silicon carbide (SiC), CVD (growth on metals and substrate free), and miscellaneous methods, that is, building of graphene from small atoms and molecules. *Top-down* methods are oppositely, based on cleavage, separation, or peeling of graphite or carbon compound, including micromechanical cleavage, electrochemical exfoliation, graphite intercalation compound (GIG) exfoliation, solvent-based exfoliation, graphite oxide exfoliation, unzipping carbon nanotubes, and arc discharge [9].

Top-down synthesis approaches for graphene are based on the breaking of the van der Waals forces to separate carbon or graphite bulk materials into separate single layers. However, there are disadvantage of this synthesis approach such as less amount of synthesized product and necessity in using of a number of synthesis steps [10]. Electrochemical exfoliation of graphite has been considered as a potentially scalable method for production of graphene and graphene-based materials. It involves the use of an electrolyte (e.g., aqueous or nonaqueous solution) and an electrical current. Due to the charge of intercalating ions, the graphite electrode works as an anode or cathode, representing oxidation or reduction reactions. In contrast to other exfoliation processes, this method is not equipment-intensive and is typically performed under ambient conditions. Moreover, it is ecofriendly compared to other chemical/sonication routes, which often involve hazardous reagents or solvents. Various graphite precursors (natural and synthetic graphites), powder, foil, rod, flake, or plate, have been investigated in electrochemical exfoliation. These processes can be classified into: (i) anodic exfoliation in the mixture of water and ionic liquids, aqueous solution of inorganic salts or mineral acids; and (ii) cathodic exfoliation in organic solvents (e.g., of propylene carbonate, dimethyl sulfoxide, N-methyl-2-pyrrolidone, etc.) containing lithium or alkylammonium salts [11].

5.5.6 Characterizations of Graphene

Graphene and graphene-based materials can be characterized by microscopic and spectroscopic analyses. Here, transmission electron microscopy (TEM), HRTEM, and AFM characterizations of graphene are briefly described. TEM provides the opportunity to necessarily determine, in basic view, the shape, size, and morphology of graphene materials. Sheet-like structure of graphene can be observed by TEM analysis. Sample preparation for TEM analysis can be achieved by sonication of tiny amounts of graphene nanomaterial in organic solvents, for example, ethanol or acetone. Preferable length of time of sonication is 3–10 min, without heating. Then, sonicated sample is placed on the sample grid and dried in order to evaporate the dissolving liquid. HRTEM characterization of graphene is analogous to those of TEM characterization, but with possibility to obtain high-resolution scaled image. At 1 nm scale of HRTEM, hexagonal carbon lattice structure can be clearly seen for sp^2-bonded carbon nanomaterials. It is found that graphene sheets have a size of 0.006–0.36 mm^2 and some are stacked together. Figure 5.36 shows size distribution of a total of 93 distinguishable graphene sheets calculated from TEM images using ImageJ software. Sheet sizes of 0.006–0.0125 mm^2 are dominant, representing 50% of the total distribution. Around 22% of sheets have sizes of 0.022–0.038 mm^2, and only a few larger sheets with sizes up to 0.3 mm^2 are present. High-resolution TEM analysis of the graphene edges reveals that majority of the graphene sheets are made of 2–5 layers, with a lattice spacing of 0.342 nm (see Figure 5.36d–f). No other carbon phases such as amorphous carbon or fullerene are found at the edges. The corresponding electron diffraction pattern of single sheets (Figure 5.36b) has a typical sixfold symmetry, confirming that the graphene sheet is of high-quality single-crystal nature.

AFM is a technique that allows acquisition of information about height of the layered graphene sheets and topography distance profile. The nanodots are dispersed on Si or freshly cleaved mica surfaces and measured by an AFM operating in the tapping mode. The nanodots exhibited an average diameter of 29 nm for a grinding time of 30 min. When the grinding time is increased to 1 and 4 hours, the average diameter of the nanodots reduces to 20 and 9 nm, respectively. Besides the diameter, the height of the nanodots also decreases

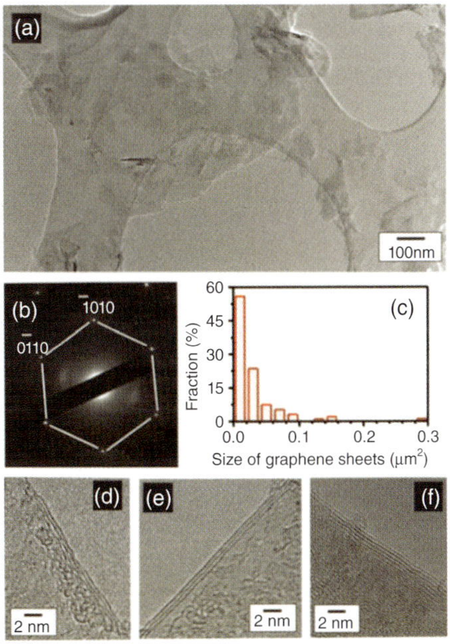

Figure 5.36 (a) Typical low-magnification TEM image of graphene sheets; (b) corresponding electron diffraction pattern of (a); (c) size distribution of graphene sheets; HRTEM images of (d) bilayer, (e) trilayer, and (f) 4–5-layer graphene sheets. (Shang *et al.* 2012 [12]. Reproduced with permission of Royal Society of Chemistry.)

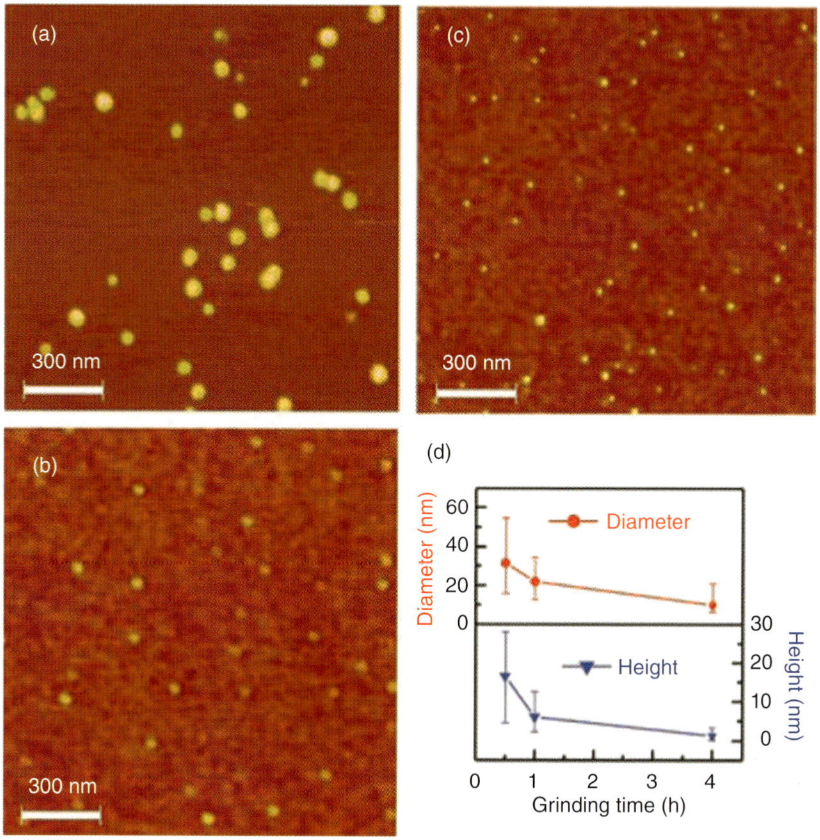

Figure 5.37 AFM images of nanodots, produced with grinding times of (a) 30 min, (b) 1 h, and (c) 4 h and a ratio of 1 : 2 of graphite (mg) to ionic liquid (ml); (d) height and diameter distributions of nanodots. (Shang *et al.* 2012 [12] [12]. Reproduced with permission of Royal Society of Chemistry.)

as the grinding times increase (Figure 5.37). For 30 min grinding, the average height of the nanodots is approximately 16 nm [12].

Raman spectroscopy is an integral part of graphene research. It is used to determine the number and orientation of layers, the quality and types of edge, and the effects of perturbations, such as electric and magnetic fields, strain, doping, disorder, and functional groups. This, in turn, provides insight into all sp^2-bonded carbon allotropes, because graphene is their fundamental building block. Raman spectroscopy can also probe scattering of photons by electronic excitations. The Raman spectrum of graphite was first recorded more than 40 years ago, and, by the time the Raman spectrum of graphene was measured for the first time in 2006, it had become one of the most popular techniques for the characterization of disordered and amorphous carbons, fullerenes, nanotubes, diamonds, carbon chains, and poly-conjugated molecules. Raman techniques are particularly useful for graphene since the absence of a bandgap makes all incident wavelengths resonant, so the Raman spectrum contains information about both atomic structure and electronic properties. The number of graphene layers in a sample can be determined by elastic light scattering/Rayleigh spectroscopy, but this approach only works for exfoliated samples on optimized substrates and does not provide other structural or electronic information. Raman spectroscopy, on the other hand, works for all graphene samples. Moreover, it is able to identify unwanted by-products, structural damage, functional groups, and chemical modifications introduced during the preparation, processing, or placement of graphene [13].

5.5.7 Applications of Graphene

Graphene have a number of applications due to its unique and interesting properties. One of graphene applications in the battery and supercapacitor devices can be achieved by deposition of graphene sheets on to nickel foam substrates which have 3d structure. Such graphene-nickel composite showed specific areal capacitance and electron charge transfer resistance properties [14]. Figure 5.38 is depicted to show the chemical reactions occurring on the graphene cathode and the graphene oxide anode, respectively, which are fixed within the battery layers.

Case Study 1: Structural Features of Graphene, Lattice Directions, Edge Location, Crystal Structure, and Energy in Reciprocal Space

- Influence of lattice orientation on growth and structure of graphene on Cu(001) was studied [16], using the hexagonal lattice directions in graphene structure, armchair and zigzag edges as represented in Figure 5.39.

The graphene edge perpendicular to the fast-growth direction was named the "fast-growth edge" where new carbon is being incorporated most rapidly and similarly to the armchair and zigzag edge configurations. Graphene and Cu lattice alignment was described as perfect when a C<10> direction is parallel to either one of two equivalent in-plane orientations, Cu [110] or Cu $[1\bar{1}0]$. However, the lattices of most graphene domains are rotated some degrees away from such ideal alignment, resulting in an entire range of different graphene configurations on the Cu surface.

- Twofold rotation was determined by symmetry of the combined structure characterized by symmetry elements common to the graphene lattice and Cu surface.
- Structure of hexagonal carbon lattice crystal structure was studied by Goerbig [17] based on location of vectors along the graphene edges and the energy in reciprocal space.

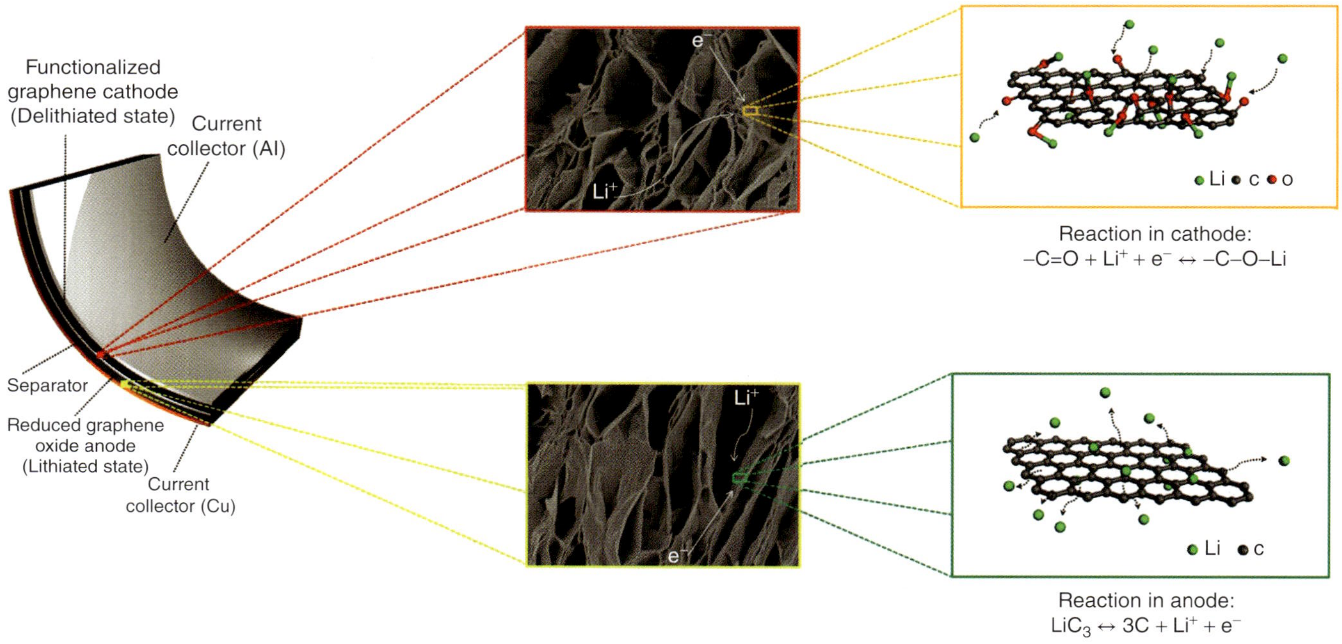

Figure 5.38 Schematic illustration of all-graphene battery and its electrochemical reaction. In the functionalized graphene cathode, Li ions and electrons are stored in the functional groups on the graphene surface at a relatively high potential. On the other hand, Li ions and electrons are stored on the surface of graphene with low potential, in the reduced graphene oxide anode. (Kim *et al*. 2014 [15]. Reprinted with permission from Nature Publishing Group.)

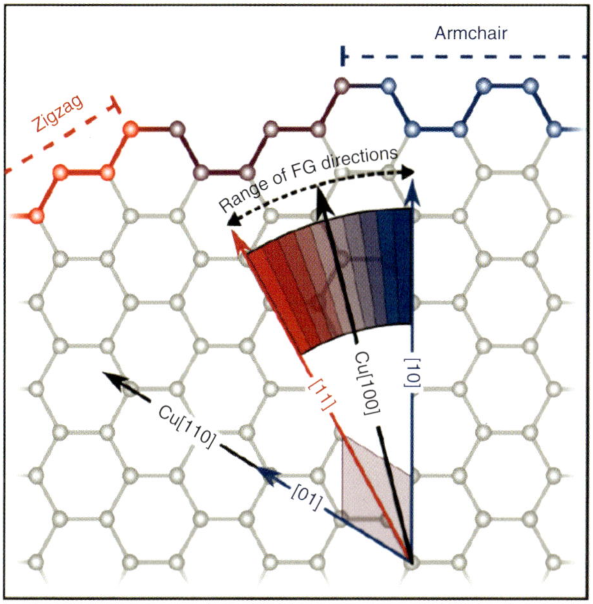

Figure 5.39 Schematic diagram illustrating lattice directions and edges of the graphene lattice (the purple diamond is the graphene unit cell). Because the fast-growth direction remains near a Cu⟨100⟩ direction, a rotation of the graphene lattice changes the lattice direction along which fast-growth direction occurs. When the lattice of a graphene domain approaches perfect alignment with the Cu(001) surface (i.e., C[6]||Cu[110] or Cu⟨1$\bar{1}$0⟩; see arrows on the left of unit cell), the fast-growth direction is directly between C⟨10⟩ and C⟨11⟩ directions. Any rotation away from alignment moves the fast-growth direction toward either the C⟨10⟩ or the C⟨11⟩ direction. A graphene edge perpendicular to a C⟨10⟩ direction (blue) has the armchair structure, while an edge perpendicular to a C⟨11⟩ direction (red) has the zigzag structure. The purple edge section is a mix of these two high-symmetry edge structures. (Wofford *et al.* 2015 [16]. Reproduced with permission of Elsevier.)

Control Questions

1) Describe the ferromagnetic properties of nanomaterials.
2) Discuss single-domain condition of nanomaterials. What is the difference between single-domain and multi-domain conditions?
3) Determine superparamagnetism and its characteristics in nanomaterials.
4) Describe types of size dependences in nanomaterials and their effects on magnetic property.
5) Describe size dependence on the heat conductivity for nanomaterials.
6) What kind of heat characteristic features exist in nanomaterials?
7) Describe the role of Mössbauer spectroscopy in the determination of materials' magnetic properties.
8) Describe the heat conductivity of crystal lattice in nanomaterials.
9) Describe the influence of morphology and polydispersity on the optical properties of nanomaterials.
10) Determine extinction and its types in nanomaterials.

11) Discuss extinction phenomenon in metallic nanoparticles.
12) What is the difference between diffusion in nanomaterials and that in nanopowders?
13) Describe the structure of graphene and topology of hexagonal carbon lattice.
14) Discuss the basic physical property and characteristics of graphene.
15) Describe the microscopic characterization of graphene by TEM, HRTEM, and AFM.
16) Describe the importance of Raman spectroscopy in the characterization of carbon, graphite, and graphene materials.
17) Discuss applications of graphene-based materials.

References

1 Ryzhonkov, D.I., Levina, V.V., and Dzidziguri, E.L. (2008) *Nanomaterials, BINOM*, BKL Publishers, Moscow.

2 Novoselov *et al.* (2012) A roadmap for Graphene. *Nature*, **490**, 192–200, doi:10.1038/nature11458.

3 Patelis, N., Moris, D., Matheiken, S., and Klonaris, C. (2016) The potential role of graphene in developing the next generation of endomaterials. *BioMed Res. Int.*, **3180954**, 7, https://dx.doi.org/10.1155/2016/3180954.

4 Abdullaeva, Z., Kelgenbaeva, Z., Tsushida, M., Hirano, M., Nagaoka, S., and Shirosaki, T. (2016) Graphene sheets with modified surface by sodium lauryl sulfate surfactant for biomedical applications. *Graphene*, **5**, 155–165.

5 Wang, W., Wu, X., and Zhang, J. (2015) Graphene and other 2D material components dynamic characterization and nanofabrication at atomic scale. *J. Nanomat.*, **198126**, 6, https://dx.doi.org/10.1155/2015/198126.

6 Nair, R.R., Blake, P., Grigorenko, A.N., Novoselov, K.S., Booth, T.J., Stauber, T. *et al.* (2008) Fine structure constant defines visual transparency of graphene. *Science*, **320**, 1308.

7 Fathi, D. (2011) A review of electronic band structure of graphene and carbon nanotubes using tight binding. *J. Nanotechnol.*, **471241**, 6, https://dx.doi.org/10.1155/2011/471241.

8 Bloss, D.F. (1971) Crystallography and Crystal Chemistry, Mineralogical Society of America, ISBN-13: 978-0939950379.

9 Edwards, R.S. and Coleman, K.S. (2013) Graphene synthesis: relationship to applications. *Nanoscale*, **5**, 38–51. doi: 10.1039/C2NR32629A.

10 Skoda, M., Dudek, I., Jarosz, A., and Szukiewicz, D. (2014) Graphene: one material, many possibilities-application difficulties in biological systems. *J. Nanomat.*, **890246**, 11, https://doi.org/10.1155/2014/890246.

11 Yang, S., Lohe, M.R., Müllen, K., and Feng, X. (2016) New-generation graphene from electrochemical approaches: production and applications. *Adv. Mater.*, **28**, 6213–6221. doi: 10.1002/adma.201505326

12 Shang, N.G. *et al* (2012) *Chem. Commun.*, **48**, 1877–1879.

13 Ferrari, A.C. and Basko, D.M. (2013) Raman spectroscopy as a versatile tool for studying the properties of graphene, *Nature Nanotechnology*, **8**, 235–246.

14 Khamlich, S., Abdullaeva, Z., Kennedy, J.V., and Maaza, M. (2017) High performance symmetric supercapacitor based on zinc hydroxychloride nanosheets and 3D graphene-nickel foam composite. *Appl. Surf. Sci.*, **405**, 329–336, https://dx.doi.org/10.1016/j.apsusc.2017.02.095.
15 Kim, H., Park, K.-Y., Hong, J., and Kang, K. (2014) All-graphene-battery: bridging the gap between supercapacitors and lithium ion batteries. *Sci. Rep.*, **4**, 5278. doi: 10.1038/srep05278.
16 Wofford, J.M. *et al* (2015) *Carbon*, **90**, 284–290.
17 Goerbig, M.O. (2011) *Rev. Mod. Phys.*, **83** (4), 1193–1243.

Further Reading

Abergel, D.S.L., Russell, A., and Fal'ko, V.I. (2007) *Appl. Phys. Lett.*, **91**, 063125.
Andreoni, W. (2000) *The Physics of Fullerene-Based and Fullerene-Related Materials*, Springer, Berlin.
Blake, P., Novoselov, K.S., Castro Neto, A.H., Jiang, D., Yang, R., Booth, T.J., Geim, A.K., and Hill, E.W. (2007) *Appl. Phys. Lett.*, **91**, 063124.
Calandra, M. and Mauri, F. (2007) *Phys. Rev. B*, **76**, 199901.
Calizo, I., Bao, W., Miao, F., Lau, C.N., and Balandin, A.A. (2007) *Appl. Phys. Lett.*, **91**, 201904.
Casiraghi, C., Hartschuh, A., Lidorikis, E., Qian, H., Harutyunyan, H., Gokus, T., Novoselov, K.S., and Ferrari, A.C. (2007) *Nano Lett.*, **7**, 2711.
Castro Neto, A.H. *et al* (2009) The electronic properties of graphene. *Rev. Mod. Phys.*, **81**, 109–162.
Charlier, J.-C., Blase, X., and Roche, S. (2007) *Rev. Mod. Phys.*, **79**, 677.
Das, A., Chakraborty, B., and Sood, A.K. (2008) *Bull. Mater. Sci.*, **31**, 579.
Dresselhaus, M.S., Dresselhaus, G., Fischer, J.E., and Moran, M.J. (1983) *Intercalated Graphite*, North-Holland, New York, p. A401.
Dresselhaus, M.S. and Dresselhaus, G. (2002) *Adv. Phys.*, **51**, 1.
Faugeras, C., Nerriere, A., Potemski, M., Mahmood, A., Dujardin, E., Berger, C., and de Heer, W.A. (2008) *Appl. Phys. Lett.*, **92**, 011914.
Geim, A.K. and MacDonald, A.H. (2007) *Phys. Today*, **60**, 35.
Giovannetti, G., Khomyakov, P.A., Brocks, G., Kelly, P.J., and van der Brink, J. (2007) *Phys. Rev. B*, **76**, 073103.
Glukhova, O. Carbon Nanoclusters, Structure, Classification Size Effects, Lecture Notes, http://theor.jinr.ru/~diastp/winter09/lectures/glukhova/glukhova_1_2.pdf (accessed 17 January 2017).
Gogotsi, Y. (2015) *MRS Bull.*, **40** (12), 1110–1121.
Leenaerts, O., Partoens, B., and Peeters, F.M. (2008) *Phys. Rev. B*, **77**, 125416.
Martins, T.B., Miwa, R.H., da Silva, A.J.R., and Fazzio, A. (2007) *Phys. Rev. Lett.*, **98**, 196803.
Novoselov, K.S., Geim, A.K., Morozov, S.V., Jiang, D., Zhang, Y., Dubonos, S.V., Gregorieva, I.V., and Firsov, A.A. (2004) *Science*, **306**, 666.
Pauling, L. (1972) *The Nature of the Chemical Bond*, Cornell University Press, Ithaca, NY.

Peres, N.M.R., Klironomos, F.D., Tsai, S.-W., Santos, J.R., Lopes dos Santos, J.M.B., and Castro Neto, A.H. (2007) *Europhys. Lett.*, **80**, 67007.

Petroski, H. (1989) *The Pencil: A History of Design and Circumstance*, Knopf, New York.

Saito, R., Fujita, M., Dresselhaus, G., and Dresselhaus, M.S. (1992) *Phys. Rev. B*, **46**, 1804.

Schedin, F., Geim, A.K., Morozov, S.V., Jiang, D., Hill, E.H., Blake, P., and Novoselov, K.S. (2007) *Nat. Mater.*, **6**, 652.

Stephan, O., Ajayan, P.M., Colliex, C., Redlich, P., Lambert, J.M., Bernier, P., and Lefin, P. (1994) *Science*, **266**, 1683.

Tanuma, S. and Kamimura, H. (1985) *Graphite Intercalation Compounds: Progress of Research in Japan*, World Scientific, Singapore.

Uchoa, B., Lin, C.-Y., and Castro Neto, A.H. (2008) *Phys. Rev. B*, **77**, 035420.

Uchoa, B. and Castro Neto, A.H. (2007) *Phys. Rev. Lett.*, **98**, 146801.

Varchon, F., Feng, R., Hass, J., Li, X., Nguyen, B.N., Naud, C., Mallet, P., Veuillen, J.Y., Berger, C., Conrad, E.H., and Magaud, L. (2007) *Phys. Rev. Lett.*, **99**, 126805.

Wehling, T.O., Novoselov, K.S., Morozov, S.V., Vdovin, E.E., Katsnelson, M.I., Geim, A.K., and Lichtenstein, A.I. (2008) *Nano Lett.*, **8**, 173.

Zhou, S.Y., Gweon, G.-H., Fedorov, A.V., First, P.N., de Heer, W.A., Lee, D.-H., Guinea, F., Castro Neto, A.H., and Lanzara, A. (2007) *Nat. Mater.*, **6**, 770.

6

Chemical Properties and Mechanical Characteristics of Nanomaterial Characterization Tools in Nanotechnology

Translated materials from the original work of Ryzhonkov, D.I., Levina,V.V., and Dzidziguri, E.L. were used in this chapter.

> *....and by the help of Microscopes, there is nothing so small as to escape our inquiry....*
>
> Robert Hooke, Fellow of the Royal Society (1635–1703)

6.1 Chemical Properties of Nanomaterials

Use of dispersive mediums showed that nanomaterials possess critically high chemical activity, which is observed during temperature change, speed, heat effect of interaction, transformation level at given conditions, and increased pyrophoric and specific catalytic properties.

Nanoparticles are able to interact effectively with other inert substances, including inert gases and noble metals. For example, it was found that during grinding of the surfaces of nanopowders, irreversible adsorption of inert gases will occur wherein bind between gas molecule and surface atoms is extremely rugged.

Also, high catalytic activity of gold nanoparticles was determined in such processes as low temperature burning of various substances, oxidation of hydrocarbons, hydrogenation of unsaturated compounds, and reduction of nitrogen oxides.

In this case, it can be concluded that there is no inert medium for nanomaterials due to developed surface and excessive energy of surface atoms. Aside from further development of materials' nanostate, a study of chemical properties of nanomaterials allowed their practical applications, which are of fundamental interest. This is important for evaluation of nanopowders flammable and detonation properties and monitoring the time with expiration due dates for development of technological application processes.

6.1.1 Size Effects in Chemical Processes

The effect of size during chemical process appears in the interaction change. The reaction speed for a large number of heterogeneous chemical processes with

Nano- and Biomaterials: Compounds, Properties, Characterization, and Applications,
First Edition. Zhypargul Abdullaeva.

participation of solid phases is determined by diffusion in hard material. However, when the radius of interacting particle R is significantly larger than the characteristic diffusion time [1],

$$\delta = \sqrt{Dt} \tag{6.1}$$

where D is diffusion coefficient and t is time. If $\delta \geq R$, then the limiting stage of process is usually a chemical reaction. Hence, for heterogeneous reactions, changes in kinetic laws will occur due to existence of the boundary particle sizes.

However, the influence of particle sizes or grains on kinetic parameters is very complex for experimental study. First of all, it is related to the polydispersive state of nanomaterials, which cause an average size effect and, often, makes it impossible to provide meaningful interpretation of experimental data. In addition, a range of factors from which kinetics of any chemical reaction depend on do not remain unchangeable upon decrease in geometrical sizes of the interacting substances and often relate to the presence of oxide film on the surface, thickness, presence of adsorption layers, adsorption energy, coefficients and diffusion types, quantity of potential nucleation centers, and many others. In other words, achieving a chemical reaction in pure form is very complicated. Due to this, studies of the effect of size on chemical reactions employ mathematical modeling as an effective method. Study of some size effects providing an adequate description of a system can possibly exist, which can be obtained experimentally.

For example, the set of reactions were studied by imitational modeling method during carbide formation in the iron particle located on inert substrate. The reaction volume was imitated by traditional cubic lattice, consisting of finite number of cells $N = n^3$, where n is the geometric size of the cube.

As calculations showed, by a decrease in particle size, the reaction speed grows exponentially. The result is illustrated in Figure 6.1, where dependence of reaction speed maximum W_{m} on the particle size at thickness of iron carbide nuclei is 0.23. Estimations also showed increase in line slope upon increase in the coverage degree level of particle by nuclei. At the same time, with reducing in the particle size, the maximum reaction speed $t_{\max}$ is shortened as ln(n) (Figure 6.2).

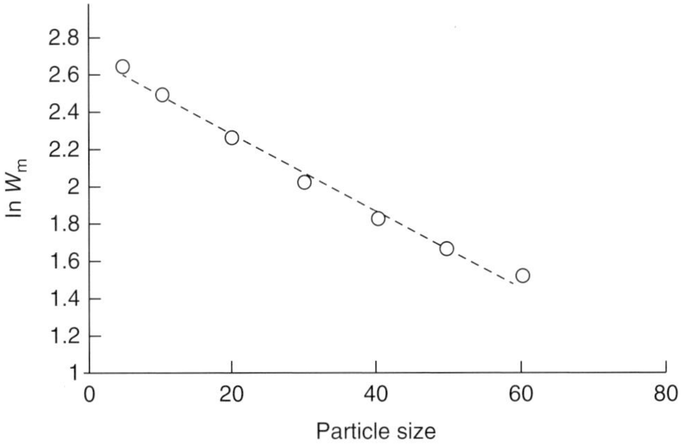

Figure 6.1 Dependence of maximum reaction speed W_{m} on particle size at fixed nuclei thickness of 0.23. (Reproduced with permission of BKL Publishers.)

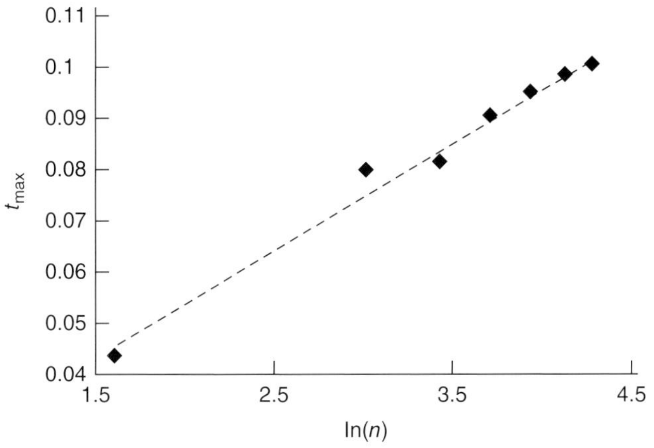

Figure 6.2 Dependence of time reaching the maximum speed W_m on particle size. (Reproduced with permission of BKL Publishers.)

One of the size effect manifestations in chemical processes is the decrease in temperature of chemical reaction flow. In particular, in double-layer films, MgO/Nb_2O_5 reaction with type

$$MgO + Nb_2O_5 = MgNb_2O_6$$

occurs simultaneously at temperatures below 800–1000 K than in the case of large grain oxides.

In nanosized systems, chemical reactions are possible than in bulk materials. For example, the reaction between hydrothermal pair ($Al + H_2O$) and nitroaromatic compounds occurring by scheme

$$Al + H_2O + NO_2C_6H_4NH_2 \rightarrow NH_2C_6H_4NH_2$$

is possible only in case the particles of Al powder have nanodiapason sizes.

6.1.2 Oxidation Processes in Nanomediums

As a rule, based on oxidation reaction, the general level reaction ability of a substance at dispersive condition can be determined. As an example, the kinetics of Fe and Mo nanopowder oxidation in air for 180 days is presented in Figure 6.3.

Particle sizes were 70 and 100 nm for Fe and Mo, respectively. In Fe nanopowder, oxidation process occurs intensively than that in Mo nanopowder. As a result, Fe will oxidize significantly during 180 days. This experimental fact can be explained by the features of Fe nanoparticle oxide film. Coincidence of an air temperature increase with Fe nanopowder mass change as shown in Figure 6.3, leads to assume that sharp mass increase and, hence, the specimen oxidation are caused by exfoliation of an oxide film by coherence irregularities in crystal lattices of oxide and metal phases. In the initial region of Fe specimen mass change curve, it can be concluded that in the absence of oxide film exfoliation, oxidation will continue to occur for 40–50 days.

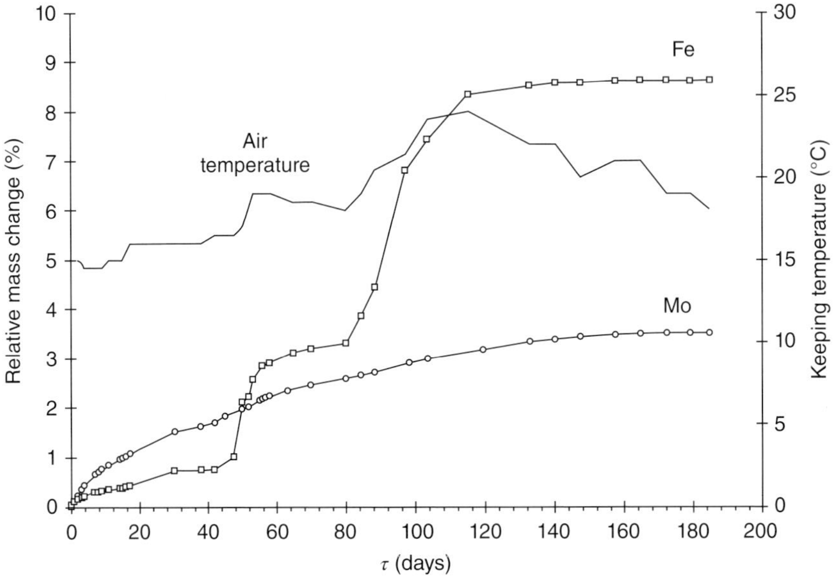

Figure 6.3 Oxidation kinetic of Fe and Mo nanopowders while in air. (Reproduced with permission of BKL Publishers.)

Oxidation process of Mo nanopowder in air practically stops for 140 days; after its synthesis, the change in the air temperature has little influence on the mass of the powder mass.

At repetitive increase of keeping temperature, as seen from Figure 6.3, the speed of the oxidation process for nanopowders will not change if the previous maximum temperature was not in excess.

As a result of conducted experiments, it can be concluded that without special protecting layers, metal nanopowders exhibit significantly high stability against oxidation in air. However, this is appropriate for certain threshold temperature, which lies in range of 200–500 °C for metals. Approvement of given is specific oxidation speed dependence on temperature for iron nanopowders obtained by chemical dispersion method (Figure 6.4).

As seen from the graph, specimen is fully not oxidized until 200 °C, as the increase in mass at temperature interval of 20–200 °C is around 1.5%. Oxidation

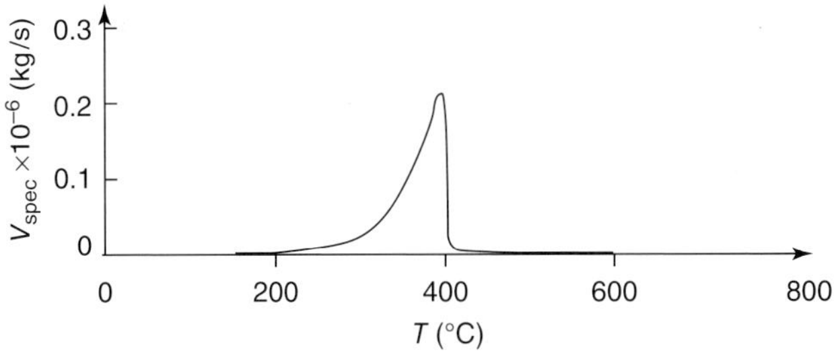

Figure 6.4 Dependence of oxidation speed on temperature of Fe nanopowder during linear heating. (Reproduced with permission of BKL Publishers.)

Table 6.1 Temperature of starting oxidation in air for ultra-disperse and large metal powders [1].

Metal	Specific surface ($m^2\,g^{-1}$)	Nanoparticle size (nm)	Temperature of NPs starting oxidation (°C)	Large nanopowder particle size (μm)	Temperature of large powders starting oxidation (°C)
Aluminum	18.5	120	420	<20	870
Iron	4.6	160	310	<45	480
Copper	6.8	105	170	<60	260
Zinc	12.9	65	220	<71	410
Tin	10.2	80	180	<45	270

speed at an interval of 200–420 °C increases and reaches a maximum at around 400 °C. By further heating, the oxidation speed sharply decreased, but insignificant growth in the mass of specimen continued until 600 °C.

For nickel and cobalt nanopowders obtained by chemical dispersion method, temperature dependencies on reaction speed are analogous. Nickel oxidizes at 200 °C and cobalt at 180 °C.

A study of oxidation in air for aluminum, copper, iron, molybdenum, zinc, and tin nanopowders obtained by electrodetonation and powders of usual sizes showed that nanomaterial oxidizes with distinct speed at significantly lower temperatures compared with high disperse powders (Table 6.1).

Based on the state of oxidation in air, nanopowders of the previously studied metals can be classified as follows:

a) Oxidation occurring in one stage (Figure 6.5): This type is characteristic of chemically active metals, reacting with large heat generation – Al, Zn, and Mo.
b) Oxidation occurring in two stages (Figure 6.6): This process is observed for polyvalent metals, forming oxides with variable composition – Fe, Cu, and Sn.

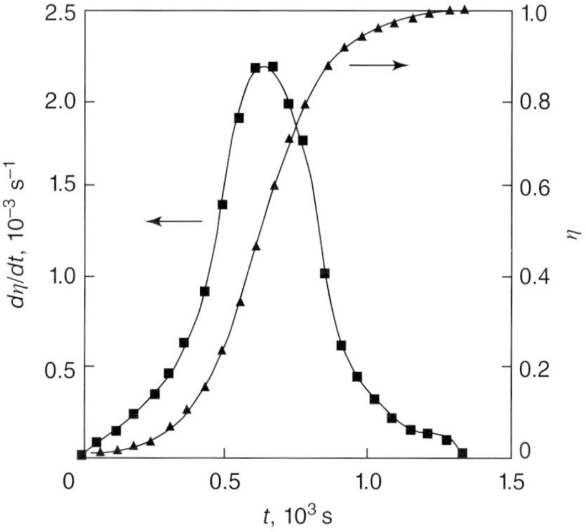

Figure 6.5 Kinetic oxidation curves of zinc nanopowder at heating speed of 10 K min^{-1}: η (oxidation level); $d\eta/dt$ (its speed). (Reproduced with permission of BKL Publishers.)

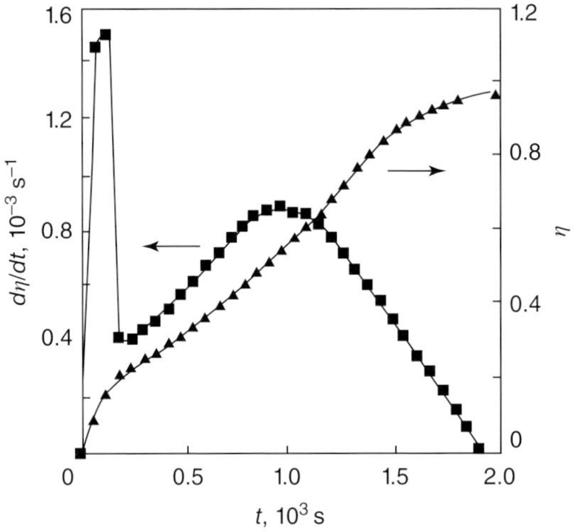

Figure 6.6 Kinetic oxidation curves of iron nanopowder at heating speed of 10 K/min. (Reproduced with permission of BKL Publishers.)

Depending on the process conditions, metals are oxidizing only by sequential, or only by logarithmic law interactions with the latter substitutions during certain interaction. The total kinetic equation of process in the dimensionless form can be presented as

$$\upsilon = k_0 \exp(-E/RT)\eta^{-\eta} \exp(-k_1\eta) \tag{6.2}$$

where υ is the reaction speed; η is the oxidation level of metal determined from thermogravimetric data due to mass change of nanopowder during heating; k_0 is the pre-exponential factor; E is the activation energy of reaction; R is the universal gas constant; T is the temperature; η is the exponent of the power law oxidation; and k_1 is the logarithmic coefficient for oxidation.

From the total equation it is found that in the case of aspiration of experimental data in coordinates of $\text{In}(\upsilon_1/\upsilon_2)$, $(\eta_2 - \eta_1)$, oxidation process obeys the logarithmic law ($n = 0$, $k_1 > 0$). In the experimental results, aspiration in coordinates of $\text{In}(\upsilon_1/\upsilon_2)$, $\text{In}(\eta_2/\eta_1)$ to power law ($0 < n < 2$, $k_1 = 0$). In turn, the tilt of the tangent of right angles tilt allows to determine the values for k_1 and n.

In Figure 6.7 and in Table 6.2, mathematical processing results of experimental data and low temperature kinetic oxidation parameters for metals are presented.

Value E for nanomaterials in a number of cases is close or near to values for large crystal metals existing in the literature. However, values of pre-exponential function for nanopowders as a rule are 2–5 times higher.

Study results allow to establish oxidation mechanism. The process, starting at $T = 400$–700 K, obeys linear law until transformation degree 0.1–0.3. The reaction speed at this stage at $n = 0$ does not depend on oxidation degree, and the process is analogical to monomolecular reaction. At this stage, fast oxidation of particles surface will take place. At the second stage, strong inhibition of process is observed, which appears in exchange of oxidation law with logarithmic. Apparently, this binds with formation of continuous oxide films.

The existence of as-called threshold temperature is caused by the following reasons. During contact with air, oxide film will form on the nanopowders' surface. The content of oxide phases is not great, not more than 5–7%. Surface oxide films with adsorbing gaseous layer provide stability of nanomaterials in

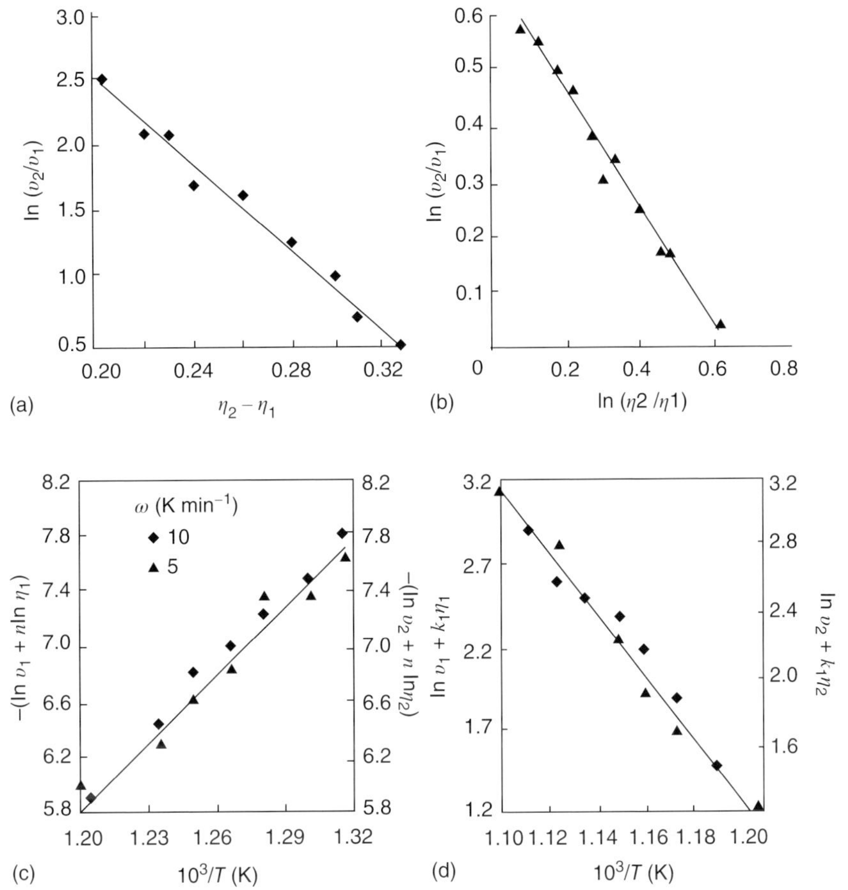

Figure 6.7 Determination for type of kinetic law and Arrhenius oxidation parameters for metal nanopowders on separate stages: (a) molybdenum, $T = 490–920$ K, logarithmic law; (b) tin, $T = 670–920$ K, parabolic law; (c) aluminum, $T = 700–830$ K, linear law; and (d) aluminum, $T = 830–1000$ K, logarithmic law.

air until reaching definite temperatures. Upon reaching some temperature, fast desorption of gases occurs, generating excessive energy in the form of heat and sharp increase in the reaction ability of nanopowder. This temperature is the threshold temperature. Consequently, it can be assumed that low temperature stability of nanopowders against oxidation is determined by the properties of adsorbed gaseous layer, not by oxide film.

As studies show, oxidation temperatures with distinct speed in nanostate of such metals as Zn, Sn, and Cu significantly are lower than that for active metals. This can be explained by the fact that intensive reaction of nanopowders with air is determined by desorption temperatures of gaseous layers with particle surface, which is lower for less active metals, due to weaker bond in gas–metal system.

6.1.3 Spontaneous Combustion and Pyrophoricity of Nanomediums

Spontaneous combustion phenomenon and pyrophoricity are very undesirable and they strongly complicate the process of obtaining and utilization of nanomaterials.

Table 6.2 Kinetic oxidation parameters of metal nanopowders in air [1].

Metal	T (K)	Nanoparticle size (nm)	k_1	k_0	E (kJ mol^{-1})
Al	700–830	Linear	—	2.2×10^6	155
	>830	Logarithmic	11	4.0×10^9	155
Mo	580–670	Linear	—	2.2×10^9	170
	670–920	Logarithmic	16	2.3×10^{37}	550
Fe	530–770	Linear	—	6×10^7	125
	>770	Logarithmic	12.5	8.2×10^{11}	84
Zn	460–620	Linear	—	5.2×10^5	100
	>620	Logarithmic	5.4	1.5×10^6	100
Sn	420–490	Linear	—	3.5×10^5	88
	>490	Parabolic	—	0.475	42
Cu	400–460	Linear	—	9.5×10^{14}	160
	460–510	Logarithmic	20	1.0×10^{17}	160
	510–560	Linear	—	3.8×10^{-2}	19
	>560	Logarithmic	13.5	1.2×10^6	48

Spontaneous combustion resulted from spontaneous heating of flammable solid materials.

It is appearing because of larger heat generation from reaction, comparing to heat removal from the environment. Depending on its nature spontaneous combustion can be divided into chemical, biological and heat combustion.

Spontaneous combustion temperature: T_c is a temperature at minimal experimental conditions by which heat generation is detected. It is determined at the start of simultaneous combustion process. Upon reaching simultaneous combustion at definite temperature T_B, called self-ignition, burning of material takes place, which can be achieved by smoldering or flame burning. Lastly, simultaneous combustion temperature is equal to self-ignition temperature. According to physical essence, simultaneous combustion and self-ignition are similar and differ only by type of burning.

During change of process parameters, in particular, by increase in mass of specimen or heating speed, the difference of $\Delta T = T_B - T_c$ is reduced, and, in extreme case, $T_B \approx T_c$.

Pyrophoricity is a phenomenon of simultaneous chemical combustion of some substances via their contact with air without heating. The specific feature of pyrophoric materials is that their simultaneous combustion temperature is lower than room temperature. Pyrophoric materials include substances such as high-dispersive metals, alkali metal carbides, silicon hydrides, boron, white phosphorus, and metal-organic compounds.

Materials cannot always be pyrophoric. This depends on the chemical nature and mass of a substance, its dispersity and shape of particles, surface development, and the presence of protective films. In particular, dispersive Fe powder with bulk thickness of 1 g cm^{-3} tends to be pyrophoric. However, at bulk thickness of 0.5 g cm^{-3} iron powder undergoes simultaneous combustion at higher temperature than the room temperature. As a rule, increase in mass of metal nanopowders up to 100–200 mg provides more heat, which leads to their simultaneous combustion in air.

From the physical point of view, self-heating is determined by balance in heat flows, that is, supply and generation of heat inside the system, and offset. At enough mass of nanopowder and the heating speed, strong self-ignition of specimen leads to self-ignition.

Obtained experimental data for oxidation kinetic of nanopowders with a linear law of interaction evaluating minimally possible self-ignition of nanosized metals.

Heating with a linear speed ω determines the heat flow to the specimen from outer source Φ_1 of the following value [1]:

$$\Phi_1 = c\rho\omega \tag{6.3}$$

where ρ is the thickness of metal and c is its heat capacity.

In turn, heat generation of specimen due to chemical reaction Φ_2 at $n = 0$ is estimated by the relation [1]:

$$\Phi_2 = Q\rho k_0 \exp(-E/RT) \tag{6.4}$$

where Q – is the oxidation heat effect and k_0 is the pre-exponential factor.

At the beginning, before reaching the threshold temperature, materials are heated only on the account of outer heat removal, and $\Phi_2 \approx 0$. At beginning of the oxidation process, equation $\Phi_2 > 0$ is realized. As soon as reaction speed will grow, self heat generation of specimen heating is occurring independently on outer heat removal: $\Phi_2 > \Phi_1$. Condition of self-heating and self-acceleration of reaction is determined by equation of heat flows. Hence, the determination of minimal self-ignition temperature in system of nanopowder in air is agree with the following equation [1]:

$$T_c = -E/\{\ln[(c\omega)/(Qk_0)]R\} \tag{6.5}$$

Values T_c and T_B are dependent on kinetic parameters, in particular $k_{0,}$ and the relation of metal heat capacity to its oxidation in acid medium $-c/Q$. At enough specimen mass and small heat removal, reaction with heat will lead to self-ignition.

Estimation and experimental results were compared for self-heating temperature (Table 6.3). In estimations kinetic parameter values obtained from thermogravimetric experiments were used.

As it is seen from Table 6.3, estimation values of self-heating temperature are in good agreement with those of determined by experimentally independent method. More easily flammable among nanosized materials is copper but less active in usual condition: its self-ignition temperature is equal to approximately 160 °C.

Based on experimental results, the correlation between value T_c and oxidation heat of metal Q (Figure 6.8) can be made. The latter is determined by thermodynamic strength of metal–oxygen bond. Hence, large value Q provides

Table 6.3 Kinetic oxidation parameters of metal nanopowders in air [1].

Metal	Self-heating	Temperature, T_c (K)
	Estimation	Experiment
Al	690	720
Mo	600	630
Fe	555	570
Zn	480	520
Sn	425	450
Cu	450	430

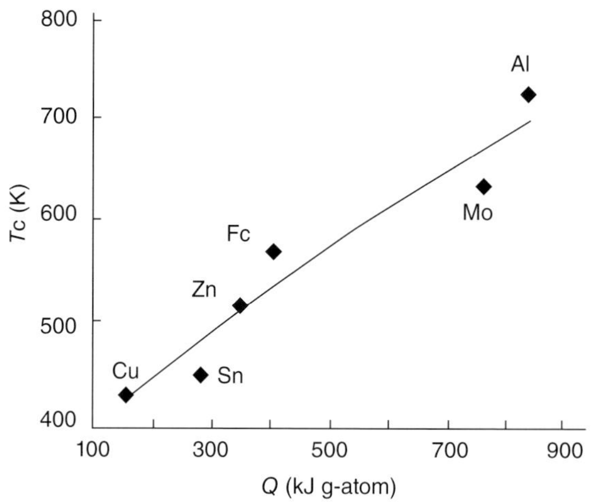

Figure 6.8 Correlation between oxidation heat and self-heating temperature during oxidation of metal nanopowders. (Reproduced with permission of BKL Publishers.)

weak interaction of adsorption gases with basic metal, followed by less active metal nanopowders, which start to oxidize and ignite at significantly lower temperatures.

6.1.4 Catalysis Involving Nanomaterials

Effectivity of nanoparticle application in catalysis is determined by quantum size and geometric and kinetic phenomena. In general case, for implementation of catalysis, number of conditions are necessary, such as: reagent molecules should faster absorb on material surface and desorb slowly, and at the same time, exhibit high surface mobility and the large reaction speed on the specimen surface. In this case, when these conditions are realized with high probability in nanosystems compared with macroscopic material, nanocatalyst will have increased activity.

At the same time, due to a number of reasons, catalytic activity of nanomaterial might be reduced. In particular, at size of nanoparticles less than path length on the surface of adsorbed molecules, the probability of reagents meeting will decrease. Nanocrystal ribs also can prevent the molecules' movement from one edge to another.

Same as with other properties, in catalysis geometrical effect bind with that, there are large amount of surface atoms in nanoparticles.

From the view of quantum size effect, the largest catalytic effect in nanoparticle should be observed when the distance between the energetical levels of electrons δ is close to the heat energy $k_B T$, where k_B – is the Boltzmann constant and T – is the absolute temperature. The given condition lets us evaluate particle sizes at which its catalytic properties are expressed significantly stronger. As it is known, Fermi energy for metals is around 10 eV. Hence, at temperature of 300 K, $\delta = k_B T \approx 0.025$ eV. Thus, $N \approx 400$ atoms, which corresponds to particle diameter of 2 nm. The given evaluation matches well matches with experimental data, according to which the maximum of particle catalytic activity is equal as determined by size of 2–8 nm.

Studies show that for each definite reaction, an optimal catalyst size exists. In particular, in experiments with rhodium catalysts, it was established that dependence of reaction speed of benzene hydrogenation on Rh particle size holds extremal character. Nanoparticles with diameter of 0.8–1.2 nm have no influence on the reaction. At catalyst sizes more than 1.2 nm, its activity starts to grow, reaching a maximum of 1.7 nm. At further diameter increase of particles up to 2 nm, catalyst activity again reduces.

But specific catalytic activity (SCA) of nickel and palladium for this reaction will increase with a decrease in particle size (Figure 6.9).

SCA is a catalytic activity referring to one surface atom in a substance.

Increase in SCA is 2–3 times for the nanoparticles of nickel during decrease in their size, and use of this metal as catalyst in hydrolysis reaction of ethane is observed (Figure 6.10).

Oppositely, in the hydrogen oxidation reaction, the growth in catalytic activity of Pt deposited on aluminum oxide with increase in metal particle size was observed (Figure 6.11).

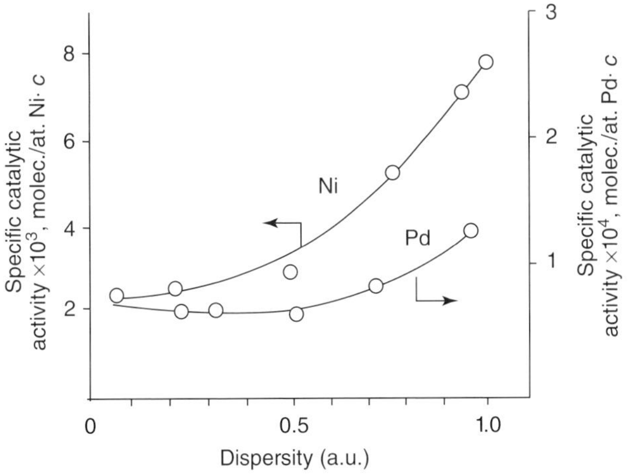

Figure 6.9 Influence of Ni and Pd nanoparticle dispersity on specific catalytic activity in hydrogenation reaction of benzene. (Reproduced with permission of BKL Publishers.)

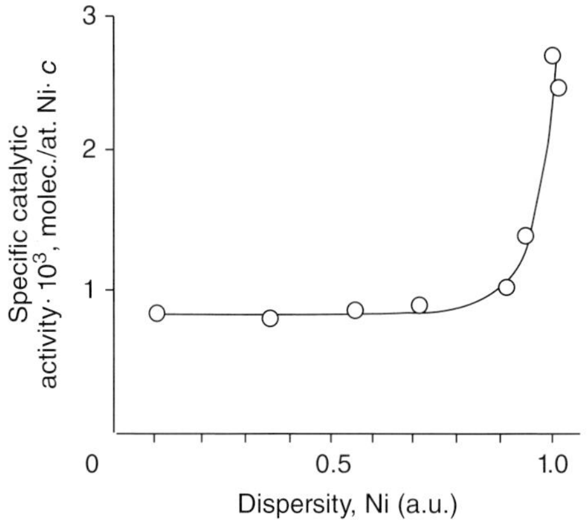

Figure 6.10 Influence of the dispersity of nickel nanoparticles on specific catalytic activity in hydrogenolysis of ethane. (Reproduced with permission of BKL Publishers.)

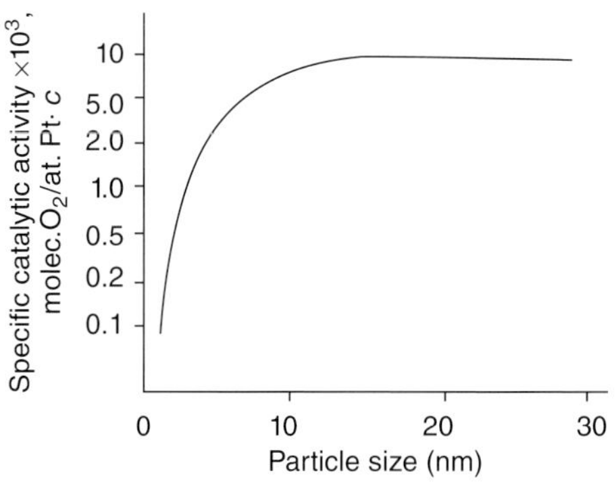

Figure 6.11 Influence of Pt particle size on specific catalytic activity in hydrogen oxidation reaction. (Reproduced with permission of BKL Publishers.)

Nanosized catalysts are always used in the form of powders, rarely in the form of solutions (suspensions) and sometimes in the form of fibers or films. Most commonly used catalyst are metal powders and alloys, which are in their turn's sediment on carrier with developed surface: zeolites, silica gel, silica, pumice, glass, and so on. The first and primary function of carrier is to contribute to the achievement of smallest size of sediment particles and prevent their spontaneous coalescence. However, in nanosystems carrier can play very important role in catalysis, which is explained as follows. Catalyst atoms can change their electronic structure due to formation of bonds with interacting carriers. Wherein, as much number of atoms are in contact with carrier, as more its influence on the catalytic activity. For large particles, their role as carriers is comparably insignificant; however, by reducing the material size, it grows and becomes more distinct.

As catalysts, nanosized metal oxides and salts are also used. For example, by decreasing the temperature from 1300 to 400 °C, nanosized hexaaluminate of barium showed high catalytic activity in methane burning reaction. Besides, alkaline earth metal catalysts, in particular calcium oxides, were successfully applied in deactivation reaction of mustard gas and other chemical war gases.

In lithium batteries, oxide nanoparticles of Co, Ni, Cu, and Fe with a size of 1–5 nm were used as electrode materials. It should be noted that the development of the given techniques becomes principally possible due to use of various nanosized materials. In electrode batteries functioning as catalyst in the given case, Li_2O formation and degradation reactions will occur by the following scheme [1]:

$$2Li - 2e \leftrightarrow 2Li^+$$

$$CoO_{spec} + 2Li^+ + 2e \leftrightarrow Li_2O + Co$$

$$CoO_{spec} + 2Li \leftrightarrow Li_2O + Co^0$$

From a thermodynamical point of view, a first reaction is possible. However, a second reaction in large crystal materials does not occur as lithium oxide is electrochemically not active. This reaction became possible due to the participation of nanosized material and its electrochemical activity growth during decrease in particle size.

6.2 Mechanical Characteristics of Nanomaterials

From the point of view of mechanical behavior, the formation of nanostructures in material can lead to high-strength condition and formation of low temperature and high speed plasticity. During the study of mechanical properties of nanosubstances, a new effect was detected based on simultaneous increase of strength and plasticity. These properties predetermine the possibility of manufacturing new high-strength, wear-resistant superplasticity materials, which is of great interest for studying and obtaining bulk materials with nanostructures.

As it is known, mechanical properties are significantly depend on material structure, and in their turn, in close relation with their obtaining methods. Microcracks, inner microstress, structure defects, change in grain size during deformation, and other factors have influence on the values above.

During observation, polycrystal is usually presented as a complex of simultaneously oriented monocrystal, separated from each other by high angle boundaries. By this model, at the initial stages of load overlay, deformation inside each grain should be the same as if each grain was deformed separately. As grain orientation in relation to overlay stress is different, then deformation did not start concurrently and developed heterogeneously. Thus, it is considered that mechanical properties in large grain polycrystals are related to two initial factors: presence of high angle boundaries and grain disorientations.

Nanostructured material can also be presented as a complex of very small crystals, separated from each other by large angle grain boundaries. The mechanical properties and behavior of nano- and large crystal materials under load influence should be the same. Experiments show that this assumption proved until definite grain sizes.

6.2.1 Hardness, Strength, and Plasticity in Nanomaterials

Hardness is one of the basic mechanical properties of a material. This property is used for the study of phase and structure transformations, as well as for product quality control.

Hardness is defined as resistance of material against indentation.

A large number of experiments showed that dependence of hardness on grain size value $H(d)$ is determined by the Hall–Petch law [1]:

$$H(d) \approx H_0 + Kd^{-1/2} \tag{6.6}$$

where H_0 is the hardness of grain body in pascal, K is the coefficient, and d is the grain size in meter.

The relation shows that a decrease in grain size can lead to the strengthening of the material. At room temperature, nanomaterial hardness is 2–7 times higher than in large crystal analogs. As it is known, material deformation is related to dislocation transformations wherein grain boundaries served as effective barriers for their movement. It is understandable that the smaller the grain is, the more common these barriers on the way of moving dislocations and hence more high stress is required for materials' initial stage plastic deformations. As a result, as grain refines, hardness grows. However, by reaching some critical value of crystals, a decrease occur in most cases (Figure 6.12).

Experimental data shows that as grain sizes of nanocopper reduce from 5 μm to 16 nm, hardness increases approximately to 2.5 times; however, with grain size from 16 to 8 nm, hardness is reduced approximately to 25%. Reduction in hardness was observed during grinding of nanostructured Pd from 13 to 7 nm and nanoalloys of Ni–P, TiAlNb, TiAl, and NbAl from 100 to 6–10 nm. As and example, Figure 6.13 shows dependence of grain hardness on grain size for nanostructured alloy Ni–25 at.% W, obtained by electro sedimentation.

It is necessary to note that deviation from the Hall–Petch law is not always observed. For example, nanostructured alloys of various compositions are obtained by crystallization from amorphous state, hardness dependencies from $d^{-1/2}$ which were presented in Figure 6.14. It is seen from the figure that Hall–Petch dependence is suitable for all studied alloys at grain sizes from 100 to ~ 10 nm. At lower value d, Hall–Petch law is performed only for Fe—Cu—Nb—Si—B alloy (Figure 6.14, curve 1). For other studied compositions, decrease in grain size is lower than 10 nm accompanied by reducing in hardness.

Determination of yield limit and yield strength during single-axis stretching is possible, when cross-section size of nanomaterial is much exceeds transverse dimensions, which are in their turns, significantly larger than average grain size.

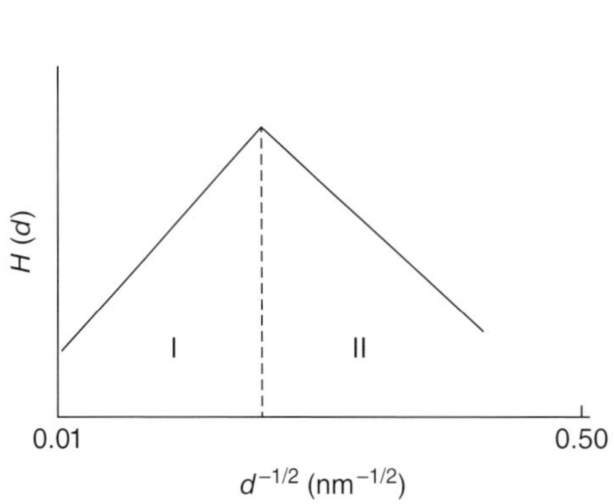

Figure 6.12 Schematic of material hardness dependence on grain size: I – region obeying Hall–Petch's law; II – anomalous dependence region. (Reproduced with permission of BKL Publishers.)

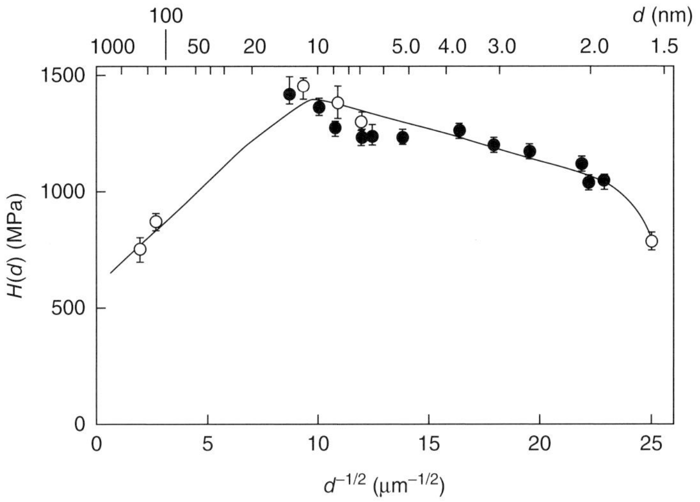

Figure 6.13 Dependence of grain hardness on grain size for nanostructured alloy Ni–25 at.% W, obtained by electrosedimentation and further annealing at various temperatures in vacuum (o) or in air (•). (Reproduced with permission of BKL Publishers.)

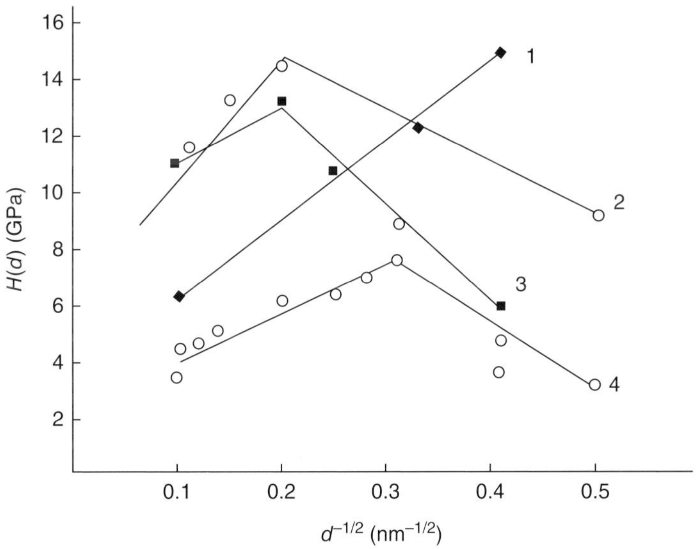

Figure 6.14 Dependence of hardness on dispersive phase's grain size, generated in alloys, obtained by crystallization under amorphous condition: 1 – $Fe_{73.5}CuNb_3Si_{13.5}B_9$, 2 – $Fe_{81}Si_7B_{12}$, 3 – $Fe_5Co_{70}Si_{15}B_{10}$, and 4 – $Pd_{81}Cu_7Si_{12}$. (Reproduced with permission of BKL Publishers.)

During this, increase in given strength characteristics for materials are analogous to increase in hardness.

Hardness is defined as resistance against destruction (rupture) and is characterized by hardness-tension, consistent to maximal (until specimen destruction) load values.

The resistance to plastic deformation is also referred to strength. Plastic deformation is characterized by tensions necessary for achieving of some given value of remaining deformations. Thus, yield strength is determined by tensions caused by stretching of plastic deformations equal to 0.2%.

In theory of polycrystals, the dependence of yield strength on grain size is important. Vickers hardness is related to the yield strength δ at temperature lower than $(0.4–0.5)T_{\text{melt}}$, in approximate relation to $H/\sigma_{\text{T}} \approx 3$. By this way, for nanomaterials yield strength $\sigma(d)$ expression analogous to formula (6.7) is rightful:

$$\sigma(d) = \sigma_0 + K_y d^{-1/2} \tag{6.7}$$

where σ_0 – is the resistance necessary for the transfer of dislocations inside the grain in pascal and K_y is the coefficient determining the complexity of deformation transfer from grain to grain.

Let us give a few examples. Hardness and titanium bending test (Figure 6.15) showed that after intensive plastic deformation, nanomaterial hardness and strength reach maximum values are three times higher compared with annealed large grain. Further annealing of specimen up to temperatures of 300–350 °C, result in no change of the yield strength. However, higher than 350 °C, when grain growth is starting, it sharply reduces. At this time, yield strength value σ_{T} (Figure 6.15) significantly reduces after annealing at 250 °C, which is related to structure change initiations.

Defective grain structure also can influence the hardness properties of nanomaterials. A diagram of the "resistance–deformation" for copper specimen undergoing equichannel pressing and additional 3 min annealing at 473 K is presented in Figure 6.16.

Plasticity is a property of solid materials to irreversibly deform under the effect of outer forces or inner stress, without destruction. It is characterized by elongation (relative change in length during stretching) and change in the cross section of specimen after stopping of uniform removal and neck formation. In large grain materials, increase in plastic deformation level from the beginning of specimen

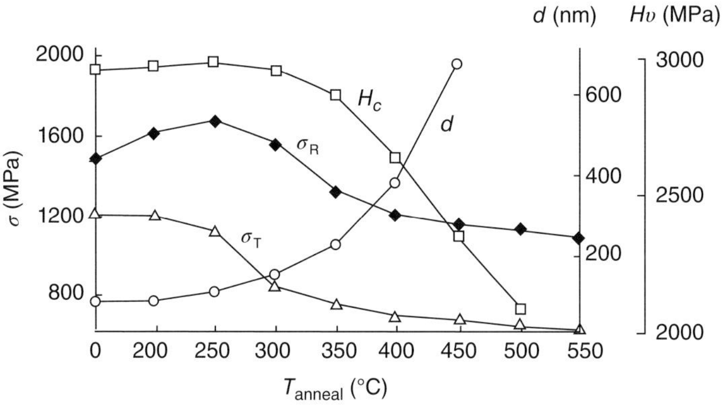

Figure 6.15 Dependence of hardness H_{υ},, strength limit ∫ B, yield strength ∫ T, and grain size of nanostructured Ti on annealing temperature. (Reproduced with permission of BKL Publishers.)

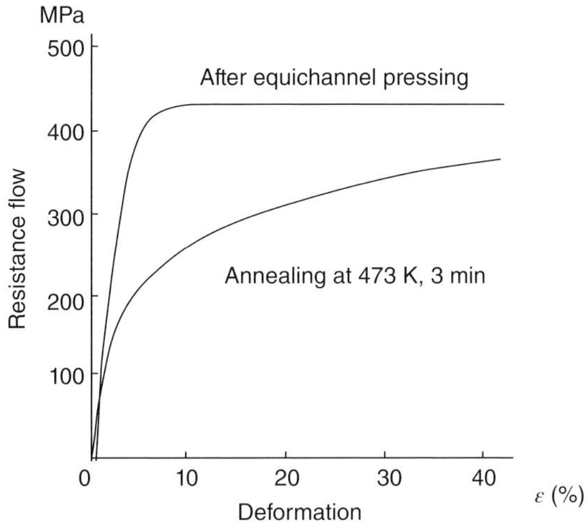

Figure 6.16 Real resistance–deformation curves during tests for nanostructured copper specimens at room temperature. (Reproduced with permission of BKL Publishers.)

destruction moment is accompanied by increase in material resistance growth against imposed stress. This phenomenon is called deformation strengthening. It is caused by dislocation braking. In turn, the more difficult the dislocation movement in material, the larger the deformation strengthening coefficient (tension derivative to deformation), characterized by deformation curve bending.

In nanomaterials the given process is slightly different. Particularly, comparative studies on copper, titanium, and intermetallic Ni_3Al specimens were done. Intensive plastic deformation was achieved at room temperature. The results of mechanical elongation for each of these materials are shown in Figure 6.17.

The specimen of final Cu with grain size around 30 μm is shown to be typical for this material behavior resulting from low elasticity limit, insignificant deformation strengthening, and high plasticity (Figure 6.17, curve 1). A great increase in the Cu strength is observed after cold working wherein plasticity is significantly lowered (Figure 6.17, curve 2). Such dependency remains for copper, subjected to two passages of equichannel pressing, when deformation value is near 2 (Figure 6.17, curve 3). The behavior of materials is principally changing when a number of equichannel passages reach 16 (Figure 6.17, curve 4). In this case, not only further growth in strength grow is observed but also significant increase in plasticity for Cu.

Similar regularity was observed in titanium. A graph of "tension–deformation" of initial large crystal condition with average grain size of 20 μm is presented in Figure 6.17, curve 5. The strengthening of material is observed after deformation by twisting in one circle (real logarithmic deformation is close to unit) and further extension at 250 °C. However, during this time, plasticity will decrease (Figure 6.17, curve 6). Further deformation level grows up to five rotations, reaching a record strength for Ti (Figure 6.17, curve 7). At this time growth in plasticity will occur when extension until breaking will exceed even maximal extension for initial annealed specimen.

As seen from Figure 6.17, curve 8, the intermetallic compound Ni_3Al obtained by hot extrusion, with grain size of 6 μm, exhibits limited plasticity. Extension

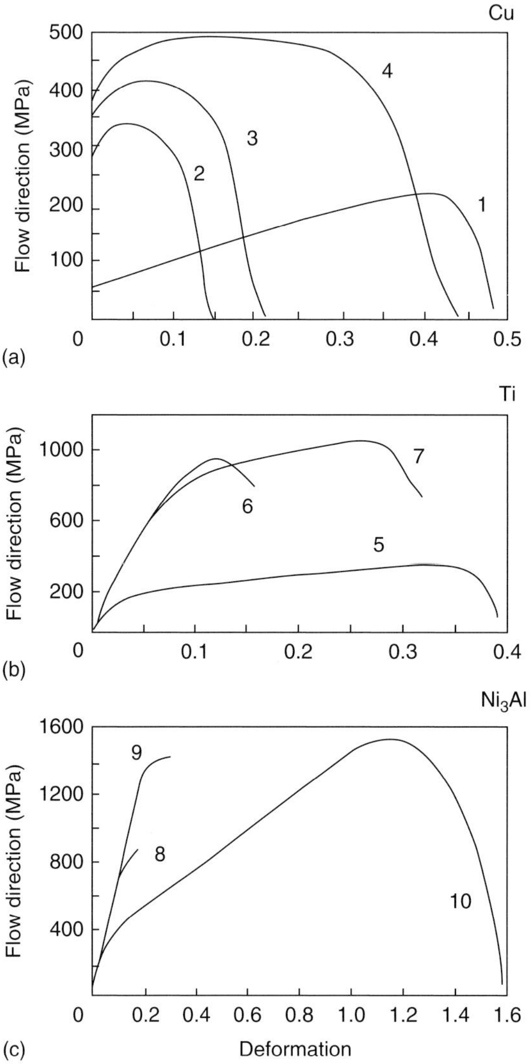

Figure 6.17 Real deformation curves for various materials. (Reproduced with permission of BKL Publishers.)

at 650 °C will not change the typical behavior for the given material. Intensive deformation by twisting to one circle increases strength, but plasticity remains insignificant (Figure 6.17, curve 9). However, intensive deformation to five rotations qualitatively changes the situation. The materials demonstrate very high strength, at the same time with record plasticity (Figure 6.17, curve 10). During this process, extension until destruction will be more than 300%.

Test results of three different materials showed that under the influence of intensive plastic deformation, which leads to structure grinding, their behavior qualitatively changes: they demonstrate very high strength and plasticity at the same time.

For strength, hardness, and plasticity features of nanomaterials, several hypotheses are proposed.

In particular, in one of the theories, dependency (6.6) is explained from the grain boundary position as barriers of dislocation movements wherein coefficient K_y is a value determined by transparency level of grain boundaries for dislocations.

In other models, the given dependency is caused by flat accumulations of dislocations in grain boundaries, accumulating movement tensions during activation of dislocation sources in the neighboring grains. As significant increase in volume fraction of triple junctions in polycrystal system might positively impact on plastic deformation processes relief, then one of ways for explanation of anomalies, bind with their determinative role.

In the model it is assumed that growth in the volume fraction of triple junctions leads to polycrystal softening and increase in volume plasticity. During this time, plastic deformation of nanomaterials is achieved as a result of grain rotations, and misalignment causes generation of partial disclinations in the joints of grain boundaries. Finally, process occurs by race disclination–dislocation mechanism of deformation, which includes radiation, adsorption, and further reradiation of dislocations by disclinations, concentrated in the triple joint places.

An explanation of the strength and plasticity features of nanomaterials from the position of double-phase structure of substance is very common in recent times. In the given model, nanomaterial is presented in the form of composite, consisting of two phases: inner grain crystal and amorphous grain boundary. Mechanical properties of given system are determined by cumulative effect of both phases wherein it is considered that hardness of crystal phase obeys the Hall–Petch law (Eq. (6.6)) and grain boundary phase has a stable strength, appropriate with strength of amorphous state. Unfortunately, the given model does not explain the transfer to anomalous dependency region of hardness from the value $d^{-1/2}$.

One more variant of the plastic deformation of nanomaterials is called combined mechanism: in relatively large grains, plastic shift occurs by classical dislocation model, obeying the Hall–Petch law, while in relatively small grains, this occurs by grain boundary slipping.

Also a model based on assumption was developed wherein the initial low temperature stage of polycrystal plastic deformation, included in general dislocations, is preceded by grain boundary slipping.

In turn, the main mechanism for grain boundary slipping is considered a transfer along the surface of grain boundary dislocations. Latter generation of dislocations can occur by sources existing on nonflat atomic surface of boundary and by effect of stress moving along this surface. Such process leads to a shift of one atom relative to another.

Grain boundary slipping theory is completely proven by computer modeling of plastic deformation process of nanomaterials. Estimation was done for nanostructured copper, consisting of free dislocation crystallites with sizes from 3.3 to 6.6 nm with simultaneous shape, separated by grain boundaries. The initial structure of nanomaterial and configuration after single-axis deformation to 10% are presented in Figure 6.18. After implementing computer deformation, a significant widening in grain boundaries can be seen, which indicates distinct contribution of grain boundary regions to plastic flow process. Computer modeling proves that

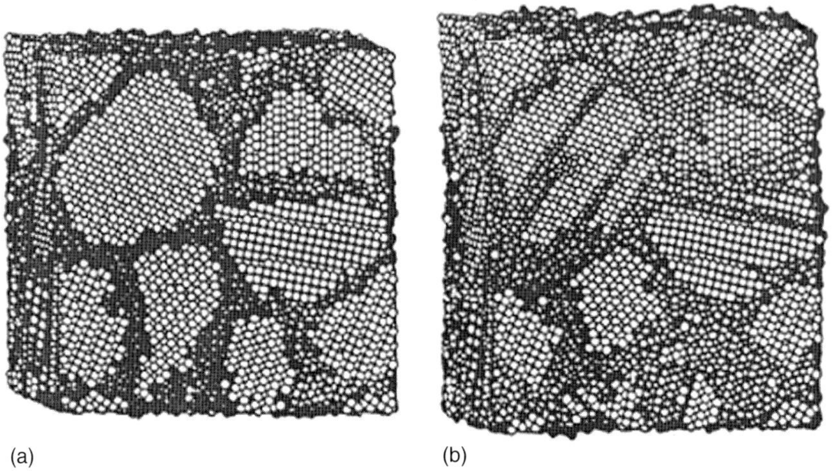

Figure 6.18 Computer image of nanostructured copper: (a) at initial state and (b) after plastic deformation with 10% level. (Reproduced with permission of BKL Publishers.)

nanomaterials after deformation are presented as double-phase system, consisting of approximately equal crystal and grain boundary phases. Aside from this, in grains there are dislocation slipping processes, with formation of stacking fault strip defects. By estimation it was established that dependency of deformation stress and yield strength on crystal sizes at given equation obey inverse relationship of Hall–Petch. At the end, based on studies, it can be argued that plastic deformation process is caused by grain boundary slipping.

6.2.2 Superplasticity Phenomenon in Nanomaterials

As experimental data shows, nanosized materials are characterized by very large values of superplasticity, significantly exceeding values that are characteristics for micro-grain condition. As this mechanical property has a large practical importance, it's paying much attention to study of this phenomenon in nanomaterials.

Superplasticity is an anomalous change in the resistance to plastic deformation based on sharp fall in strength and very strong increase in plasticity.

In other words, superplasticity is exponentially large component of hundreds and thousands percent, relative to elongation of material during stretching. Usually this property is observed in polycrystal materials with a grain size of less than 10 μm at deformation under definite temperature–speed interval. As a rule, these are temperatures equal to $(0.5\text{–}0.6)T_{\text{melt}}$ and deformation speed of $10^{-4}\text{–}10^{-3}\ \text{s}^{-1}$.

Superplasticity for the first time was observed in 1934 in Sn—B alloy during its elongation to more than 20 times. Superplasticity in ceramics was detected in 1985 in polycrystal tetragonal ZrO_2 oxide, stabilized by yttrium oxide Y_2O_3. This phenomenon is very important for obtaining products from ceramic materials by shaping, hard-phase annealing, or hot-pressing at fairly low temperatures. Due to superplasticity, high precision in size is achieved for ceramic products with very complex shape, having pores and surface with varying curvature. An exact mathematical description of superplasticity flow microcrystal materials is a difficult problem, as deformation value depends on a number of factors. However, more general law of this process was found, which can be described by the following condition:

$$\varepsilon \sim [DGb^{p+1}/(\hbar T)] \cdot 1/d^p \tag{6.8}$$

where ε is the deformation speed (s^{-1}); D is the coefficient of grain boundary diffusion ($m^2\ c^{-1}$); G is the shift module (Pa); b is the Burgers vector (m); T is the test temperature (K); d is grain size (m); and p is an exponential depending on grain size (usually equal to 2).

According to suggested dependency, it can be expected that decrease in grain size brings a sharp increase in superplasticity and achieves superplasticity at low enough temperatures and at high speed of deformation.

During the study a number of microcrystalline systems increase in plasticity to 100% at mildly high temperatures: 650–725 °C for Ni_3Al, 700 °C for TiO_2, and 1150–1250 °C for ZrO_2. Due to transfer of these materials to nanostate, superplasticity temperature was decreased to about 300–400 °C. Use of plastic deformation methods for Al- and Ti-structure grinding allowed great shift speed interval of superplastic deformation manifestations to the region of large values (Figure 6.19) by decreasing the deformation temperature at the same time. Use of this unique property of nanostructured alloys gives meaningfully widen possibilities of high speed and low temperature superplasticity practical applications for effective shaping of various details and complex shape products.

Superplasticity at low temperatures and at high deformation speeds is based on unequal state of grain boundaries in nanostructured materials, which led to acceleration of dynamic processes on boundaries (e.g., grain boundary slipping).

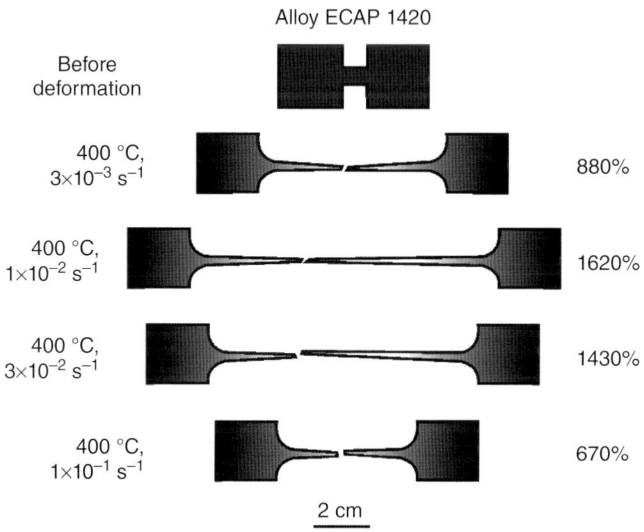

Figure 6.19 Manifestation of high-speed super-plasticity in nanostructures aluminum alloy during the stretching test. (Reproduced with permission of BKL Publishers.)

It is necessary to mention that influence of average grain size on superplastic behavior is not unambiguous. Recently obtained results prove that decrease in average grain size until 100 nm leads to increase in superplasticity. However, further role of structure grinding appearing in this effect requires more clear studies wherein in nanosized materials with grain size unit less than any critical value, generation of dislocations can be complicated, which might lead to decrease in superplasticity level.

6.3 Concept Map of Characterization Tools in Nanotechnology

Characterization tools in nanotechnology are unceasingly diversified. A number of precision characterization techniques and equipment were developed recently. Concept map illustrated in the Figure 6.20 is illustrating main units in nanomaterials characterization, classified by purpose and kind of characterization tools, such as microscopical, spectroscopical, and X-ray diffraction (XRD) appliance technique. Under part is characterization software and computer programs assigned for calibration and analysis of various data obtained after nanomaterials characterization.

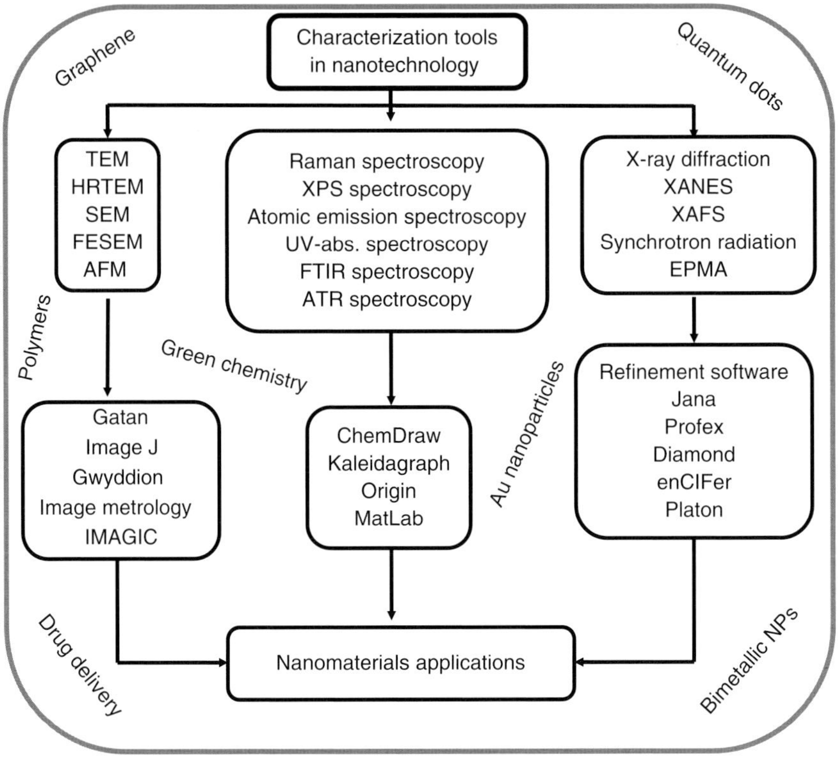

Figure 6.20 Concept map of characterization tools in nanotechnology.

6.4 Diffraction Methods for Nanomaterial Characterization

There are a number of diffraction methods for nanomaterials characterization, such as XRD, synchrotron radiation, neutron diffraction, electron diffraction, neutronography, small-angle X-ray scattering (SAXS), and small-angle neutron scattering (SANS). The XRD method is used for determination of phase compositions of various materials and crystalline structures, and have been considered as very basic and fundamental technique for identification of materials [2]. The discovery of X-ray dates back to 1912 when M. Laue observed X-rays during his works on crystals and diffraction grafting experiments [3]. Each material has its unique diffraction beam, which can be defined and analyzed using the Joint Committee on Powder Diffraction Standards (JCPDS) library database. Current applications of XRD method spread to number of items such as pharmaceuticals, environment, geology, materials science, polymer, nanocomposites, and frontier sciences [4]. The XRD pattern of the nanoparticles is depicted in Figure 6.21. As can be seen from the figure, it represents a system of strongly broadened and overlapped lines. The grain sizes were calculated from the (113) line of the basic γ-Fe_2O_3 maghemite phase by the Warren–Averbach method using the approximation by the Voigt function.

To allow for the overlapping of neighboring lines and to correctly describe the diffraction pattern background, two additional components (212) and (202) and the overlapped lines of the α-Fe_2O_3 hematite phase, the amount of which in the

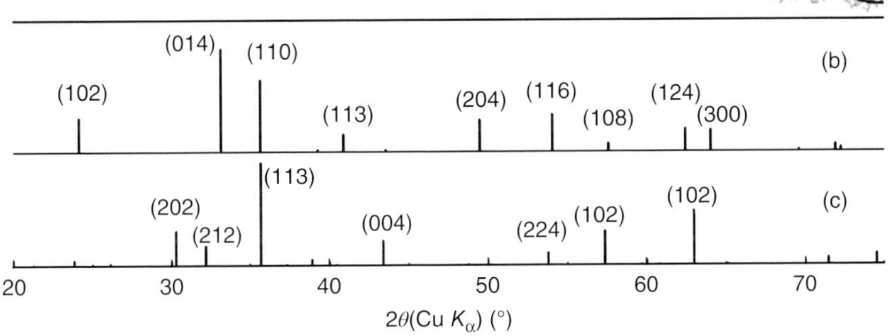

Figure 6.21 (a) X-ray diffraction pattern of Fe_2O_3 nanoparticles; (b) and (c) stroke diffraction patterns of constituent phases: (b) α-Fe_2O_3 (1.6 at.%) and (c) γ-Fe_2O_3 (98.4 at.%). The inset shows the result of approximation of line (113) by the Voigt function [5] reproduced with permission of Springer.

sample was 4 at.% (Figure 6.21, inset), were taken into account. The following results were obtained: $\langle L \rangle a = 2.9$ nm and $\langle L \rangle v = 5.8$ nm. From this, under the assumption of a spherical shape of the particles, their average particle diameters were found to be $\langle D \rangle a = 4.3$ and 7.7 nm. The close values of the average particle size obtained from the analysis of the diffraction patterns and TEM images show the applicability of the Warren–Averbach method using the approximation by the Voigt function to the estimation of the sizes of nanograins based on the analysis of a single diffraction line (reproduced from Colloid Journal, Determination of Nanoparticle Sizes by X-ray Diffraction, 74, 6, 2012, p. 675–685, Dorofeev, G.A. *et al.*, with permission of Springer).

6.5 Microscopical Characterization of Nanomaterials

Microscopical characterizations are considered as one of the most important tools in nanomaterial analysis, which lets us know about morphological characteristics, including the structure, size, and shape of nanomaterials.

The main characteristics of electron microscopy methods used for nanomaterial characterization are dependent on the recorded radiation type. There are several types of electron microscopy methods. For example, scanning electron microscopy (SEM) is based on the radiation type by reflected electrons, secondary electrons, characteristic X-rays, braking, and thermal radiations. Transmission electron microscopy (TEM) is based on radiation type by non-scattered electrons, and scanning transmission electron microscopy (STEM) is based on radiation type by elastically and inelastically scattered electrons. Ultra-high voltage electron microscopy (UHVEM) is based on radiation by non-scattered electrons, and emission electron microscopy (EEM) is based on radiation through electrons emitted by the object under external influence. Mirror electron microscopy (MEM) is based on radiation by electrons reflected from "electronic mirror" in the immediate proximity to the surface of the object, which is applied to the negative voltage [2]. General descriptions with principles for (S)TEM, HRTEM, AFM, and SEM were described further in this section.

6.5.1 TEM Characterization of Nanomaterials

In transmission electron microscopy, a beam of high-energy electrons (typically 100–1000 keV) is directed at a very thin specimen (a few 100 nm at most), and the image is formed from electrons that pass through the specimen. Three contrast mechanisms may contribute to the image: absorption, diffraction (sometimes known as amplitude), and phase contrast. To create images using phase contrast, more than one electron beam must pass through the objective aperture: usually the zero-order (undiffracted beam) and at least one diffracted beam. The interference between these beams creates lattice images, and the technique is also known

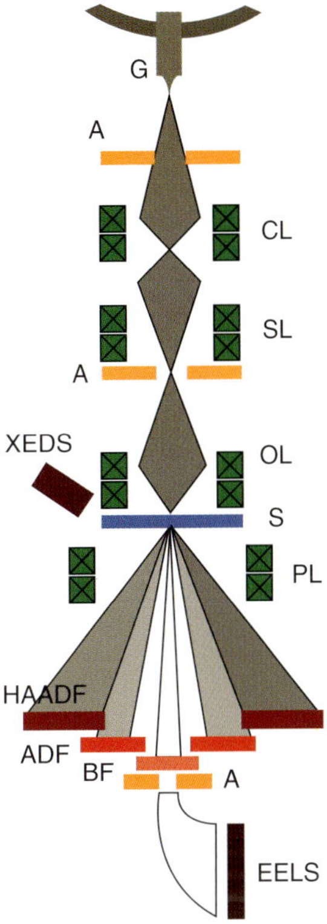

Symbol	Component
G	Electron gun
A	Apertures
CL	Condenser lenses
SL	Scanning lenses
OL	Objective lens
S	Sample
PL	Projector lenses
BF	Bright field detector
ADF	Annular dark field detector
HAADF	High-angle ADF detector
XEDS	X-ray detector
EELS	EELS spectrometer

Figure 6.22 Schematic diagram of a STEM that depicts the main detectors and standard positions of the spectrometers. (Stroppa *et al.* 2012 [6]. Reproduced with permission of John Wiley and Sons.)

as high-resolution electron microscopy (HREM). Using two beams from a single set of lattice fringes and using three or more beams (not lying on the same row) form cross-lattice fringes, giving the impression that the crystal structure is being imaged. Because of the complex way the images are formed in phase-contrast HREM, a technique that has been developed to form lattice images in the scanning transmission electron microscope (STEM) by using high-angle incoherent scattering with very poor probes. Schematic of STEM is presented in Figure 6.22.

This gives images that are essentially independent of focus, with the added benefit of atomic number contrast. Scanning transmission electron microscopes are variant of TEMs with scanning coils added to the column – sometimes known as (S)TEMs. The advantages of STEM over TEM include the following:

- The focus does not change as the magnification is changed (in TEM the image needs refocusing each time the magnification is changed).

- The signal can be amplified to produce a highly visible image on the CRT (in TEM the image on the phosphor screen may be very faint, particularly at high magnifications).
- Many different signals can be collected (such as secondary and backscattered electrons, cathodoluminescence and energy loss spectra, and transmitted electron and X-rays) [7].

In low-energy STEM, the specimen response will be proportional to the average scattering power of atoms which will give rise to mass–thickness contrast, or absorption contrast. For a good Z-contrast, it is necessary to use large scattering angles in transmission. In the transmission mode of SEM, the aperture can be increased to obtain a high transmission and signal-to-noise ratio (SNR). SEM remains one of the most flexible tools for high-resolution imaging (resolution down to 1 nm), however 1 nm resolution is sometimes not achieved when characterizing ordinary samples due to limitations arising from the nature of beam–sample interactions when secondary electron signal is used. STEM-in-SEM is one method that can overcome these limitations and enable imaging with high resolution. As the samples investigated are thin in comparison with SEM, the interaction volume is rather small. For this reason, in STEM mode, the resolution is only limited by the spatial broadening of the electron probe at the exit surface of the sample, whereas structures at the entrance surface are resolved with a resolution of approximately same as the diameter of the electron probe. This beam-broadening phenomenon is called the "top–bottom effect" (Golla-Schindler, 2004). For illustration, Figure 6.23 shows the investigation of small indium cluster on a formvar film with a polystyrene sphere placed on the indium layer (reproduced from Micron, 38, 4, p. 390–401, A history of scanning

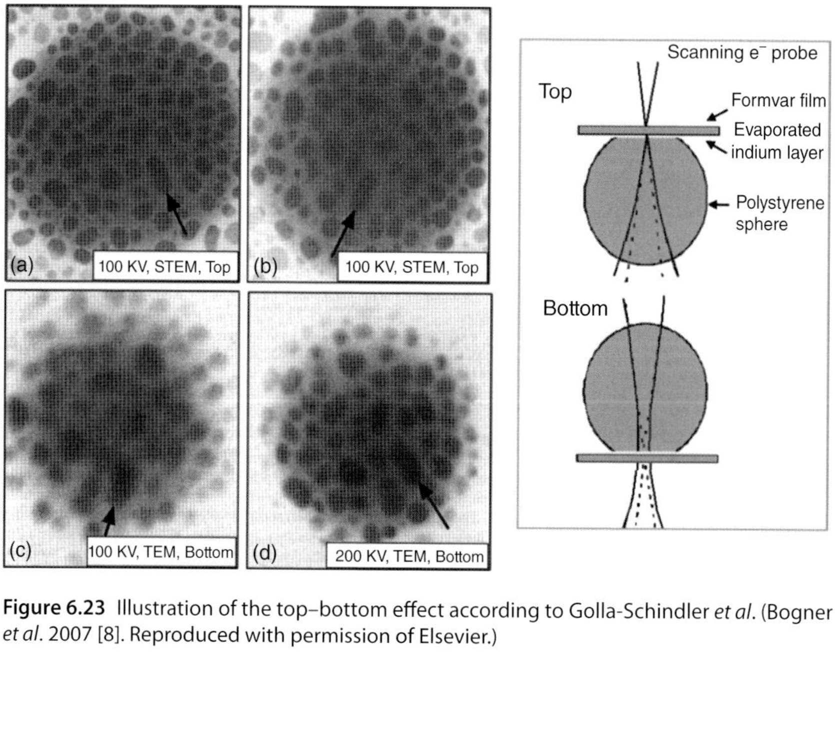

Figure 6.23 Illustration of the top–bottom effect according to Golla-Schindler *et al.* (Bogner *et al.* 2007 [8]. Reproduced with permission of Elsevier.)

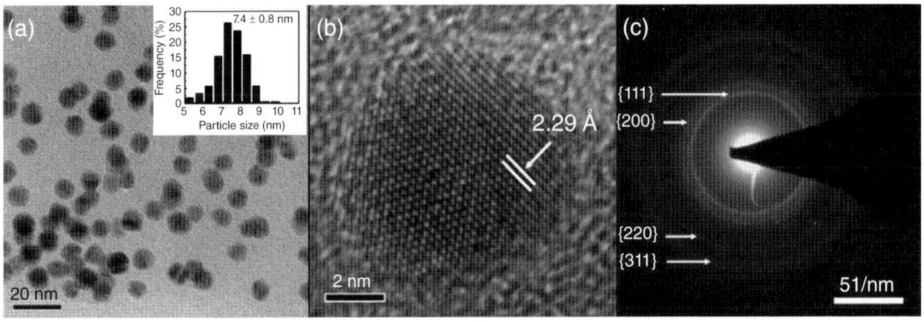

Figure 6.24 TEM image (a), high-resolution TEM image (b), and SAED patterns (c) of the Au–Pd bimetallic NPs. The inset in (a) indicates the size distribution of the NPs. (Zhan *et al.* 2011 [9]. Reproduced with permission of Elsevier.)

electron microscopy developments: Towards "wet-STEM" imaging by A. Bogner *et al.*, Copyright (2007), with permission from Elsevier).

6.5.2 HRTEM Characterization of Nanomaterials

A lot of incredible possibilities can be provided by using high-resolution transmission electron microscope for nanomaterial analysis and characterizations. The main one is obtaining high-resolution image information about the location of atoms in the given nanomaterial and determination of elemental compositions in atomic and weight percent, which is called EDX analysis. Moreover, lattice distances can be calculated by special operating functions installed within microscope. Difference between HRTEM and TEM is in their lens resolutions, dominant in the case of HRTEM. For example, let us refer to microscopical characterizations of bimetallic nanoparticles. High-resolution and TEM image of the Au–Pd bimetallic NPs are shown in Figure 6.24. It showed a well-defined spherical shape with fairly uniform size of 7.4 ± 0.8 nm. The d-spacing of the adjacent (111) lattice of the bimetallic NPs was 2.29 Å (shown in Figure 6.24b), while those of the individual Au NPs and Pd NPs were 2.36 and 2.25 Å, respectively. Such a value conforms to the reported value of Au–Pd alloy structure. Moreover, SAED pattern of Au–Pd bimetallic NPs (Figure 6.24c) showed four diffraction rings corresponding to four different crystal planes in the face-centered cubic structure. They could be identified as polycrystalline bimetallic NPs since two phase-segregated metals produce eight diffraction rings [9].

6.5.3 AFM Characterization of Nanomaterials

Atomic force microscope (AFM) consists of a vibrating microcantilever with a nanoscale tip interacting with a sample surface by short- and long-range intermolecular forces [10].

Initial piezoresistive self-sensing cantilevers primarily used doped silicon resistors followed by cantilevers with polysilicon and thin metal film strain-sensing resistors. Piezoresistors measure strain through a change in resistivity (effect dominant in semiconductors) and a change in geometry (effect

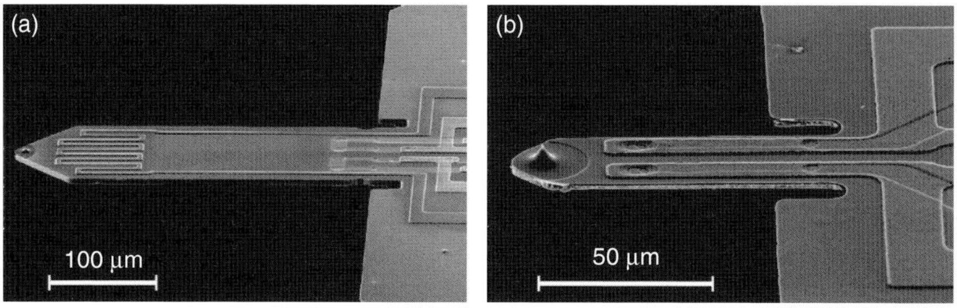

Figure 6.25 SEM images of representative (a) 300 μm × 100 μm and (b) 70 μm × 30 μm silicon piezoresistive cantilevers used for noise measurements and AFM imaging. (a) The large-sized piezoresistive cantilever has a meander-like patterned heater resistor for thermal actuation (close to the free end, not used in measurements) and two active piezoresistors (close to the fixed end). (b) The small-sized piezoresistive cantilever has two active piezoresistors along its length. (Dukic *et al.* 2015 [11]. https://www.ncbi.nlm.nih.gov/pmc/articles/PMC4647226/. Used under: https://creativecommons.org/licenses/by/4.0/.)

dominant in metals). Piezoresistive cantilevers are made using standard silicon manufacturing processes and can use a simple measurement setup. The sensors are usually configured in a Wheatstone bridge with differential amplification where the measured voltage is directly proportional to the cantilever deflection. Concurrent to piezoresistive cantilevers, piezoelectric self-sensing cantilevers using various materials (PZT, ZnO, AlN) were developed. Numerous other self-sensing techniques were also demonstrated in the past although none became preferable over optical sensing in routine AFM imaging due to the comparatively lower SNR, detection speed, or complexity of integration. The cantilevers used in the measurements were 300 μm × 100 μm and 70 μm × 30 μm piezoresistive silicon cantilevers (PRSA and PRS probes, SCL-Sensor. Tech. Fabrication GmbH, Austria) presented in Figure 6.25a,b [11].

AFM observation results depend on a number of factors, such as nanoparticle agglomeration, self-ordering on substrate, type, and roughness of substrate on which observed nanomaterial was deposited during sample preparation [12]. Sample preparation is a crucial process requiring significant thin sample in order to obtain single layer under observation. Data after observation further can be analyzed by computer software (Blaga L. *et al.*, 2014).

AFM operates in an environmentally controlled medium with acoustic isolation chamber (Figure 6.26).

6.5.4 SEM Characterization of Nanomaterials

Scanning electron microscopy (SEM) can provide information on surface topography, crystalline structure, chemical composition, and electrical behavior of the top 1 μm or so of specimen. Various specialized stages (e.g., hot, cold, or designed to permit *in situ* mechanical testing) can be attached to enable behavior under various conditions to be examined. For example, cathodoluminescence (emission of light) at temperatures near absolute zero is much stronger than at room temperature, so images formed from the light emitted by a cold specimen are

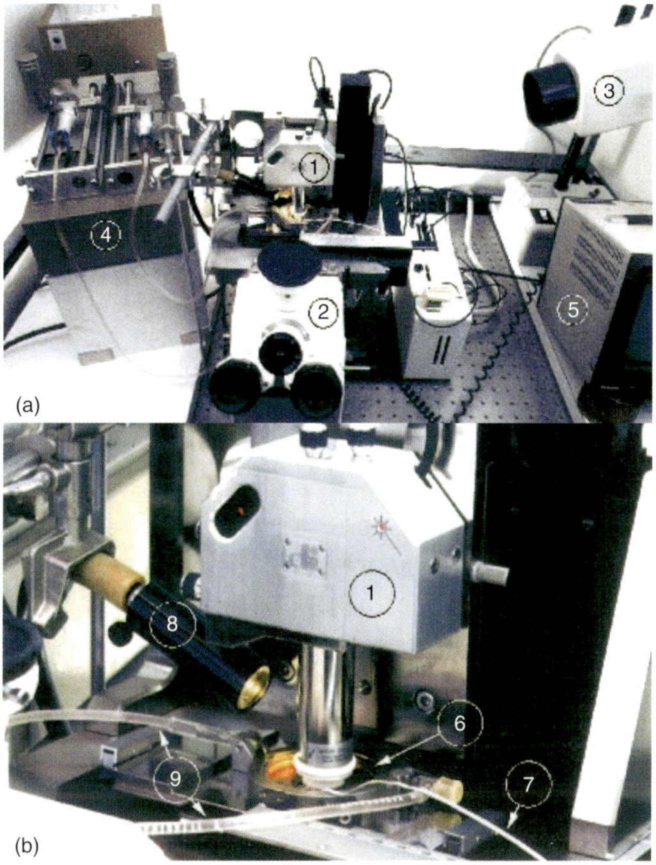

Figure 6.26 The setup of AFM and LM in the environmentally controlled, acoustic isolation chamber. (a) Overview of the integrated LM–AFM system. (b) Close-up view of Dvorak–Stotler controlled-environment culture chamber in place on the BioScope AFM scanner table. (1) DIAFM scanner head; (2) Zeiss Axiovert light microscope; (3) Nevtek airstream incubator; (4) Harvard infusion/withdrawal pump; (5) video monitor; (6) Dvorak–Stotler controlled-environment culture chamber; (7) YSI thermistor temperature probe; (8) fiber-optic illuminator for transmitted LM; (9) medium perfusion tubing 10. (Nagao and Dvorak 1998 [13]. Reproduced with permission of Wiley.)

much less noisy. Further advantages of SEM over optical microscopy include the following [6]:

- SEM benefits from a large depth of field so most of the specimen surface is simultaneously in focus whatever the surface roughness. Optical microscopes operating at high magnification have a very small depth of field, so image quality is very dependent on the surface being smooth.
- Much higher magnifications can be achieved (up to 1 000 000×), with an ultimate resolution of 1 nm. The maximum useful magnification in an optical microscope is around 1000×.

- The possibility of getting more information than just the surface topography, for example, crystal structure, chemical composition, and electrical properties. Switching between different imaging techniques enables information to be cross-correlated with confidence.

Basic SEM Optics and Operations

In an SEM the incident electrons (from an electron gun) typically have energies of 2–40 keV. There are three types of electron gun in general use: the most common is the tungsten hairpin filament which is heated (by passing a current through it) to over 2500 °C to produce thermal emission of electrons from its tip. Lanthanum hexaboride (LaB_6) filaments also work by thermionic emission, but advantages include a larger maximum beam current, that is, a "brighter" beam (because LaB_6 has a lower work function than tungsten) and a longer working lifetime. However, these filaments are more expensive.

Field emission guns (not heated, so also known as "cold cathode" emitters) provide the brightest beam with very small deviations in electron energy by applying a very high electric field to a finely pointed tip until quantum mechanical tunneling of electrons occurs. Whereas thermionic guns need a vacuum near the gun of only 10^{-6} Torr, field emission guns need better than 10^{-10} Torr to preserve the tip, increasing the cost of FEG microscopes [14].

Four examples of nanoparticle materials have been selected to be highlighted here as representative with respect to their accurate morphological characterization by SEM/T-SEM as well as their qualitative elemental analysis by high-resolution EDX. The first material consists of SiO_2 nanoparticles of sizes ranging from the micrometer down to below 100 nm (Figure 6.27). The attention of the reader shall be drawn on the sensitivity of the "top" observation by the in-lens detection as far as details in nanometer range on the sample surface are concerned and on in-depth structural details, which are provided by the transmission "channel," respectively. Because of its high sensitivity to even slight sample surface charging, edge effects are visible in the in-lens imaging mode.

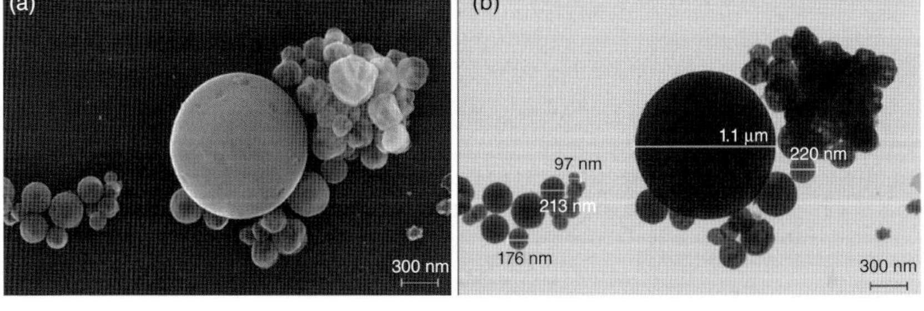

Figure 6.27 SEM micrographs of SiO_2 particles obtained with (a) a high-resolution in-lens detector and (b) the conventional *E–T* detector of the transmitted electrons coming from the same scanned area as in (a). (Hodoroaba *et al.* 2014 [15]. Reproduced with permission of John Wiley and Sons.)

However, operating the in-lens mode at low beam voltages shall diminish the edge effects and improve surface topographic information in the images. This becomes challenging at very high magnifications as in the case of nanoparticles of sizes well below 100 nm. Furthermore, as systematically described in the literature, accurate and traceable dimensional results, that is, of the nanoparticles diameter down to below 10 nm, can be gained by T-SEM [15].

6.6 Spectroscopical Characterization of Nanomaterials

Spectroscopical characterization methods are divided into several classes based on energy type and region of electromagnetic wavelength used. Figure 6.28 illustrates hierarchical schematics of spectroscopical characterization methods for nanomaterials. For example, according to energy type, there are laser and electromagnetic wavelength radiation-based spectroscopical tools. Laser based is Raman spectroscopy characterized by determination of structure of nanomaterials, mainly of carbon materials and minerals. Electromagnetic wavelength energy-based types of spectroscopical tools include FTIR, electron spectroscopy, UV absorption, magnetic nuclear resonance, and so on.

According to interaction character between specimen and electromagnetic wavelength, there are X-ray, ultraviolet, visible, infrared, microwave and radio wavelength spectroscopy tools.

6.6.1 FT-IR Spectroscopy of Nanomaterials

Fourier transform infrared (FTIR) spectroscopy is useful in determination of structure and surface characteristics of nanomaterials. Different organic materials including chemical bonds with vibration modes and type of functional groups can be detected by FTIR spectroscopy tool. FT-IR spectra was applied for analysis of substance named as "Bisphenol A" along with DTF (Density Functional Theory or the B3LYP), and represented in Figure 6.29. Here CH out of plane bending motion is clearly seen. B3LYP is showing two distinct peaks at 825 cm^{-1} and 826 cm^{-1}. Moreover, peak for CH is out of plane bending, and does not come from the single atoms of carbon or hydrogen. High absorption

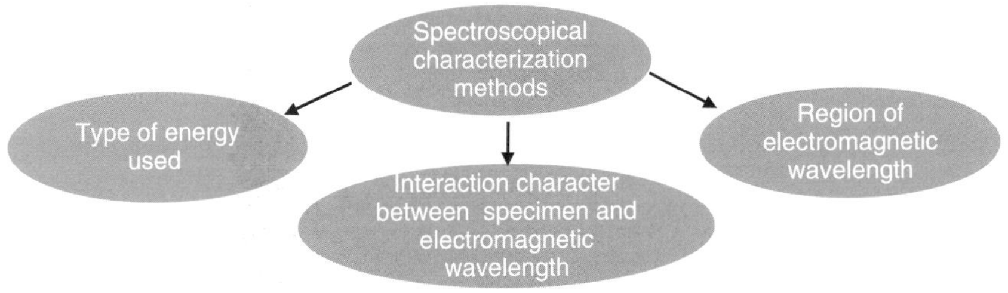

Figure 6.28 Hierarchical schematics of spectroscopical characterization tools for nanomaterials.

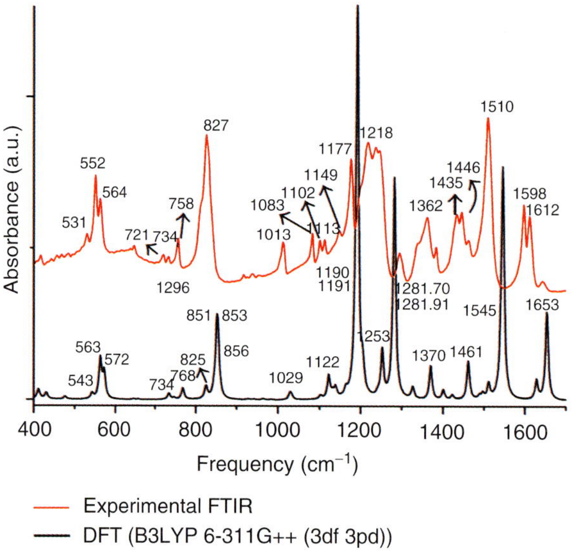

Figure 6.29 FTIR (400–1700 cm^{-1}) spectra of "Bisphenol A" along with DFT spectra. Values of some peaks are given near the tip of the respective peak (Ullah *et al.* 2016 [16], https://creativecommons.org/licenses/by/4.0/).

peak of 827 cm^{-1} is assigned to four simulated vibrational modes of 844, 851, 853, and 856 cm^{-1} due to their closeness. The major contribution in 844 cm^{-1} mode is appearing from CO stretching and CC stretchings (Ullah *et al.* 2016 [16], reproduced under https://creativecommons.org/licenses/by/4.0/).

6.6.2 X-ray Photoelectron Spectroscopy of Nanomaterials

X-ray photoelectron spectroscopy (XPS) has been used for qualitatively determination of surface components and composition of the samples as represented in Figure 6.30. The XPS survey is presenting narrow scan spectra of $Ca_{10-x}Agx(PO_4)_6(OH)_2$ substance. In the XPS spectrum of Ag:HAp, the binding energies for compound elements were as following: Ag (3d, 368.09 eV), Ca (2p, 347.3 eV), O (1s, 532.1 eV), and P (2p,133.09 eV) can be obviously found, XPS narrow scan spectra of Ag element is presented in Figure 6.30b. XPS results provide the additional evidence for the successful doping of Ag^+, in Ag:HAp. (Ciobanu *et al.* 2013 [17], https://creativecommons.org/licenses/by/3.0/.)

Case Study 1: Oxidation of Fe Nanoparticles

- Oxidation process of iron nanoparticles and their spectroscopical, magnetic, and microscopic evidence was studied by Kumar, N. *et al.* [18]. According to this study, oxidation behavior of nano-Fe^0 particles in an anoxic environment was determined using different state-of-the-art analytical approaches, such as high-resolution transmission electron microscopy (HR-TEM) combined with energy-filtered transmission electron microscopy (EFTEM), X-ray absorption spectroscopy (XAS), and magnetic measurements. Oxidation of iron nanoparticles in controlled experiments was compared for standard

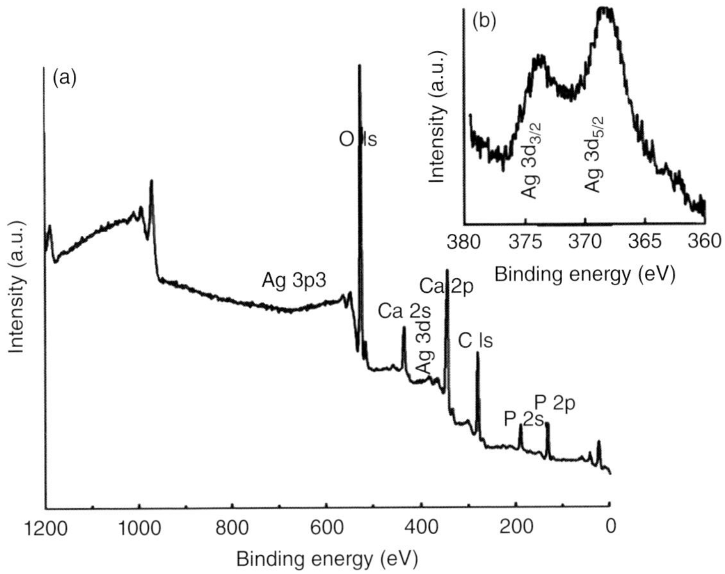

Figure 6.30 (a) XPS general spectrum of $Ca_{10-x}Ag_x(PO_4)_6(OH)_2$ powder with $x_{Ag} = 0.4$ and (b) narrow scan spectra of Ag element. (Ciobanu *et al.* 2013 [17], https://creativecommons.org/licenses/by/3.0/.)

double-distilled (DD) water, DD water spiked with trichloroethene (TCE), and TCE-contaminated site water.

- Growth and oxidation of iron (Fe) nanoparticles was studied during synthesis by chemical reduction in aqueous phase [19], where formation mechanisms for iron oxides such as Fe_2O_3 and Fe_3O_4 nanoparticles were also described. Oxidation of Fe to Fe_3O_4 and finally to Fe_2O_3 was carried out by oxidative etching process, based on decreasing the amount of stabilizer agent. Then obtained structures were characterized by high-resolution (HRTEM) and scanning/transmission (STEM) electron microcopies, energy dispersive spectroscopy (EDS), and optical spectroscopy (UV-Vis and IR). The magnetite oxidation to maghemite is described by the following chemical scheme [19]:

$$(Fe_8^{3+})_t(Fe_8^{2+}Fe_8^{3+})_0O_{32} \rightarrow (Fe_8^{3+})_t(Fe_{5.33\,2.67}^{2+}Fe_8^{3+})_0O_{32} \qquad (6.9)$$
$$\text{Magnetite}\,Fe_3O_4 \rightarrow \text{Maghemite}\,Fe_2O_3$$

Case Study 2: Microscopical Characterization of Nanomaterials and Sample Preparation

- Nanomaterials characterized by microscopical analyses, consisting of transmission electron microscope (TEM), high-resolution transmission electron microscope (HRTEM), AFM, and scanning electron microscope (SEM), have to fulfill the requirements to achieve observation results. In general, sample should be prepared for analysis by subjecting onto metal (copper, carbon) sample holder grid. Sonication prior to microscopical observation will provide

de-agglomeration of particles and their good distribution in solvent, hence a better possibility during observation.
- The size of nanomaterial specimen is different depending on the observation equipment type and observation purpose. For example, in the case of HRTEM, the size of the specimen should be significantly tiny (nanometer size), whereas, in the case of SEM observation, the specimen might be of larger size (micrometer size).
- During microscopical observation, specimen and electron beam efflux from microscope will interact, causing changes in the specimen.
- By the course of time, specimen position will undergo change; hence, image data obtained will be varied depending on time in which the given image was obtained.

Case Study 3: Nanomaterials Strength

- Strength in nanomaterials, for example, in carbon nanotubes, was shown by graph in a study by Stach [20]. Figure 6.31 presents the strength graph for carbon nanotubes, which have been found indeed as strong as theory suggests.
- Due to small size, mechanical properties of carbon nanotubes were measured by Ruoff and his colleagues as carefully attached nanotube ropes between two AFM tips inside a scanning electron microscope. Elastic modulus and failure strength were measured for nanotubes.

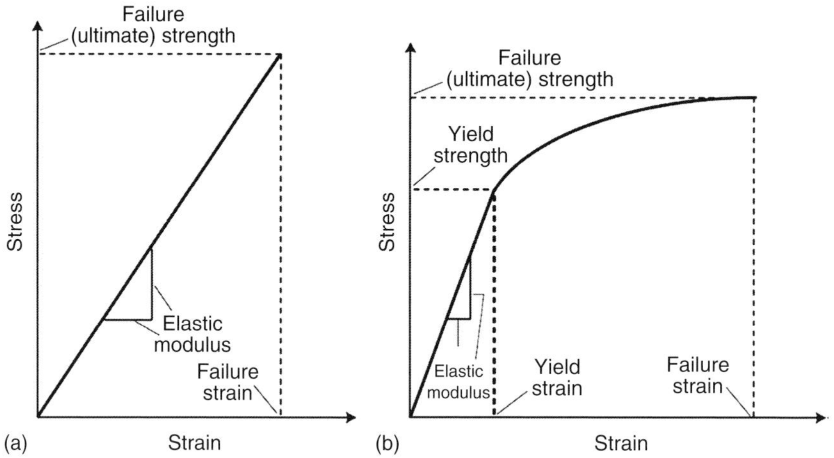

Figure 6.31 Schematic of stress–strain curves for a brittle material (a) and a plastic material (b) showing how the elastic modulus and other mechanical properties of a material can be determined. Experiments measure the displacement caused by an applied load, and these two quantities are then converted into strain and stress via simple relations, respectively. Plastic materials (such as metals) start to deform at the yield stress or strain before eventually failing at higher values of stress/strain, whereas brittle materials (like ceramics) fail without going through a deformation phase. The experiments of Espinosa and coworkers suggest that nanotubes behave like brittle materials, although in many calculations they display some plastic-like behavior. (Stach 2008 [20]. Reproduced with permission of Nature Publishing Group.)

Control Questions

1) Describe the chemical properties of nanomaterials.
2) Determine the size effect in nanomaterials and its relation with diffusion coefficient.
3) Describe the dependence of maximum reaction speed W_m on particle size at fixed nuclei thickness.
4) Determine the specific catalytic activity of nanomaterials and its relation with particles dispersity.
5) Discuss the mechanical properties of nanomaterials and features such as microcracks, inner microstress, structure defects, change in grain size during deformation, and other factors.
6) Determine hardness, strength, and plasticity in nanomaterials.
7) Discuss superplasticity and its features in microcrystalline materials.
8) Describe spontaneous combustion and pyrophoricity of nanomediums.
9) Describe the characterization tools in nanotechnology and their variety for nanomaterial analysis.
10) Describe the microscopical characterizations of nanomaterials and superiority in their properties for providing better observation results.
11) Describe the basic operation of scanning electron microscope (SEM).
12) Describe the spectroscopical characterization tools in nanotechnology and their hierarchical divisions.
13) What is the difference between FESEM and AFM techniques?
14) Describe the features in FTIR spectroscopy analysis of nanomaterials.
15) What is the difference between XPS and FTIR measurement techniques for nanomaterials characterization?
16) Describe the X-ray photoelectron spectroscopy analysis features in characterization of nanomaterials.
17) Describe the features of atomic force microscope for nanomaterial characterization.
18) Explain the stress–strain curve for nanotubes strength and other mechanical properties.

References

1 Ryzhonkov, D.I., Levina, V.V. and Dzidziguri, E.L. (2008) *Nanomaterialy, uchebnoe posoibie, Moskva, BINOM, Laboratorya znanyi*, BKL Publishers, ISBN 978-5-94774-724-9.

2 Vinokurov, A.L. and Eliseev, A.A. (2011) Metody issledivanya veschestv v nanokristallicheskom sosotoyanii, Moskva 2011, Moskovskyi gosudartstvennyi universitet M.V. Lomonosova, http://www.nanometer.ru/2009/10/24/12563591295716/.../%CF_.

3 Borisov, S.V. and Podberezskaya, N.V. (2012) X-ray diffraction analysis: a brief history and achievements of the first century. *J. Struct. Chem.*, **53**, 1.

4 Das, R., Ali, E., and Abd Hamid, S.B. (2014) Current applications of X-Ray powder diffraction. *Rev. Adv. Mater. Sci.*, **38**, 95–109.
5 Dorofeev, G.A., Streletskii, A.N., Povstugar, I.V. *et al* (2012) Determination of nanoparticle sizes by X-ray diffraction. *Colloid J.*, **74**, 675.
6 Stroppa, D.G., Zagonel, L.F., Montoro, L.A., Leite, E.R., and Ramirez, A.J. (2012) High-Resolution Scanning Transmission Electron Microscopy (HRSTEM) techniques: high-resolution imaging and spectroscopy side by side. *ChemPhysChem*, **13**, 437–443.
7 Vernon-Parry, K.D. and Wright, A.C. (2001) TEM: An introduction, part 2, III Vs Review, *The Advanced Semiconducting Magazine*, Vol **14** (1–2), 48–51.
8 Bogner, A., Jouneau, P.H., Thollet, G., Basset, D., and Gauthier, C. (2007) A history of scanning electron microscopy developments: towards "wet-STEM" imaging. *Micron*, **38** (4), 390–401.
9 Zhan, G. *et al* (2011) Green synthesis of Au–Pd bimetallic nanoparticles: single-step bioreduction method with plant extract. *Mater. Lett.*, **65** (19–20), 2989–2991.
10 Raman, A., Melcher, J., and Tung, R. (2008) Cantilever dynamics in atomic force microscopy. *Nano Today*, **3** (2), 20–27.
11 Dukic, M. *et al.*, (2015) Piezoresistive AFM cantilevers surpassing standard optical beam deflection in low noise topography imaging, *Sci. Rep.*, **5**, 16393, p. 1–11.
12 Klapetek, P., Valtr, M., Nečas, D., Salyk, O., and Dzik, P. (2011) Atomic force microscopy analysis of nanoparticles in non-ideal conditions. *Nanoscale Res. Lett.*, **6**, 514.
13 Nagao, E. and Dvorak, J.A. (1998) An integrated approach to the study of living cells by atomic force microscopy. *J. Microsc.*, **191**, 8–19.
14 Vernon-Parry, K.D. and Wright, A.C. (2000) Analysis, scanning electron microscopy: an introduction. *III Vs Rev.*, **13** (4), 40–44.
15 Hodoroaba, V.-D., Rades, S. and Unger, W.E.S. (2014) Inspection of morphology and elemental imaging of single nanoparticles by high resolution SEM/EDX in transmission mode. *Surf. Interface Anal.*, **45**, 945–948.
16 Ullah, R., Ahmad, I., and Zheng, Y. (2016) Fourier transform infrared spectroscopy of (Bisphenol A). *J. Spectrosc.*, Article ID 2073613, 5 pages, http://dx.doi: 10.1155/2016/2073613.
17 Ciobanu, C.S., Iconaru, S.L., Chifiriuc, M.C., Costescu, A., Coustumer, P.L., and Predo, D. (2013) Synthesis and antimicrobial activity of silver-doped hydroxyapatite nanoparticles. *BioMed Res. Int.*, Article ID 916218, 10 pages, http://dx.doi.org/10.1155/2013/916218.
18 Kumar, N. *et al* (2014) Oxidation Process of Iron Nanoparticles and their spectroscopic, magnetic, and microscopic evidence. *Environ. Sci. Technol.*, **48** (23), 13888–13894.
19 Ruíz-Baltazar, A., Esparza, R., Rosas, G. and Pérez, R. (2015) Effect of the surfactant on the growth and oxidation of iron nanoparticles. *J. Nanomater.*, Article ID 240948, 8 pages, http://dx.doi.org/10.1155/2015/240948.
20 Stach, E.A. (2008) NANOMATERIALS Nanotubes Reveal Their True Strength, Paper 340, Birck and NCN Publications, pp. 586–587.

Further Reading

Hasegawa, K. (2012) Introduction to single crystal X-Ray analysis. *Rigaku J.*, **28** (1) pp. 14–18.

Roiter, Y. and Minko, S. (2005) AFM single molecule experiments at the solid–liquid interface: in situ conformation of adsorbed flexible polyelectrolyte chains. *J. Am. Chem. Soc.*, **127**, 15688–15689.

Rao, A., Schoenenberger, M., Gnecco, E., Glatzel, T., and Meye, E. (2007) Characterization of nanoparticles using atomic force microscopy. *J. Phys. Conf. Ser.*, **61**, 971–976.

Online Sources

Assmus A. Early History of X Rays, http://www.slac.stanford.edu/pubs/beamline/25/2/25-2-assmus.pdf (accessed 17 January 2017).

Iowa State University. http://www.mse.iastate.edu/research/laboratories/sem/microscopy/how-does-the-sem-work/high-school/how-the-sem-works/ (accessed 17 January 2017).

Nature Publishing Group. Invention of Microscope, http://www.nature.com/milestones/milelight/full/milelight01.html (accessed 17 January 2017).

NIST Database for Spectral Identification, http://srdata.nist.gov/xps/ (accessed 17 January 2017).

PURDUE University. https://www.purdue.edu/ehps/rem/rs/sem.htm (accessed 17 January 2017).

7 Introduction to Biomaterials

There are no gains without pains.

Ben Franklin, author (1706–1790)

7.1 Biomaterials: Subject, Purpose, and Problems

Dealing with biological and implant materials, as well as interaction between both of them in the living body, the purpose of biomaterials science is to improve the quality and length of life by support of artificial implants and artificial organs. Biomaterials science focuses on the manufacturing process of novel biomaterials, implants, drugs, nanoscale techniques, and nanobiomedical products. Tissue engineering (TE) is one of the developing areas in biomaterials science. Nowadays progress and success in technology allows the managing and controlling of a number of biochemical and metabolic processes in the living organism. The latest progress, 3D bioprinting, can allow the use and implantation of artificial organs, carefully produced by the application of various purpose-based printers and via passage of several steps [1]. Besides past works and challenges, research efforts in biomaterials development are currently shifting to the use of increasingly complex material systems to facilitate the *de novo* design and synthesis and fabrication of novel biomaterials holding properties tailored to specific biological needs and clinical applications [2].

The main problems of biomaterials science are:

- Selection of appropriate source materials for implants, artificial organ design, and manufacturing in order to improve life span and implant-tissue adaptation
- Tissue reconstruction, depending on the use of scaffolds made of complex 3D polymer structures that have been built from 2D layers, and implants
- Application and use of natural biomaterials for TE and 3D bioprinting
- Considerations of physicochemical and mechanical stability features for implants

7.1.1 Current Goals of Biomaterials Field

The use of biomaterials such as ceramic led to the improvement of the quality and length of life, compared with the discovery of fire in the ancient times. These

Nano- and Biomaterials: Compounds, Properties, Characterization, and Applications,
First Edition. Zhypargul Abdullaeva.

ceramic materials used for reconstruction and replacement of damaged body parts were named bioceramics [3].

The *field of biomaterials* is in the midst of a revolutionary change in which the life sciences are becoming equal in importance to materials science and engineering as the foundation of the field. Simultaneously, advances in engineering (for example nanotechnology) are greatly increasing the sophistication with which biomaterials are designed and have allowed fabrication of materials with increasingly complex functions. Such sophisticated materials are often designed to mimic a subset of the physicochemical properties of natural materials. Increasingly, nature inspires not only the materials themselves but also the means by which they are made. Whereas synthetic materials are typically engineered on the scale of millimeters or larger and then milled to have micrometrical or nanometer-scale features, natural materials are constructed on these smaller scales by self-assembly, a bottom-up means of fabrication that facilitates the construction of information-rich, complex structures in a highly reproducible manner with minimal energy input.

Knowledge gained from fundamental studies is being used in conjunction with fabrication methods such as self-assembly to design biomaterials that interface with the biology of the host. This is typically done by means of binding interactions with cell surface receptors, to regulate the maintenance, regeneration, or even destruction of specific tissues in the body. Key aspects of this line of research include the following: the rich information content of new materials that mimic cellular and extracellular materials, with particular emphasis on presentation of signals in a controlled spatiotemporal manner; provision of non-chemical (for example electrical or mechanical) signals to elicit structural changes in the material or to manipulate cell fate directly; the finding that the physical properties of the materials are probably just as important as their chemistry in terms of the biological response they elicit; and the notion that materials can be designed to regulate host biology at a distance, either by controlling cell trafficking or by trafficking of the material itself in the body [4] (reprinted by permission from Macmillan Publishers Ltd: [Nature 462, review article: Inspiration and application in the evolution of biomaterials, p. 426–432, N. Huebsch, D.J. Mooney] copyright (2009).

7.2 General Requirements for Biomaterials

There are still a number of requirements for biomaterials intending for use in the human body, such as novel and improved properties able to perform correctly with good compatibility and satisfactory longevity [5]. Shape memory is an important property for metal alloy biomaterials, characterized by their ability to remember and recover their original shapes [6].

Recently, however, research suggests that the field of biomaterials might be witnessing the emergence of a powerful set of new design parameters. Increasingly, scientists are seeking physics-derived solutions for controlling biological responses. For example, methods have been developed for fabricating polymeric particles with controlled shape, mechanical properties, surface topology, and compartmentalization. Particles with unique physical properties have been shown to influence many vital interactions within the body including phagocytosis, circulation, targeting, and adhesion.

The tissues of the human body have selective mechanical properties ranging from soft (brain, about 0.5 kPa), to moderately stiff (skin and muscles, around 10 kPa), to stiff (precalcified bone, >30 kPa). The narrow specifications of elastic moduli create mechanically defined microenvironments that effectively support the development of cellular architecture. For example, mesenchymal stem cells (MSCs) showed strikingly different morphologies when cultured on polyacrylamide (PAAm) substrates with varying elasticities. Particle diameter can often be controlled through physical properties of the materials, such as polymer and surfactant concentration, or through the experimental parameters of the fabrication method, for example, the mixing method (vortexing, sonication, stirring), nozzle/capillary diameter, and material flow rate.

Particles with sizes ranging from less than a nanometer to a few tens of micrometers have been fabricated and tested for biomedical applications. Several important *in vivo* functions of particles (drug carriers) depend on particle size: these include circulation times, extravasation, targeting, immunogenicity, internalization, intracellular trafficking, degradation, flow properties, clearance, and uptake mechanisms (Figure 7.1). Particle diameter dictates their transport and adhesion in blood vessels, airways, or gastrointestinal tract. There exist a variety of size-based clearance mechanisms in the blood. Microparticles are captured by Kupffer cells in the liver or physically trapped in the capillary beds, whereas nanoparticles smaller than 100 nm leave the blood vessels through fenestrations in the endothelial lining [7].

7.3 Biomaterials in Body Systems

Biomaterials are used to replace diseased or damaged part of the body (artificial hip, joint, and kidney), assist healing (suture, bone screw, and bone plates), improve function (cardiac pacemaker and contact lens), correct functional abnormality (e.g., Harrington's spinal cord), correct cosmetic concerns, and aid diagnosis and treatment [8]. Types and variety of biomaterials utilized for manufacturing of body replacements range from metals (Ti, Cr, Mo, and their alloys), polymers (nylon, rubber, polyester, etc.), and ceramics (HAP, Al_2O_3, glass, etc.) to composites (carbon, fiber-reinforced bone cement (BC)), characterized by their advantages and disadvantages [9].

There are a number of factors including stability, corrosion resistance, biocompatibility, and bioinert properties as requirements for biomaterials being used in the living body. The implanted biomaterial should not cause any negative effects such as allergic reaction, inflammation, and toxicity either immediately after implantation or under postoperative conditions. Also, biomaterials for

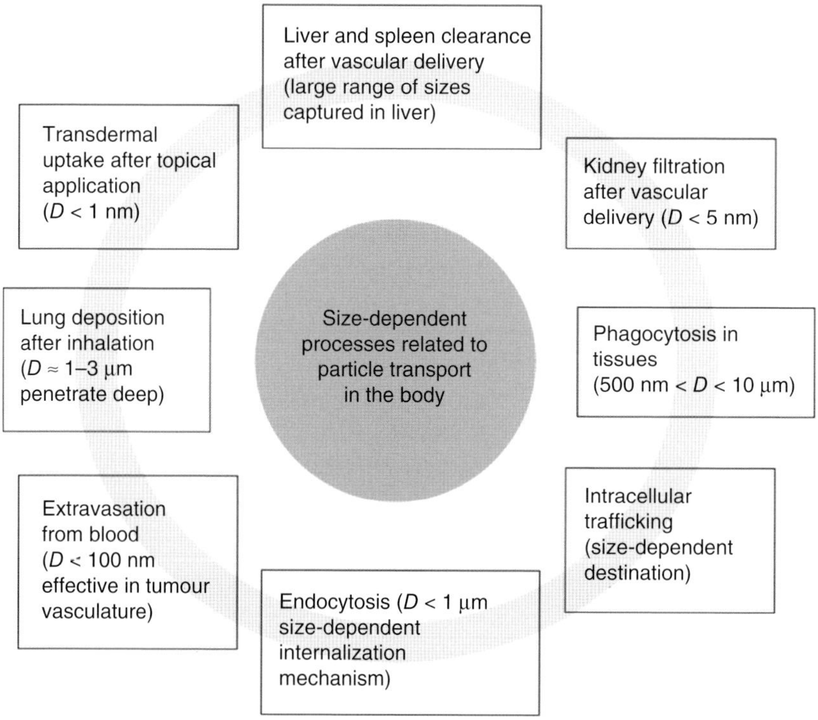

Figure 7.1 Size-dependent processes of particle transport in the human body. Particles can pass through biological barriers by a number of different processes. These include passive (diffusive) and active processes ranging from extravasation to transdermal uptake. Most of these processes affect distribution and clearance of micro- and nanoparticles in the human body, and they strongly depend on particle size [2]. (Mitragotri *et al.* 2009 [7]. Reproduced with permission of Nature Publishing Group.)

use in the human body should hold sufficient mechanical properties, such as strength, force sustainability, and corrosion and wear resistance, apart from fatigue strength and fracture toughness [10].

Recently, a variety of biomaterials are used in the human body, including brain and nerve tissue scaffolds; ear and teeth implants; contact lens; heart valve replacements and pacemakers; blood vessel stents; artificial BC; muscle suture; hip, knee, and joint replacements; and 3D bioprinted materials. Figure 7.2 shows a schematic of some types of biomaterials used in the human body.

7.4 Types and Classification of Biomaterials

Biomaterials are developing rapidly in chemical engineering and are classified into several types based on their structure, composition, and application purposes. According to the classification by H. Suh [11], there are three classes of biomaterials in medical use: class I (no direct contact with body tissue), class II (intermittent or instant contact with body tissues), and class III (constant contact with body tissue). Also, biomaterials were classified into *artificial* and *natural*

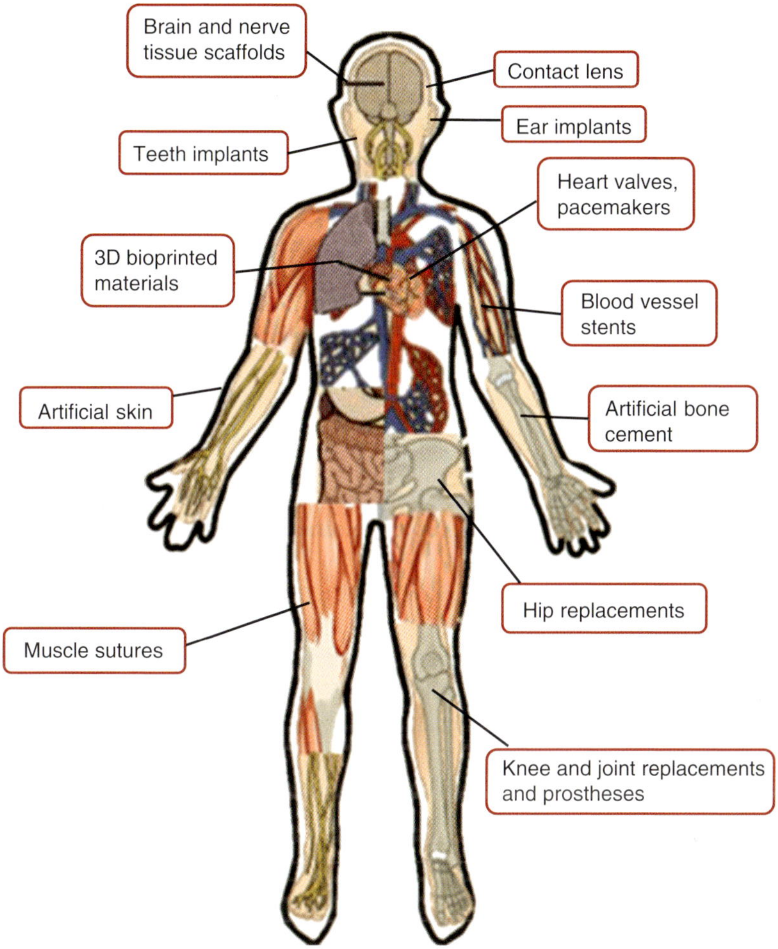

Figure 7.2 Schematic illustration of biomaterials types used in the human body.

biomaterials for body restoration based on composition criteria. In turn artificial materials are separated into *inorganic* (metal, ceramics) and *organic* (synthetic polymers). Natural biomaterials are divided into natural polymers, cultured cells, and preserved tissues.

The industry of biomaterials includes organizations and companies that design, produce, and manufacture materials used in health and biological sciences. The biomaterials can be classified as *biomedical*, that is, with an artificial origin (metals, ceramics, polymers), and *biological*, that is, with a natural origin (vegetal, animal, or human) [12].

Biomaterials classification reported recently is shown in Figure 7.3.

7.4.1 Metallic Biomaterials

Metallic biomaterials are widely used as biomedical materials and have significant contribution to medicine; they cannot be replaced by ceramics or polymers

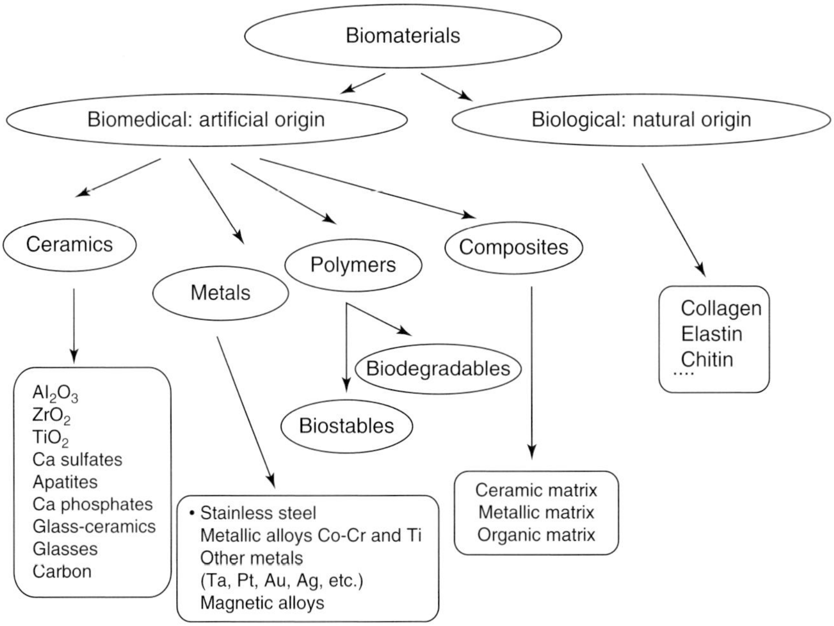

Figure 7.3 Classification of biomaterials. (Vallet-Regí 2001 [12]. Reproduced with permission of Royal Society of Chemistry.)

presently because of their unique properties such as high strength and toughness. Since safety is the most important property of biomaterials, corrosion-resistant materials such as stainless steel, Co–Cr–Mo alloy, and commercially pure (cp) Ti and Ti alloys are currently used as biomaterials [13]. Microrough surfaces with roughness below 50 μm prepared recently allow better early adhesion of mineral ions and atoms, biomolecules and cells, and connective tissue or bone which result in thinner tissue reaction with inflammatory cells [13].

FeMn Alloys

Metals are generally considered more suitable than polymers for stent applications, mainly due to their superior mechanical properties, close to those of SS316L, which is widely considered as the gold standard for stent implants. Recently, magnesium alloys and iron have been proposed for biodegradable stents. A number of Mg alloys have been proposed, including AE21, AM60B, AZ91, and WE43. Stents of WE43 alloy were even tested preclinically in lower limb of adult patients, implanted in the left pulmonary artery of a preterm baby and in the aorta of a newborn. Stent prototypes made of pure iron ($Fe > 99.8\%$) were also implanted in the descending aorta of porcine. In general, both metals showed favourable biological performance. However, the degradation rates were considered too rapid for Mg alloys and slow for pure iron for stent applications. Rapid accumulation of degradation products onto vessel walls was reported after an implantation study of WE43 in porcine arteries. Meanwhile, a long-term

Table 7.1 Typical mechanical property of the recently proposed metals for degradable stents compared with SS316L alloy.

Material	Yield strength (MPa)	Ultimate strength (MPa)	Elongation at break (%)
Stainless steel 316L[a)]	190	490	40
WE43 magnesium alloy[b)]	150	250	4
Iron[c)]	150	210	40

a) Stainless steel 18Cr, 14Ni, 2.5Mo, annealed plate, as specified in ASTM F138.
b) WE43B-T6, extruded bar, as specified in ASTM B107/B107M.
c) Pure iron (99.8%), annealed plate, as provided by Goodfellow Corporation, Oakdale, PA, USA.
Source: Hermawan *et al.* 2009 [14]. Reproduced with permission of Wiley.

implantation study in porcine aortas showed that the iron stent strut had not completely disappeared after to 18 months.

From a structural point of view, the mechanical properties of iron are more attractive than those of magnesium alloys, if compared with stainless steel (Table 7.1). Moreover, the properties of Fe alloys could be further improved by targeted alloying and by applying specific thermomechanical treatment (reproduced from Journal of Biomedical Materials Research Part A, Degradable metallic biomaterials: Design and development of Fe–Mn alloys for stents, 93(1), 2010, p. 1–11, Hermawan, H., *et al.*, with permission of Wiley). Chemical compositions of Fe–Mn alloys [14] are shown in Table 7.2.

CoCr Alloys

The use of CoCr alloys for surgical applications is mainly of interest for orthopedic prostheses for the knee, shoulder, and hip. For long-term requirements in arthroplasty, a high corrosion resistance combined with a good biocompatibility is needed. The fabrication process with the use of Co, Cr, and Mo allows to achieve extremely hard implants with a high corrosion resistance in body fluids. Cobalt-based alloys (e.g., CoCrW, CoCrMo) have Young's modulus of about 250 ± 10 GPa combined with a high wear and heat resistance. Despite lower biocompatibility compared with cp titanium, Co-based alloys have advantages in joint arthroplasty. In cemented titanium hip stems, an elevated rate of aseptic

Table 7.2 Chemical composition of FeMn alloys.

	Concentration (wt%)					
Alloy	Mn	C	Si	N	O	Fe
Fe20Mn	18.4	0.02	<0.006	<0.005	<0.224	Balance
Fe25Mn	24.0	0.04	<0.006	<0.005	<0.224	Balance
Fe30Mn	29.3	0.04	<0.006	<0.005	<0.224	Balance
Fe35Mn	35.3	0.04	<0.006	<0.005	<0.224	Balance

Source: Hermawan *et al.* 2009 [14]. Reproduced with permission of Wiley.

loosening and a high rate of subsidence compared with Co-based alloys are described. It has also been shown that Ti6Al4V has a lower mechanical resistance and a higher production of wear compared with Co-based femoral components in knee arthroplasty.

Ti and Ti Alloys

Since its introduction for bone plates and screws in 1965, cp titanium has found an increasing application as an implant material in medicine. Cp titanium has high corrosion resistance and an outstanding biocompatibility and, furthermore, does not cause allergic reactions. This may be due to a protective oxide layer, which forms spontaneously on the implant surface as long as oxygen is present.

To further improve mechanical strength of titanium implants, $\alpha + \beta$ titanium alloys, such as Ti6Al4V, Ti6Al4V ELI, and Ti6Al7Nb, have been developed. These titanium alloys have the greatest commercial potential and are widely used as load-bearing orthopedic implants due to their relatively good fatigue resistance and biological passivity. Implant sensitivity to titanium alloys is very seldom, despite components such as vanadium that are described to be cytotoxic. *In vivo* studies have shown that Ti–6Al–4V has similar biological compatibility with vanadium-free titanium alloys. It has been proven that cp titanium and titanium alloys have clear advantages in cell culture experiments with human osteoblasts compared with stainless steel and CoCr. The higher osteoblastic differentiation of human osteoblasts on cp titanium and titanium alloys indicates an improved biocompatibility compared with stainless steel and CoCr [15] (reproduced from European Journal of Trauma 32, Metallic Biomaterials in Skeletal Repair, 2006, p. 149–59, K.H. Frosch, K.M. Stürmer, with permission of Springer).

As an example of metal and metal alloy biomaterials, porous β-type Ti–40Nb alloy produced by hot-pressing method [16] for biomedical applications is presented in Figure 7.4. The porosity (pT) for the SLM-fabricated cylinders was $17\% \pm 1\%$ (median = 17.0%; variance: 0.4%), which is in good agreement with the value obtained using density determined by simply dividing the mass of the cylinder by its volume. As seen from the figure, porosity is mainly formed by spherical pores, which result from gas uptake by the powder during the ball milling process. These big spherical pores and such a relatively high porosity are not typical for alloys fabricated using SLM from gas-atomized powders. The relative density of Ti alloys fabricated using gas-atomized powder and SLM is of the order of 99%. For hot-pressed cylinders, the sizes of the micropores and pT were 3–12 μm and $3 \pm 0.4\%$ (median = 3.0%; variance = 0.06%), respectively. pT for SLM-fabricated cylinders was significantly higher than that for hot-pressed cylinders ($p = 0.01$).

Ti and Ti alloys are widely used as metal biomaterials. Among them, Ti alloys suggested for medical applications are five beta (β) titanium alloys, such as TMZF™, Ti–13Nb–13Zr, TIMETAL® 21SRx, Tiadyne 1610, and Ti–15Mo, which have been proposed for medical applications in the United States. The following are brief descriptions of these five titanium alloys.

TMZF™ Alloy

The Ti–12Mo–6Zr–2Fe (TMZF™) alloy was developed by Howmedica Inc. and has been approved by the Food and Drug Administration (FDA) for certain

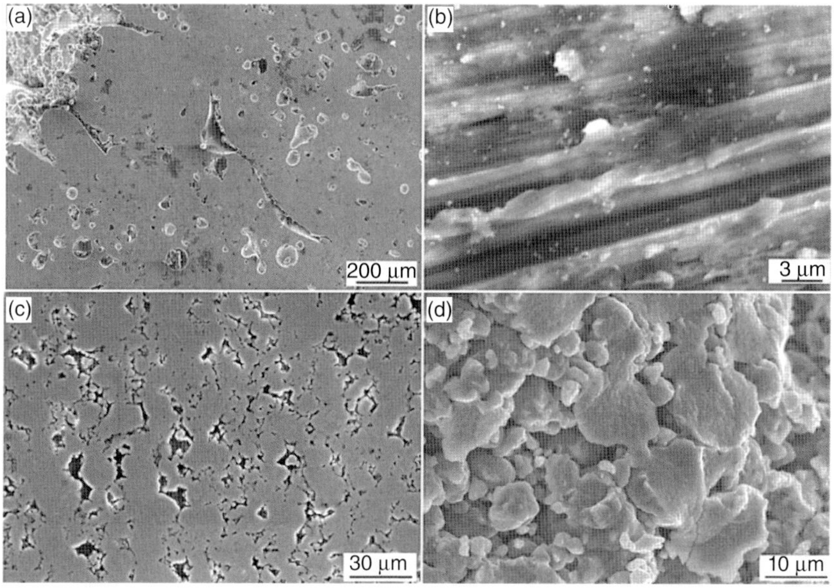

Figure 7.4 Scanning electron microscope (SEM) images of cross sections of (a) sample made by SLM of Ti–40Nb ball-milled powder and (b) its higher resolution image and (c) sample made by hot pressing of Ti–40Nb ball-milled powder and (d) its higher resolution image. (Zhuravleva *et al.* 2013 [16]. http://www.mdpi.com/1996-1944/6/12/5700/htm. Used under: https://creativecommons.org/licenses/by/4.0/.)

product applications. The chemical composition of the TMZF alloy is given in Table 7.3; TMZF™ alloy is a metastable beta alloy. It retains an all-beta structure after rapid cooling from its β-transus temperature of 754 °C or higher. The all-beta structure will precipitate fine alpha phase upon subsequent aging. The solution-annealed TMZF™ alloy having a single beta phase structure is suitable for orthopedic implants for its low modulus of elasticity, excellent strength, and ductility. The strength of solution-annealed TMZF™ alloy can be further increased through an aging treatment with a concurrent increase in modulus.

Table 7.3 Chemical composition limits for TMZF™ alloy.

Element	Min. Max. (wt%)
Molybdenum	10.0–13.0
Zirconium	5.0–7.0
Iron	1.5–2.5
Oxygen	0.08–0.28
Carbon	0.00–0.05
Nitrogen	0.00–0.05
Hydrogen	0.00–0.020
Titanium	Balance

Source: Wang 1996 [17]. Reproduced with permission of Elsevier.

Table 7.4 Chemical composition limits of Ti–13Nb–13Zr.

Element	Min. Max. (wt%)
Niobium	12.5–14.0
Zirconium	12.5–14.0
Iron	0.00–0.25
Oxygen	0.00–0.15
Carbon	0.00–0.08
Nitrogen	0.00–0.05
Hydrogen	0.000–0.012[a)]
Titanium	Balance

a) Material 0.813 mm and under may have hydrogen content up to 0.015%.
Source: Wang 1996 [17]. Reproduced with permission of Elsevier.

The TMZF™ alloy exhibits higher tensile strength, a lower modulus of elasticity, higher fracture toughness (90 MPa m^{-1}), and better wear resistance than the mill-annealed Ti–6AI–4V ELI alloy. It also has an excellent corrosion resistance and a smooth fatigue strength similar to that of Ti–6AI–4V ELI alloy. Possessing high strength, low modulus, and excellent corrosion resistance, this alloy is well suited for orthopedic applications.

Ti–13Zr–13Nb Alloy

The Ti–13Nb–13Zr alloy was developed by Smith and Nephew Richards Inc. The chemical composition is given in Table 7.4. It was reported that Ti–13Nb–13Zr is a near-β alloy and consists of hcp martensite (α') in the water quenched condition. With subsequent aging, the Ti–13Nb–13Zr alloy consists of hcp martensite (α') and submicroscopic bcc beta precipitates. The dispersed beta precipitates strengthen and harden the material [16]. Aging treatment normally results in conversion of the martensite to an $\alpha + \beta$ mixture for β-Ti alloys (metastable β and near-β alloys). The presence of martensite in the aged Ti–13Nb–13Zr alloy indicates that the alloy is more likely an $\alpha - \beta$ alloy instead of a near-β alloy. This alloy in the aged condition was reported to have higher tensile strength, a lower modulus, and higher toughness (65 MPa m^{-1}) than the mill-annealed Ti–6Al–4V alloy.

TIMETAL® 21 SRx

TIMETAL® 21SRx is a derivative of TIMETAL® 21S, an alloy developed by TIMET in the 1980s as a matrix material for metal matrix composites on the National AeroSpace Plane (NASP). Aluminum has been removed from TIMETAL® 21S to improve biocompatibility. To maintain a comparable level of alpha stabilization, the oxygen level was slightly increased in TIMETAL® 21SRx. It exhibits higher tensile strength and lower modulus of elasticity than the mill-annealed Ti–6AI–4V.

Tiadyne 1610

Tiadyne 1610 was developed by Teledyne Wah Chang Albany (TWCA) for medical applications, particularly for orthopedic implant. Only tensile properties of Tiadyne 1610 have been published. Tiadyne 1610 has a lower modulus and tensile strength than mill-annealed Ti–6Al–4V alloy.

Ti–35Nb

The Ti–35Nb alloy is being evaluated for orthopedic implant applications by Synthes USA. This metastable β-Ti alloy can retain a fine beta grain structure after solution annealing at 800 °C with rapid quenching. It was reported that Ti–35Nb has excellent corrosion resistance but much lower tensile strength than that of the Ti–6AI–4V ELI alloy and comparable to that of CP grade 4 titanium [17] (reprinted from Materials Science and Engineering A 213, Wang, K., The use of titanium for medical applications in the USA, 134–137, Copyright (1996), with permission from Elsevier).

7.4.2 Composite Biomaterials

Composite biomaterials are characterized by composition and structure parameters. Biomedical composite materials were classified into three groups based on the engineering performance. They are (i) materials that make up individual components; (ii) materials that quantity, form, and arrange their components; and (iii) materials that interact between components [18]. Another classification of composite biomaterials binds with the basis of reinforcing materials geometry: fibrous and particulate composite biomaterials [19]. *Composite material* is defined as a material consisting of fibers embedded in the matrix (McGraw-Hill Dictionary, Copyright © 2003). *Fibrous composite* materials are materials containing a single layer of fiber [20]. *Porous biomaterials* are defined as those porous biomaterials with graded/gradient pore size/porosity [21]. Composite materials were classified into *fiber-reinforced* (single-layer and multilayer) and *particle-reinforced* (random and preferred orientation) types. Single-layer composites were further subdivided into continuous fiber-reinforced (unidirectional and bidirectional) and discontinuous fiber-reinforced (random and preferred orientation) composites [22]. Natural composite material in combination with synthetic materials can be used as smart composites. Smart composite designs are possible by modulating the bulk and surface properties of materials that mimic the native tissues, either in chemical (extracellular matrix molecules) or in physical properties, for example, stiffness [23]. Composite materials also can be made by inspiration from natural biological materials (biologically inspired materials) with molecular-scale interactions optimized to direct functional features. Interest in replacing synthetic materials with natural materials due to biocompatibility and sustainability is important to understand the molecular structure and chemistry of the raw component materials [24].

Nanostructured Calcium Phosphate Cement (CPC)

Calcium phosphate cements (CPCs) are self-setting synthetic bone graft materials. The first CPC consisted of a mixture of tetracalcium phosphate

(TTCP: $Ca_4(PO_4)_2O$) and dicalcium phosphate anhydrous (DCPA: $CaHPO_4$) and was developed in 1986. CPC was approved in 1996 by the FDA for repairing craniofacial defects. When mixed with an aqueous solution to form a paste, CPC can self-harden to form hydroxyapatite (HA) *in situ*. It has good biocompatibility, *in situ* hardening and molding capabilities, and injectability properties, enabling minimally invasive applications. Recent studies enhanced the mechanical, physical, and biological properties of CPC through the introduction of absorbable fibers, chitosan, mannitol porogen, gas-foaming agents, and alginate microbeads and biofunctionalization. These approaches improved mechanical strength, setting time, degradability, macroporosity, cell attachment, and delivery of cells and growth factors [25].

7.4.3 Nanostructured CaP Composites

Composite approaches can be used to improve the mechanical properties of nanostructured CaP in order to satisfy clinical needs in load-bearing areas. Combining natural or synthetic polymers with nanostructured CaP is a promising strategy, since bone tissue itself is a nanocomposite of HA and collagen. Many degradable polymers have been explored for this purpose, such as collagen fibers, silk fibroin, gelatin, chitosan, poly-L-lactide, poly-DL-lactide-*co*-glycolide (PLGA) and poly(vinylalcohol). Each type of polymer has its own characteristics to contribute to the property improvement of the composite. Collagen is the most abundant polymer in bone tissue. By incorporating collagen into the composite, it provides more cell recognition sites and accelerates biomaterial's degradation rate, thus allowing fast replacement by new bone [25] (reprinted by permission from Macmillan Publishers Ltd: [Bone Research 2, 2014, 14017] (Bone tissue engineering via nanostructured calcium phosphate biomaterials and stem cells, Wang, P., *et al.*), copyright (2014)).

Bone and Nacre

As described in several recent review articles, bone and nacre (abalone shell) are prime examples of natural materials that combine strength with toughness, making them truly damage tolerant. Also described in this subsection are other natural materials that have evolved efficient strategies for developing exceptional damage tolerance, including teeth, the dactyl clubs of stomatopod shrimps, and bamboo. Bone is composed of cells embedded in an extracellular matrix, which is an ordered network assembled from two major nanophases: collagen fibrils made from type I collagen molecules (~300 nm long, ~1.5 nm in diameter) and HA ($Ca_{10}(PO_4)_6(OH)_2$) nanocrystals (plate shaped, 50 nm × 25 nm in size, 1.5–4 nm thick) distributed along the collagen fibrils [26] (Figure 7.5a–c).

The microscale features of bone provide a channel for cell migration, nutrient delivery, and vascularization. Pores and their interconnectivity are indispensable for tissue formation. The combination of multi-scaled pore size and porosity into one structure has shown to be an effective solution for yielding improved overall performances of TE scaffolds. While macroporosity (pore size 450 μm) has a strong impact on osteogenicity, microporosity (pore size 10–100 μm) and pore wall roughness are important factors as well. Figure 7.6 shows interconnected porosity of a collagen type I–HAp scaffold. The most common fabrication

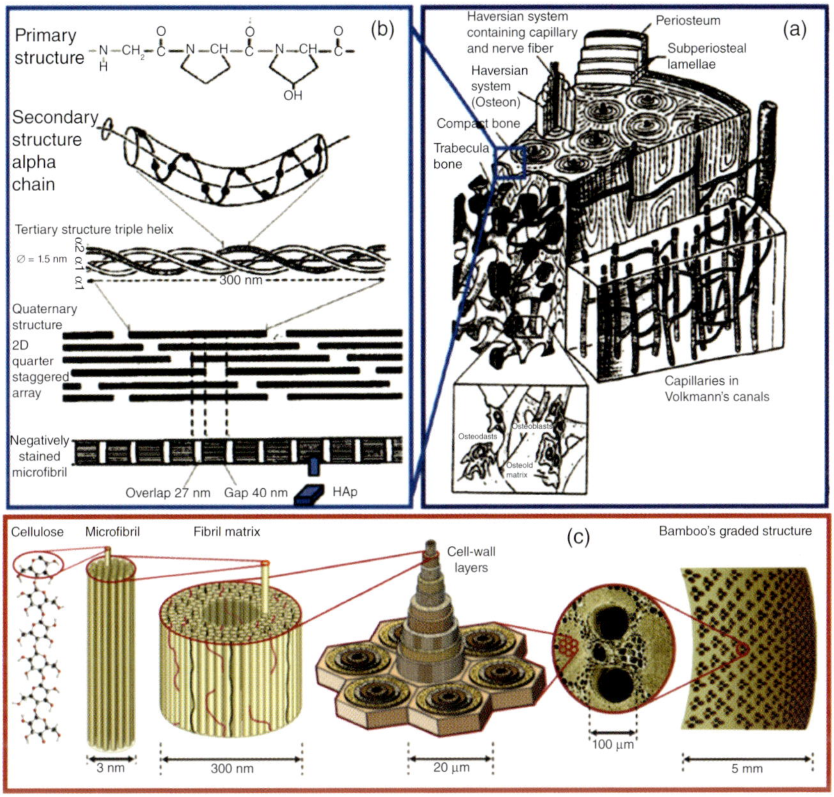

Figure 7.5 Hierarchical structure of bone and bamboo: (a) structure of bone; (b) structural components of tubercular bone [27] (http://www.oapublishinglondon.com/article/773. Used Under: CC: BY 3.0.); (c) bamboo is composed of cellulose fibers imbedded in a lignin–hemicellulose matrix shaped into hollow prismatic cells of varying wall thickness. In bamboo and palm, which have a more complex structure than wood, a radial density gradient of parallel fibers in a matrix of honeycomb-like cells increases each material's flexural rigidity. Bamboo increases its flexural rigidity even further by combining a radial density gradient with a hollow-tube cross-sectional shape. (Wegst *et al*. 2015 [26]. Reproduced with permission Nature Publishing Group.)

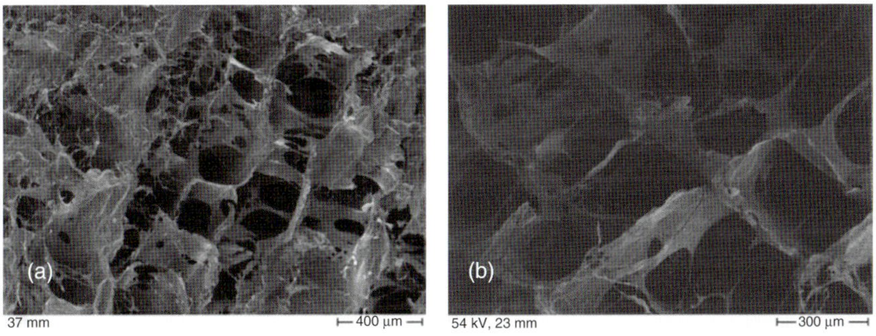

Figure 7.6 Interconnected porosity of a collagen type I–HAp (1:1 wt) scaffold manufactured by freeze-drying [27]. (http://www.oapublishinglondon.com/article/773. Used Under: CC: BY 3.0.)

methods used to re-create the microscale porosity and special organization of native bone in a biomaterial are rapid prototyping (e.g., solid-free form), salt leaching, gas foaming, phase separation, freeze-drying, and sintering depending on the scaffold material. Following a biomimetic approach to TE, choosing a natural polymer (specifically collagen) can limit the aforementioned techniques considerably. Natural polymers are protein based, which means they are susceptible to temperature (denaturation above 40) and pH; therefore, techniques using high temperature or chemicals are not suitable. Freeze-drying/lyophilization is one of the methods frequently used to generate microporosity in natural scaffolds. Here, a solution of collagen is frozen and then freeze-dried. The pores are negative replicate of ice crystals that are formed during freezing, forcing collagen into interstitial spaces, which are then removed by freeze-drying [27].

Carbon Fiber Composite

Carbon fibers (CFs), or carbon nanofibers with nanoscale diameter dramatically improve the functions of conventional biomaterials, by making possible the development of new composite materials and provide possibilities for new applications for regenerative medicine as well as for cancer treatment [27]. CF composite materials have superior properties and benefits for orthopedic surgery applications because of properties such as: excellent fatigue, radiolucency and high strength/weight ratio characteristics, easy inclusion and combination with other materials [28].

In the search of an alternative to alloys, carbon fiber-reinforced cement (CFRC) materials were preferred to carbon fiber-reinforced plastic (CFRP) materials because they do not degrade with time, are not sensitive to stress corrosion, or do not release soluble products. They have better aging properties than CFPR and can be subjected to surface densification, can be porous and allow bony ingrowth, and can be coated with osteophytic materials. CFs are prepared from polyacrylonitrile in three steps: stretching of molecular chains followed with stabilization by spared oxidation and finally carbonization at high temperature ($T \gg 1000\,°C$). The material, being porous (5–30%), needs to be densified later on by chemical vapor infiltration (CVI) of pyrolytic carbon. In addition to high mechanical strength, articular surface replacements require materials with low friction coefficient and low wear. Carbon–ceramic composites were produced with CVI of silicon carbide (SiC) into CFRC with a final 35% concentration of SiC [29].

BC nanofibers and fibrous silk (FS) film were combined to produce BC–FS composite material with enhanced mechanical properties: pure SF film had an ultimate tensile stress of 67.7 ± 3.2 MPa and was calculated to have Young's modulus of 5.1 ± 0.1 GPa, while 0.4BC/0.6SF composite plate and 0.5BC/0.5SF composite plate had Young's modulus values of 9.6 ± 1.1 and 10.9 ± 0.9 GPa, respectively, which are higher than that of pure SF film. Young's modulus of the 0.6BC/0.4SF composite plate was more than double, from 5.1 ± 0.1 to 12.0 ± 1.5 GPa [30]. Figure 7.7 presents SEM images, showing enhanced mechanical properties of silk fibroin-based composite plates for fractured bone healing.

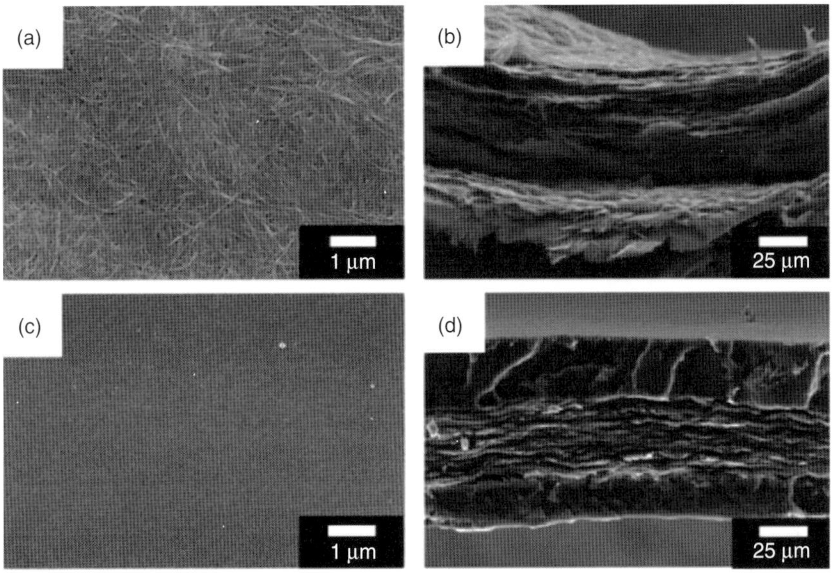

Figure 7.7 SEM photographs of surface and fractured surface of BC sheet (a, b), and of 0.6BC/0.4SF composite plate (c, d), respectively. (Choi *et al.* 2013 [30]. Reproduced with permission of Springer.)

Case Study 1: Mechanical Properties of Bone Cements and Tissue Interface Formation after Implantation

- The development of bioactive bone cement and its clinical applications was studied by Yamamuro *et al.* [31]. According to this study, mechanical property of bioactive bone (BA) cement was compared with polymethyl methacrylate (PMMA) cement, as it is shown in Table 7.5.
- Formation of interface between PMMA cement (PC) and bone (B) in the acetabulum at 6 months was observed. In the PMMA cement group, the histologic findings at the cement–bone interface were essentially the same at 1, 3, and 6 months, an intervening soft tissue layer being consistently present at the cement–bone interface, reproduced in Figure 7.8.

Table 7.5 Mechanical properties of BA cement in comparison with PMMA cement.

Mechanical properties	Bioactive Dough type	Bone cement Injection type	PMMA cement
Comprehensive strength (MPa)	270	220	95
Bending strength (MPa)	135	120	85
Tensile strength (MPa)	50	50	25
Fracture toughness (MPa $m^{0.5}$)	1.6	1.6	1.1

Source: Yamamuro *et al.* 1998 [31]. Reproduced with permission of Elsevier.

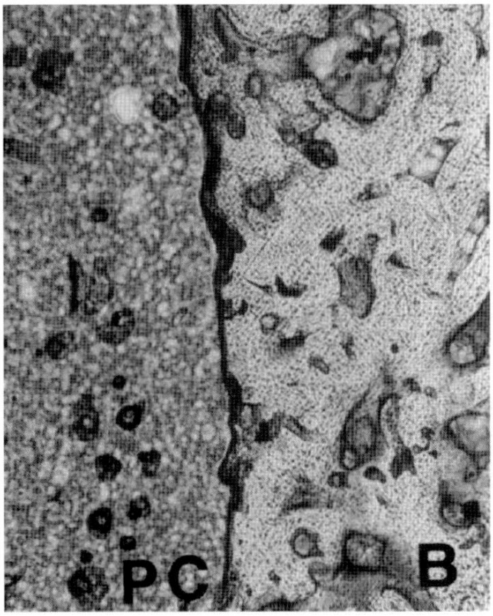

Figure 7.8 Case study: Giemsa surface staining showing an interface between PMMA cement (PC) and bone (B) in the acetabulum at 6 months. There is an intervening connective tissue layer between P and B (X20). (Yamamuro *et al.* 1998 [31]. Reproduced with permission of Elsevier.)

- Bonding strengths with BA cement at 1, 3, and 6 months after surgery were 2.6 ± 1.4, 3.2 ± 1.5, and 4.7 ± 1.0 MPa, respectively. Those with PMMA cement were 1.4 ± 1.0, 1.5 ± 1.2, and 1.0 ± 0.7 MPa, respectively. Thus, bonding strength with BA cement increased with time after surgery, while that with PMMA cement did not show significant change. Therefore, the bonding strength with BA cement became significantly greater than that with PMMA cement at 6 months.
- Affinity index was calculated for each section in % ratio and % ratio of the bone-bonding length against the total length of the cement–bone interface. The affinity indices in the BA cement group increased markedly with time in the femur as well as in the acetabulum, while those in the PMMA cement group did not show significant changes. The affinity indices in the BA cement group became greater than those in the PMMA cement group with statistical significance at 3 and 6 months after surgery [31].

Control Questions

1) Determine the subject and purpose of biomaterials science.
2) Describe the goals and problems of biomaterials science.
3) Discuss requirements for biomaterials.
4) Describe biomaterials used in the human body as damaged tissue or body part replacements.
5) Discuss about types and classifications of biomaterials. What are the main criteria on which the given classification was based?
6) Discuss the advantages of metallic biomaterials.

7) Describe the types of metallic biomaterials and metal alloys.
8) Describe the chemical composition of Ti alloys used for biomedical applications.
9) Determine composite biomaterials.
10) Describe the types of composite biomaterials used in the living body.
11) Discuss biologically inspired or materials produced by biomimetic way. What kind of advantages they possess compared with synthetic materials?
12) Discuss bone cement composite materials and their characteristics.
13) Describe hierarchical structure of bone and the main components composing bone.
14) Describe hierarchical structure of nacre. What is the difference between natural bone and nacre?
15) Describe carbon fiber composites and their characteristics.

References

1 Murphy, S.V. and Atala, A. (2014) 3D bioprinting of tissues and organs. *Nat. Biotechnol.*, **32**, 773–785.
2 Groen, N., Guvendiren, M., Rabitz, H., Welsh, W.J., Kohn, J., and de Boer, J. (2016) Stepping into the omics era: Opportunities and challenges for biomaterials science and engineering. *Acta Biomater.*, **1** (34), 133–142.
3 Hench, L.L. (1998) Bioceramics. *J. Am. Ceram. Soc.*, **81**, 1705–1728.
4 Huebsch, N. and Mooney, D.J. (2009) Inspiration and application in the evolution of biomaterials. *Nature*, **462** (26), 426–432.
5 Rahyussalim, A.J., Marsetio, A.F., Saleh, I., Kurniawati, T., and Whulanza, Y. (2016) The needs of current implant technology in orthopaedic prosthesis biomaterials application to reduce prosthesis failure rate. *J. Nanomater.*, Article ID 5386924, 9 pages, doi: 10.1155/2016/5386924
6 Wadood, A. (2016) Brief overview on nitinol as biomaterial. *Adv. Mater. Sci. Eng.*, Article ID 4173138, 9 pages, doi: 10.1155/2016/4173138
7 Mitragotri, S. *et al* (2009) Physical approaches to biomaterials design. *Nat. Mater.*, **8**, 15–23.
8 Park, J. and Lakes, R.S. (1992) *Biomaterials, An Introduction*, Springer. ISBN 978-0-387-37879-4.
9 Wong, J.Y., Bronzino, J.D., and Peterson, D.R. (2012) *Biomaterials: Principles and Practices*, CRC Press, ISBN: 9781439872512.
10 Manivasagam, G., Dhinasekaran, D., and Rajamanickam, A. (2010) Biomedical implants: corrosion and its prevention-a review. *Recent Pat. Corros. Sci.*, **2**, 40–54.
11 Suh. H. (1998), Recent advances in biomaterials, *Yonsei Med. J.* **39**(2):87–96.
12 Vallet-Regí, M. (2001) Ceramics for medical applications. *J. Chem. Soc., Dalton Trans.*, 97–108, DOI: 10.1039/B007852M.
13 Hanawa, T. (2002) Evaluation techniques of metallic biomaterials in vitro. *Sci. Technol. Adv. Mater.*, **3**, 289–295.

14 Hermawan, H., Dubé, D., and Mantovani, D. (2010) Degradable metallic biomaterials: design and development of Fe-Mn alloys for stents. *J. Biomed. Mater. Res. Part A*, **93** (1), 1–11.
15 Frosch, K.H. and Stürmer, K.M. (2006) Metallic biomaterials in skeletal repair. *Eur. J. Trauma*, **32**, 149–159.
16 Zhuravleva, K. *et al* (2013) Production of porous β-type Ti–40Nb alloy for biomedical applications: comparison of selective laser melting and hot pressing. *Materials*, **6**, 5700–5712.
17 Wang, K. (1996) The use of titanium for medical applications in the USA. *Mater. Sci. Eng., A*, **213**, 134–137.
18 Iftekhar, A. (2004) Biomedical composites, in *Standard Handbook of Biomedical Engineering and Design*, University of Minnesota, Minneapolis, The McGraw-Hill Co, Chapter 12.
19 Ramakrishna, S., Ramalingam, M., Sampath Kumar, T.S., and Soboyejo, W.O. (2010) *Biomaterials: A Nano Approach*, CRC Press, ISBN: 9781420047813.
20 Rosen, B.W. (1964) Failure of Composite Consisting of Matrix Stiffened by Uniaxially Oriented Fibers, When Subjected to Uniaxial Tensile Load Parallel to Fiber Direction, Structural Mechanics, 19650027655.
21 Miao, X. and Sun, D. (2010) Graded/gradient porous biomaterials. *Materials*, **3** (1), 26–47.
22 Agarwal, B.D. and Broutman, L.J. (1980) *Analysis and Performance of Fiber Composites*, John Wiley & Sons, Inc., New York, pp. 3–12.
23 Perez, R.A., Won, J.E., Knowles, J.C., and Kim, H.W. (2013) Naturally and synthetic smart composite biomaterials for tissue regeneration. *Adv. Drug Delivery Rev.*, **65** (4), 471–496.
24 Lapidot, S., Meirovitch, S., Sharon, S., Heyman, A., Kaplan, D.L., and Shoseyov, O. (2012) Clues for biomimetics from natural composite materials. *Nanomedicine (Lond)*, **7** (9), 1409–1423.
25 Wang, P. *et al* (2014) Bone tissue engineering via nanostructured calcium phosphate biomaterials and stem cells. *Bone Res.*, **2**, 14017.
26 Wegst, U.G.K., Bai, H., Saiz, E., Tomisa, A.P., and Ritchie, R.O. (2015) Bioinspired structural materials. *Nat. Mater.*, **16**, 23–36.
27 Tamaddon, M. and Czernuszka, J.T. (2013) The need for hierarchical scaffolds in bone tissue engineering. *Hard Tissue*, **2** (4), 37.
28 Saito, N., *et al.*, Safe clinical use of carbon nanotubes as innovative biomaterials, *Chem. Rev.* 2014, **114**, 6040–6079.
29 Christel, P., (1985) *Biomechanics: Current Interdisciplinary Research, Potential Applications of Carbon-Carbon Composite Materials for Total Joint Replacement*, vol.**2**, Developments in Biomechanics, SM Perren, E Schneider, Springer, pp 61–72.
30 Choi, Y., Cho, S.Y., Heo, S. *et al* (2013) Enhanced mechanical properties of silk fibroin-based composite plates for fractured bone healing. *Fibers Polym.*, **14**, 266.
31 Yamamuro, T. *et al* (1998) Development of bioactive bone cement and its clinical applications. *Biomaterials*, **16**, 1479–1482.

Further Reading

Bader, R. *et al* (2003) Carbon fibre-reinforced plastics as implant materials. *Orthopäde*, **32** (1), 32–40.

Badyalak, A.D. 2015, *Host Response to Biomaterials*. Academic Press, ISBN-13:978-0128001967.

Blazewicz, M. (2001) Carbon materials in the treatment of soft and hard tissue injuries. *Eur. Cells Mater.*, **2**, 21–29.

Brunski, J. (1996) in *Biomaterials Science, An Introduction to Materials in Medicine* (eds B.D. Ratner *et al*), Elsevier Academic Press, San Diego, CA, p. 37.

Gauthier, O., Khairoun, I., Bosco, J., Obadia, L., Bourges, X., Rau, C., Magne, D., Bouler, J.M., Aguado, E., Daculsi, G., Weiss P., (2003), Noninvasive bone replacement with a new injectable calcium phosphate biomaterial, *J. Biomed. Mater. Res. Part A*, **66**(1), 47–54.

Griffith, L.G. and Naughton, G. (2002) Tissue engineering-current challenges and expanding opportunities. *Science*, **295** (5557), 1009–1014.

Ikada, Y. (2006) Challenges in tissue engineering. *J. R. Soc. Interface*, **3** (10), 589–601.

Leaversuch, R. (2003) New twist in thermoplastic composites makes high-strength, net-shape fasteners. *Plast. Technol.*, **49**, 49.

Longo, J.A., Koeneman, J.B., Orthopedic applications of carbon fiber composites, Chapter, *Biomaterials Engineering and Devices: Human Applications*, DL Wise, DJ Trantolo, K-U Lewandrowski, JD Gresser, MV Cattaneo, MJ Yaszemski, eds. Humana Press, 2000, pp. 203–214.

Mano, J.F. *et al* (2004) Bioinert, biodegradable and injectable polymeric matrix composites for hard tissue replacement: state of the art and recent developments. *Compos. Sci. Technol.*, **64**, 789–817.

Mayer, J. *et al.* (2000) New injection molding technologies for carbon fiber reinforced polyetheretherketone (PEEK) applied to highly loaded, anisotropic implants. Sixth World Biomaterials Congress Transactions 3, May 2000.

Moumene, M. *et al.* (2001) Carbon Fiber/PEEK composite stackable cage implants: a biomechanical evaluation. 27th Annual Meeting Transactions Society for Biomaterials, May 15–20, Society for Biomaterials, Mt. Laurel, NJ.

Poitout, D.G. (2016) *Biomechanics and Biomaterials in Orthopedics*, 2nd edn, Springer, 547 p., ISBN: 1848826648, 9781848826649..

Scotchford, C.A. *et al* (2003) Use of a novel carbon fibre composite material for the femoral stem component of a THR system. In vitro biological assessment. *Biomaterials*, **26**, 4871–4879.

Wen, X., Wang, X., and Zhang, N. (1996) Microrough surface of metallic biomaterials: a literature review. *Bio-Med. Mater. Eng.*, **6** (3), 173–189.

8

Properties of Biomaterials

The body is a big wisdom, a plurality with one sense, a war and a peace, a flock and a shepherd.

Friedrich Nietzsche, expressionist (1844–1900)

8.1 Mechanical Properties of Biomaterials

Biomaterials exhibit a number of mechanical properties, such as *stress shielding*, which can be prevented by matching the modulus of elasticity of biomaterials to that of bone, which varies from 4 to 30 GPa. Additionally, the material should have a low modulus combined with high strength to prolong the service period of the implant and prevent loosening, thereby preventing the need for revision surgery.

High wear resistance: The material should have a high wear resistance and exhibit a low friction coefficient when sliding against body tissues. An increase in the friction coefficient or a decrease in the wear resistance can cause the implant to loosen. Moreover, the wear debris generated can cause inflammation that is destructive to the bone supporting the implant.

Long fatigue life: The material should exhibit a high resistance to failure by fatigue to prevent implant failure and stress shielding from fatigue fracture. The failure of implants by fatigue has been reported for hip prostheses [1].

8.1.1 Mechanical Properties of Biomaterials

The mechanical properties of materials describe their ability to withstand applied loads and displacements. *Stiffness* is related to the elastic modulus, and defines the force required to produce elastic deformation; as such, Young's modulus E is defined by the initial slope of the uniaxial stress–strain curve, where the strains are recoverable (elastic). *Strength*, defined by the yield stress at the onset of permanent (plastic) deformation or by the maximum strength at the peak load before fracture, is a measure of the force per unit area that the material can withstand. *Hardness* – another measure of strength – is estimated from the extent of penetration of an indenter into the surface of the material under an applied load. *Ductility* is a measure of the maximum strain before fracture,

Nano- and Biomaterials: Compounds, Properties, Characterization, and Applications,
First Edition. Zhypargul Abdullaeva.

and is generally assessed as the per cent elongation of the sample or its relative change in cross-sectional area. *Toughness* measures resistance to fracture; it can be assessed in terms of the area under the load–displacement curve, but is better evaluated using the methodologies of fracture mechanics. *Fracture mechanics*: To evaluate fracture resistance quantitatively, fracture mechanics is used. In linear elastic fracture mechanics (LEFM), the material is considered to be nominally elastic, with the plastic zone remaining small compared with the in-plane specimen dimensions. The local stresses, σ_{ij}, at distance r and angle θ from the tip of a crack, can be expressed (as $r \rightarrow 0$) by $\sigma_{ij} \rightarrow (K/(2\pi r)^{1/2}) f_{ij}(\theta)$, where $f_{ij}(\theta)$ is an angular function of θ and K is the stress intensity, which is defined in terms of the applied stress, σ_{app}, crack length a and a geometry function Q. Hence the stress intensity, $K = \sigma_{\text{app}}(\pi a)^{1/2}$, represents the magnitude of the local stress (and displacement) fields. Provided that K characterizes these fields over dimensions relevant to local fracture events, it is deemed to reach a critical value – the fracture toughness – at $K = K_c$, provided that small-scale yielding prevails; for plane-strain conditions, the plastic zone must also be small compared with the thickness dimension. An equivalent approach involves the strain-energy release rate, G, which is defined as the rate of change in potential energy per unit increase in crack area. For linear elastic materials under mode I (tensile opening) conditions, G and K are simply related by $G = K^2/E$ [2]. (reprinted by permission from Macmillan Publishers Ltd: [Nature Materials, 14, p. 23–36] (Bioinspired structural materials, Wegst, U.G.K., *et al.*), copyright (2014))

The mechanical properties of metallic biomaterials such as Young's modulus, yield strength, tensile strength, and fatigue limit were compared for stainless steel Co–Cr alloys, titanium (Ti), Ti–6Al–4V, and cortical bone in Table 8.1.

Concerning *Young's modulus*, the level of the value of Young's modulus, which is effective to prevent stress shielding between the implant made of low Young's modulus β-type titanium alloy and bone, should be proved. The effect of Young's modulus on bone atrophy has previously been investigated using implants made of titanium alloys with different Young's moduli. Figure 8.1 shows the relationships between the tensile properties and working ratio of TNTZ subjected to cold working by general cold rolling or swaging. The tensile strength and 0.2% proof stress increase with an increase in the working ratio and become almost equal to those of Ti–6Al–4V ELI (having tensile strength of around 800 MPa) with good

Table 8.1 Comparison of mechanical properties of metallic biomaterials with bone.

Material	Young's modulus, *E* (GPa)	Yield strength (MPa)	Tensile strength (MPa)	Fatigue limit (MPa)
Stainless steel	190	221–1213	586–1351	241–820
Co–Cr alloys	210–253	448–1606	655–1896	207–950
Titanium (Ti)	110	485	760	300
Ti–6Al–4V	116	896–1034	965–1103	620
Cortical bone	15–30	30–70	70–150	

Source: Hussein *et al.* 2015 [1]. http://www.mdpi.com/1996-1944/8/5/2749/htm. Used under: https://creativecommons.org/licenses/by/4.0/.

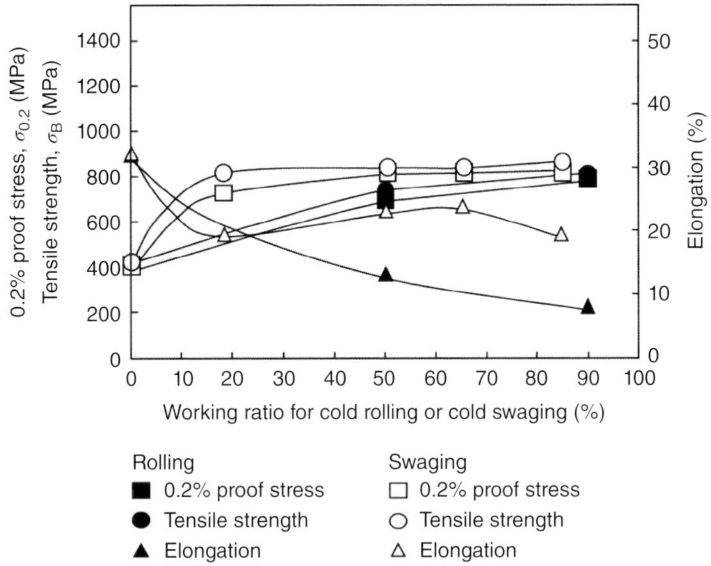

Figure 8.1 Tensile properties of TNTZ subjected to cold rolling or old swaging as a function of working ratio. (Niinomi and Nakai 2011 [3]. https://www.hindawi.com/journals/ijbm/2011/836587/abs/. Used under: https://creativecommons.org/licenses/by/3.0/.)

elongation of TNTZ subjected to both cold rolling and cold swaging. Young's modulus of TNTZ subjected to cold rolling or cold swaging is almost constant with increasing working ratio and tends to decrease when the working ratio is high because the trend of the formation of the texture becomes significant.

8.1.2 Titanium Alloy with Self-Adjustable Young's Modulus

While using low modulus titanium alloys, some surgeons specializing in spinal diseases, such as scoliosis, spondylolisthesis, and spine fracture, pointed out that the amount of spring back in the implant rods should be small so that the implant offers better handling ability during surgeries. The implant rods undergo bending when they are manually handled by surgeons within the small space inside the patient's body for *in situ* spine contouring. It is considered that the amount of spring back depends on both the strength and Young's modulus of the implant rod. If two implant rods having the same strength but with different Young's moduli are used, the implant rod having lower Young's modulus shows greater spring back. Implant rods made of low modulus titanium alloys exhibit lower Young's modulus, resulting in greater spring back. Thus, low Young's modulus, which is one of the key features of β-type titanium alloys such as TNTZ as a metallic biomaterial, is obviously a desirable property for patients but becomes an undesirable property for surgeons. Titanium alloys, which satisfy the requirements of both surgeons and patients with regard to Young's modulus of the implant rod, are currently being developed. The amount of spring back is considered to be small for the alloy having higher Young's modulus as compared with that of one having low Young's modulus as schematically shown in Figure 8.2. Therefore, the

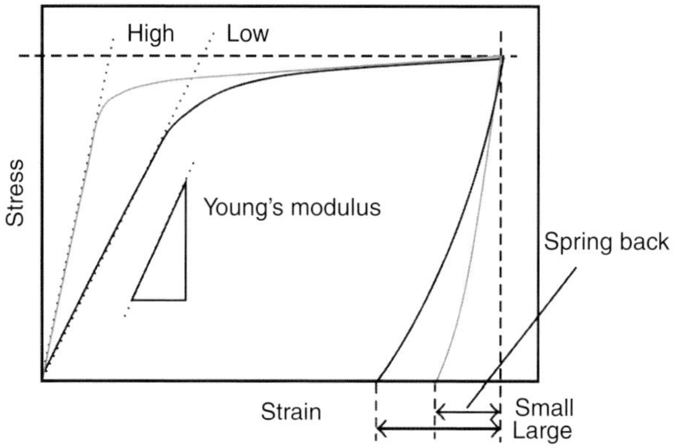

Figure 8.2 Schematic of relationship between Young's modulus and spring back. (Niinomi and Nakai 2011 [3]. https://www.hindawi.com/journals/ijbm/2011/836587/abs/. Used under: https://creativecommons.org/licenses/by/3.0/.)

low Young's modulus β-type titanium alloy, whose Young's modulus varies and becomes high only at the deformed part, is considered to reduce spring back and satisfy the low Young's modulus condition as well. This concept is called self-adjustment of Young's modulus. In general, Young's modulus of metals and alloys does not drastically change by deformation. However, in the case of certain metastable β-type titanium alloys, nonequilibrium phases such as α′, α″, and ω phases appear in the β matrix during deformation. If Young's modulus of the deformation-induced phase is higher than that of the original β phase, Young's modulus of only the deformed part of the implant rod increases, whereas that of the nondeformed part remains low. In orthopedic operations performed for the treatment of spinal diseases, the implant rod is bent by the surgeons so that it corresponds to the curvature of the spine.

Therefore, if a suitable titanium alloy is employed as the implant rod material, spring back can be suppressed by the deformation-induced phase transformation that occurs during bending in the course of operation, while low Young's modulus can be retained for patients. In general, Young's modulus of ω phase is much greater than those of the α, α′, α″, and β phases. Among these phases, the ω, α′, and α″ phases can be induced by deformation in β-type titanium alloys with certain chemical compositions [3].

8.1.3 Wear Resistance of Biomaterials Used in the Living Body

Table 8.2 lists various developed materials and their fabrication techniques, the types of wear tests, and the parameters used to characterize wear, along with a summary of the results obtained by various researchers.

There are some techniques for improving the wear resistance of metallic biomaterials:

- *Ion implantation (physical deposition)* is considered a simple technique for significantly modifying the physical and/or chemical properties of the near surface of a material in which suitable ions are embedded into the surface of

Table 8.2 Wear studies of metallic biomaterials.

References	Material and fabrication processes	Experimental test techniques and parameters	Main results
Cvijovic'-Alagic *et al.* [36]	Ti–13Nb–13Zr Ti–6Al–4V Arc melting	A block-on-disc tribometer was used to conduct wear and friction tests in a simulated body fluid (Ringer's solution) *Temperature*: ambient *Normal load*: 20–60 N *Sliding speed*: 0.26–1.0 m s^{-1}	The Ti–6Al–4V alloy showed a higher wear resistance than the Ti–13Nb–13Zr alloy Abrasion was the primary wear mechanism
Stefano Gialanella *et al.* [37]	NiTi commercial alloy	A *block-on-disc* was used to measure dry sliding wear. A profilometer was used to quantify wear *Sliding speed*: 0.837 m s^{-1} *Sliding distance*: 1004 m *Loads*: 50–200 N	A NiTi/WC–Co coupling exhibited a high wear rate *Wear mechanism*: a transition from delamination wear to a regime featuring a mixture of delamination and oxidation wear
K.S. Suresh *et al.* [38]	Ti–13Nb–13Zr Equal channel angular pressing (ECAE)	A tribometer was used as a lubricity fretting test system for texture and wear behavior; fretting wear and 3D surface texture measurements were performed *Normal loads*: 6 N *Frequency*: 20 Hz *Temperature*: 37 ± 0.1 °C	The grain size and the texture of material affected the wear of the surface. There was no difference in the friction coefficient between the ECAE-processed and as-received samples
Li-juan Xu *et al.* [39]	β-Type Ti–15Mo–*x*Nb arc-melting vacuum-pressure casting system	A *ball-on-disc* was used for dry wear tests *Normal load*: 1 and 2 N *Test-disc rate*: 100 r min^{-1}	The lowest friction coefficient was obtained for a Ti–15Mo–5Nb alloy under a 1 N load. Adhesion was the primary wear mechanism
M. Fellah *et al.* [41]	Ti–6Al–7Nb and AISI 316L stainless steel	*Ball-on-disc* and sphere-on-plane *Load*: 3, 6, and 10 N *Sliding speed*: 1, 15, and 25 mm s^{-1}	The same mechanisms of wear and friction were found for all of the tested samples
S.J. Li *et al.* [42]	Ti–Nb–Ta–Zr and Ti–6Al–4V induction skull melting method	*Reciprocal pin-on-disc* in a 0.9% NaCl solution *Reciprocating velocity*: 45 rpm *Sliding distance*: 30 km	The wear resistance of Ti–29Nb–13Ta–4.6Zr was enhanced by incorporating Nb_2O_5 oxide particles into the diffusion-hardened surface of the alloy

(*Continued*)

Table 8.2 (Continued)

References	Material and fabrication processes	Experimental test techniques and parameters	Main results
Animesh Choubey *et al.* [45]	CP titanium, Ti–6Al–4V, Ti–5Al–2.5Fe, Ti–13Nb–13Zr, and Co–28Cr–6Mo	*Ball-on-flat fretting* wear tester: Hanks' balanced salt solution *Normal load*: 10 N for 10 000 cycles *Frequency*: 10 Hz	The primary wear mechanisms of Ti alloys were tribomechanical abrasion, transfer layer formation, and cracking
A. Iwabuchi *et al.* [46]	Co–29Cr–6Mo alloy and Ti–6Al–4V	*Fretting apparatus and a reciprocating* sliding tribometer: Quasi-body fluid, Hanks's solution *Normal load*: 5 N; *frequency*: 10 Hz *Temperature* in the solutions: 37 ± 2 °C	Co alloy exhibited good wear resistance; Ti alloy exhibited good fretting resistance
X. Luo *et al.* [47]	ASTM F1537 Co–Cr alloy	*Pin-on-disc* tribometer *Load*: 20 N *Rotation speed*: 60 rpm	The tribocorrosion properties of the Co–Cr alloy were enhanced by a layer of the S-phase
Akihiko Chiba *et al.* [48]	Co–CrMo forged	*Pin-on-disc* *Load*: 9.8 N 24 rpm	Forged CoCr exhibited a lower wear loss than a cast CoCr alloy
S. M. T. Chan *et al.* [49]	(CoCr), stainless steel (SS)	*Pin-on-disc sliding speed*: 0.5 mm s^{-1}, 5 mm wear track radius *Normal load*: 1.8 N	
Alfons Fischer *et al.* [50]	AISI 316L Co–29Cr–6Mo	Pin-on-disc for dry sliding wear tests *Load*: 5 N *Relative velocity*: 0.1 m s^{-1} *Ambient temperature*: 25 °C	Ni-free high-nitrogen steel and LC-CoCrMo alloy exhibited higher wear resistance and dry friction than Ni-containing austenitic steels
A. Igual Muñoz *et al.* [40]	Co–Cr–Mo Low and high carbon	*Tribocorrosion techniques* *Load*: 1.2 N; *frequency*: 1 Hz. *Temperature*: 37 ± 0.1 °C Simulated body fluids [NaCl and phosphate-buffered solutions (PBS) with and without albumin]	LC CoCrMo had a higher wear resistance in NaCl and PBS albumin than HC No differences were observed for the alloys in the other solutions
M. Alvarez-Vera *et al.* [51]	Co–Cr alloy with boron additions (0, 0.3, 0.6, and 1 B wt%) by casting method	Three-axial hip joint simulator	Wear resistance as the boron increased

Table 8.2 (Continued)

References	Material and fabrication processes	Experimental test techniques and parameters	Main results
L. Mohan *et al.* [52]	Commercially pure titanium (CP-Ti) parts produced using selective laser melting (SLM) and casting	A pin-on-disc at room temperature A stainless steel disc of 45 mm diameter *loads*: (15, 20, 25, and 30 N) *Sliding speed*: 0.5 m s^{-1} for 15 min	SLM CP-Ti showed better wear resistance compared to casting as a result of fine grains and higher microhardness

Source: Hussein *et al.* 2015 [1]. http://www.mdpi.com/1996-1944/8/5/2749/htm. Used under: https://creativecommons.org/licenses/by/4.0/.

a material from a beam of ionized particles. This technique has been reported to improve the wear performance of Ti–6Al–4V and Co–28Cr–6Mo alloys.
- *Nitriding* (a thermochemical surface treatment) has been used to increase the resistance of a Ti–6Al–4V alloy to dry wear.
- *Carburization and boriding* techniques are used to enhance surface hardness, which in turn improves wear resistance.
- *Plasma spray coating* has also been used to enhance the wear resistance of few biomaterials [1].

8.2 Biological Properties of Biomaterials

The physicochemical and biological properties of a novel biodegradable composite scaffold made of nano-hydroxyapatite and naturally derived polymers of chitosan (CS) and carboxymethyl cellulose (CMC), namely, *n*-HA/CS/CMC, which was prepared by freeze-drying method, were studied. CS, a deacetylated derivative of chitin, is a biodegradable and biocompatible cationic natural polymer, and CS-based materials can accelerate bone formation because of their similarity to glycosaminoglycans (GAGs) in structure. Consequently, *n*-HA/CS composite scaffold has been widely studied for bone tissue engineering. However a poor interaction exists between *n*-HA and CS phases so that the *n*-HA/CS composite scaffold has poor physicochemical properties. Fortunately, CMC is a natural biodegradable and biocompatible anionic polymer obtained from natural cellulose by chemical modification, and it is very similar to CS in structure; thus, there is strong ionic cross-linking action between CMC and CS. Besides, its biological properties such as cell biocompatibility *in vitro* and tissue biocompatibility *in vivo* by a short period implantation were also preliminarily studied [4].

8.2.1 *In Vivo* Tissue Biocompatibility

Tissue biocompatibility *in vivo* of the scaffold was evaluated by a short-time implantation in muscles of rats and harvesting after 2 and 4 weeks. During the experiment period, all rats remained in good health, and the surgical incisions healed well without any wound complications. After 2 and 4 weeks' harvest, the histological sections of the scaffold specimen were stained with H&E and Masson's trichrome. The muscle cells were normal and there were no evident foreign body reactions for the surrounding tissues at 2-week implantation. After 4-week implantation, it could be seen that the scaffold integrated well with surrounding tissues and there was no visible interface between the muscle (M) and the scaffold (S). Meanwhile, it can be found that most of the scaffold had been biodegraded and many blood vessels (BV) had grown into the pores of the scaffold where the histological sections were stained with Masson's trichrome, which was used to assess the formation of collagen and vascularization. After 2-week implantation, there was bulk collage appearing after 4 weeks; most surface of the scaffold was covered by collagen, indicating that the scaffold had good biocompatibility. Additionally, a large number of small blood vessels were also seen in the scaffold, which was favorable to deliver nutrient and ensured cells to survive and proliferate so as to construct new tissues. The information of the cell attachment and proliferation on the scaffold provided by cell culture experiment *in vitro* is often used as an important initial evaluation of cell biocompatibility (Figure 8.3).

In the present study, MG63 and MSCs are used in the cell seeding experiment; the phase-contrast microscopy observation and the MTT assay results show that the *n*-HA/CS/CMC scaffold is nontoxic and cell biocompatible, which contributed to the ideal three-dimensional porous structure and mechanical property. However, the chemical composition and the method of fabrication of the scaffold play a more important role in cell biocompatibility. Moreover, compared with other methods to develop porous scaffold, such as particulate leaching or foaming method, the method here avoided using any poisonous solvents in the process of preparation. Therefore, the scaffold is cell biocompatible, and it is suitable for implantation. Although *in vitro* test has given some preliminary indicatives of cell biocompatibility, it is still necessary to procure a much clearer idea of host tissue response to the scaffold after implantation

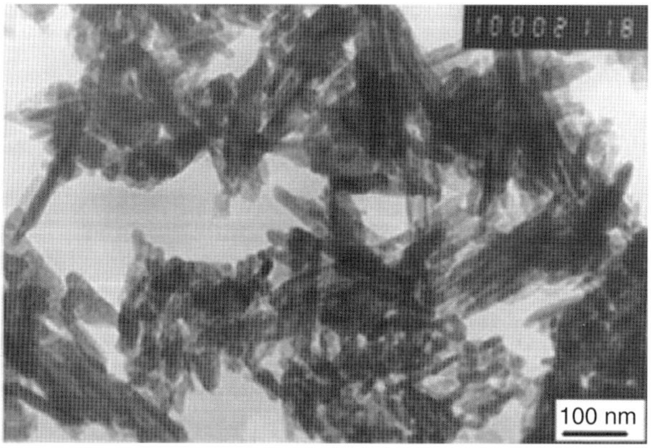

Figure 8.3 The TEM photograph of *n*-HA/CS/CMC composite. (Liuyun *et al.* 2009 [4]. http://jbiomedsci.biomedcentral.com/articles/10.1186/1423-0127-16-65. Used under: https://creativecommons.org/licenses/by/2.0/.)

in vivo. In this study, the scaffold was placed in the muscle of rats for 4 weeks. For the short period implantation, from rough observation, it was found that all experimented rats survived before harvesting, which shows that the sample of implantation is nontoxic and there was no evident feign body reaction. By observing histological sections, we find that most of the scaffold had been biodegraded after 4 weeks, which results from the biodegradable component of CS and CMC, and it is useful to blood vessels and new tissues to ingrowth [4].

The nascent field of biological-based materials science can be divided into three broad (and overlapping) areas: (i) *biological materials*, the study of natural materials (e.g., bone, feathers, skin); (ii) *biomimetics or bioinspired materials design*, the synthesis of novel materials, devices, and structures inspired on biology; and (iii) *biomaterials*, the application of materials in the biomedical arena (e.g., implants).

Biological constituents: Biological materials are composed of only a few elements. If one considers that there are approximately 100 stable elements in the periodic table, only ~10% are found as the building blocks of organic and inorganic tissues. Notable are the deficiency of metallic elements and the prevalence of the lightest elements – the first two rows of the table.

Biopolymers: The structural organic constituents of biological tissues are either protein-forming polypeptides (primarily, in biological materials, collagen, keratin, elastin, resilin, fibroin, or abductin) or polysaccharides (chitin, cellulose) as shown in Table 8.1. Structural proteins can be further divided into those that are dominated by stiff secondary structure regions (such as triple helix in collagen or β-sheet strands in silk or β-keratin) and those that mostly contain amorphous random-coil domains (as found in elastin, resilin, and abductin). The stiffness of these crystalline biopolymers is generally orders of magnitude greater than the amorphous ones, but they have strains to failure orders of magnitude lower (Table 8.3) – the elastic energy is stored in the atomic bonds in the crystalline biopolymers, whereas it is stored as entropy changes in the elastomeric biopolymers.

Proteins: Crystalline protein molecules have a few well-defined secondary structures such as the α-helix, the β-sheet, the β-turn, and the coiled coil (supercoil bundle of at least two α-helices). Proteins are long-chain amino acids whose side chains have various sizes (and hence steric constraints), charges, and hydrophobic/hydrophilic characteristics [5].

Keratins are composed of two α-helices bundling into a superhelix coiled coil. In mammals, this coiled-coil structure is the primary constituent of hair, nails, hooves, horns, and the epidermal layer of the skin. In reptiles and birds, the claws, scales, feathers, and beaks are β-keratin, tougher than the α-form, and are usually configured into a β-pleated sheet arrangement. *Elastin* is found in vertebrates (skin, arterial walls, *ligamentum nuchae* in the neck of ungulates), resilin is found in insect flight systems, abductin is found in the hinges of bivalve mollusks, and fibroin is found in spider and silkworm silk. These fibers provide extensive elasticity and resilience in tissues that undergo reversible, repetitive deformation. For elastin, there are several distinct morphologies: in the skin and lungs as rope-like networks, in blood vessels as thin concentric sheets, and in the cartilage as three-dimensional cellular structures. *Resilin* has been

Table 8.3 Stiffness, tensile strength, and strain failure for selected biological and synthetic materials.

Biopolymers	*E* (MPa)	σ_f (MPa)	ε_f	References
Abductin	1–4			[98, 99]
Cellulose	150 000	18	0.024	[99]
Collagen (along fibers)	1 000	50	0.09	[2009, 99]
Elastin	0.3–1.5		>2	[8, 99, 100]
Fibroin	10 000	70	0.09	[99]
Keratin (wool)	5 000	200	0.5	[101]
Kevlar 49 fiber	130 000	3600	0.03	[102]
PMMA	1 600	15	0.013	[103]
Resilin	0.6–1.8	3	>3	[2009, 104]
Rubber	0.01–0.1	15	8.5	
Silk				
Cocoon silk (*Bombyx mori*)	7	600		[102]
Spider silk (web frame and dragline, major ampullate) *Araneus diadematus*)	10 000	1100	0.18	[101]
Spider silk (viscid, catching spiral, *Araneus diadematus*)	3	500	0.27	[101]
Tendon	2 000–9 000	50–100	0.09	[2009, 105]
Biominerals				
Aragonite ($CaCO_3$)	72 000			[67, 106, 107]
Hydroxyapatite ($Ca_{10}(PO_4)_6(OH_2)$)	112 000	115		[108]
Hydroxyapatite (from enamel)	83 000	60		[109, 110, 111]
Magnetite (Fe_3O_4)	72 000			[106]
Radular teeth (Fe_3O_4 from chiton)	90 000–125 000			[106]
Silica ($SiO_2 \cdot nH_2O$)	600–2 000			[112]
Silicon carbide (SiC)	450 000			
Zirconia (ZrO_2)	200 000	250		
Biocomposites				
Bone				
Trabecular bone	800–14 000	1–100		[3]
Cortical bone (longitudinal)	6 000–20 000	30–150	0.03	[3]
Nacre (abalone)	40 000–70 000	160		[61]
Wood (oak)	10 000	100		

Source: Chen *et al.* 2012 [5]. Reproduced with permission of Elsevier.

hard to be examined since only small portions are available from insects. It is extremely resilient and also has excellent fatigue properties, and successful recombinant expression in bacterial cultures has been obtained. In the 1960s, Weis-Fogh first described the chemical and mechanical properties of resilin. He found that it could be stretched up to 300% and, when unloaded, regained its

Table 8.4 Comparison of mechanical properties of keratinized materials and other biological and synthetic materials.

	Elastic modulus (GPa)	Tensile strength (MPa)	Bending strength (MPa)	Toughness ($MJ\,m^{-3}$)	Work of fracture ($kJ\,m^{-2}$)	Moisture content (wt% water)	References
Oryx horn (*Oryx gazella*)	4.3		212		19	na	[20]
	6.1	137				0	[28]
	4.3	122				20	[28]
	1.8	56				40	[28]
Waterbuck horn (*Kobus ellipsiprymnus*)	3.3		245		20	na	[20]
Sheep horn (*Ovis canadensis*)	4.1		228		22	na	[20]
	9					0	[30]
	1.5					20	[30]
	2.20		127.1	56–74		10.6	a)
	0.81		3.1	12–18		34.5	a)
Bovine hoof	0.4	16.2	14.3			29.9	[12]
Equine hoof	2.6	38.9				18.2	[13]
	0.2		19.4			41% RH	[40]
	0.3–0.6	6.5–9.5				100% RH	[10]
Bovine femur bone		148				Hydrated	[41]
	13.5		246.7		1.7		[42]
Antler bone (*Cervus canadensis*)					6.2	Hydrated	[42]
	7		145				[39]
Red abalone shell (*Haliotis rufescens*)	70			12.4		Hydrated	[7]
		170					[43]
Fiberglass			197		90		[44]
	5.9	110					[45]
Polycarbonate	2.4	67			33		[46]
				33			[47]

a) This work (longitudinal direction — radial direction).
RH, relative humidity; na, not available.
Source: Tombolato *et al.* 2010 [6]. Reproduced with permission of Elsevier.

original shape. Hooves are the most similar biological material to horns and have been the subject of the largest body of scientific literature. They contain tubules ~220 μm × 140 μm in major and minor axes, respectively, with a medullary cavity of ~50 μm [5]. Bovine hooves are similar to equine hooves in both structure and properties, as shown in Table 8.4.

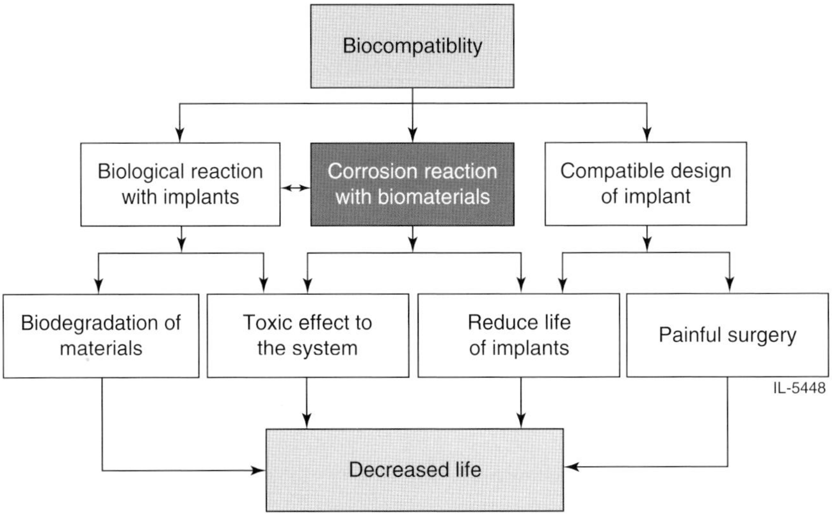

Figure 8.4 Factors affecting biocompatibility. (Singh *et al.* 2007 [7]. Reproduced with permission of Springer.)

Biocompatibility of biomaterials (or implant devices) used in the living body can be affected by three main factors, such as biological reaction of tissue with implants, corrosion reaction with biomaterials, and compatible design of implants (Figure 8.4).

Inappropriate design of implant devices, unwanted device degradation/corrosion, and/or development of adverse host tissue reaction can lead to device failure, leading to reactions that are usually undesirable and have the potential to cause chronic inflammation and/or hypersensitivity [7].

8.3 Chemical Properties of Biomaterials

One of the early examples of the use of bioclick reaction to design biomaterials was reported in 2003 by Lutolf and Hubbell, who explored Michael-type addition reactions between vinyl-sulfone-terminated 4-arm poly(ethylene glycol) (PEG) star polymers and bis-cysteine peptides to generate hydrogels. These peptide-functionalized materials were successfully designed to serve as local delivery vehicles to present signals to cells and as a matrix to promote wound healing. This synthetic strategy and approach has been greatly expanded in the drug delivery and tissue engineering communities to engineer materials with tailorable properties. Zhong and Feijen and coworkers have used Michael-type conjugation chemistries to prepare degradable hydrogels from thiol-functionalized dextran and vinyl-sulfone-conjugated dextran or acrylate-functionalized 4-arm PEG star polymers. More recently, Wagner and coworkers reported the use of Michael-type addition between thiols and acrylates and maleimides to synthesize biodegradable polyurethane urea elastomers. In addition to CuAAC and SPAAC, a number of other cycloaddition reactions are of increasing interest for the synthesis of biologically related polymers.

Many of these proceed in aqueous media at room temperature without the need for a catalyst and thus are attractive alternatives, for example, CuAAC. For example, Shoichet *et al.* prepared hyaluronic acid hydrogels via Diels–Alder click chemistry from furan-modified hyaluronic acid and PEG dimaleimide. Ninh and Bettinger used this chemistry to synthesize reconfigurable, biodegradable shape-memory elastomers. Another interesting conjugation strategy is the hetero-Diels–Alder reaction (HDA) between reactive dienes and highly electron-deficient thiocarbonyl thiol compounds. This approach is intriguing since polymers that incorporate such electron-deficient groups can be prepared by RAFT polymerization using, for example, benzyl pyridine-2-yldithioformiate. HDA cycloaddition chemistry has been used to graft poly(isobornyl acrylate) onto cellulose substrates that present cyclopentadienyl functionalities. Anseth and coworkers explored the inverse electron demand Diels–Alder click reaction between tetrazine-functionalized 4-arm PEG prepolymers and a dinorbornene peptide cross-linker to obtain cell-instructive hydrogels [8].

Faster or even very fast reaction kinetics is shown in Figure 8.5 illustrating some factors that have influence on the chemical reactivity of biomaterials [9].

Chemical behavior related to corrosion degradation and oxidation for some Ti and Ti alloys is listed in Tables 8.5 and 8.6. Different from metal and ceramic biomaterials, polymers tend to undergo degradation by wear, swelling, leaching, and chemical ways, while metal and ceramic biomaterials by corrosion and mechanical degradation [7].

As it is seen from Table 8.6, chemical oxidation occurs for metal biomaterials depending on their chemical compositions and elemental content quantities.

Titanium, which is used for dental implants and in orthopedic devices, provides a specific example. When fresh titanium is exposed to air, it reacts rapidly with atmospheric oxygen to form a surface oxide, which is typically a few nanometers thick. The composition and thickness of this oxide layer

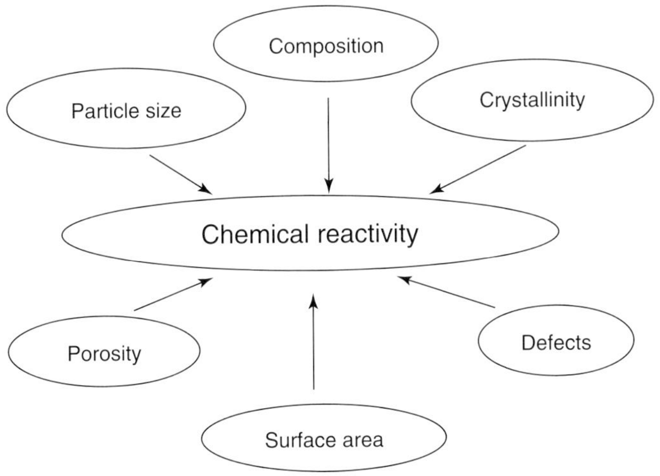

Figure 8.5 Some factors that have influence on the chemical reactivity of substances. (Vallet-Regí 2001 [9]. Reproduced with permission of Royal Society of Chemistry.)

Table 8.5 Types of biomedical materials and their applications.

Biomaterials	Objectives	Degradation mechanism	Applications
Metals/alloys SS316L, Co–Cr alloys, Ti and Ti alloys, Ni–Ti alloy	Load bearing	Corrosion and mechanical	Fracture fixations, plates, screws, pins, nails, joint replacements, orthodontic wires, femoral stems, cases for pacemakers, supports for heart valves, dental implants, dental crowns, bridges, fillings, and inner ear bone replacements
Ceramics and carbon coatings, alumina, oxides, zirconia, glass, glass-ceramics, and hydroxyapatite (HAP)	High hardness, wear resistance, and better bone bonding	Corrosion and mechanical	Carbon in heart valves, dental implants, joint implants, coatings for dental and joint implants, fill bone voids/cavities by HAP, tissue scaffolds, drug delivery systems, and inner ear implants
Polymer ultrahigh molecular weight polyethylene, polyester, polytetrafluoroethylene, PMMA, hydrogels, silicone rubber, PGA/ PLA, collagen, cellulose, and chitosan	Articulating surface	Wear, swelling, leaching, chemical	Joint replacement, vascular grafts, bone cement, orthodontic devices (e.g., plates, dentures) contact and intraocular lenses, catheters, hand and toe joints, artificial tendon and ligament, reconstructive surgery, sutures, staples, tissue scaffolds, drug delivery systems, and hemostatic bandages, pace maker leads.

Source: Singh *et al.* 2007 [7]. Reproduced with permission of Springer.

Table 8.6 Types of oxide form on titanium and titanium alloys.

Material	TiO_2	Al_2O_3	Nb_2O_5	MoO_3/MoO_2	ZrO_2
CP Ti	Yes	Yes	No	No	No
Ti–6Al–4V	Yes	Yes	No	No	No
Ti–5Al–2.5Fe	Yes	Yes	No	No	No
Ti–6Al–7Nb	Yes	Yes	Yes	No	No
Ti–15Mo–5Zr–3Al	Yes	No	No	Yes	Yes

Source: Singh *et al.* 2007 [7]. Reproduced with permission of Springer.

have been extensively analyzed for a variety of treatment conditions. The oxide stoichiometry is approximately TiO_2. For oxidation temperatures <200 °C, the oxide appears amorphous and glass-like, while thicker oxides formed at elevated temperatures or by electrochemical oxidation are more crystalline [10].

8.3.1 Ceramic Biomaterials

Ceramic biomaterials are defined as materials used for the repair of living body and are made of various metal oxides, glasses, and bone composites.

Ceramics include a variety of biomaterials such as calcium and carbon phosphates and alumina, and hydroxyapatite (HAp) is used for oral and maxillofacial surgery as bone substitute and as coating for metal and carbon implants. Sales were expected to jump from M$128 in 1987 to M$344 in 2002 [11].

Ceramics used for the repair and reconstruction of diseased or damaged parts of the musculoskeletal system, termed bioceramics, may be bioinert (alumina, zirconia), resorbable (tricalcium phosphate), bioactive (hydroxyapatite, bioactive glasses, and glass-ceramics), or porous for tissue ingrowth (hydroxyapatite-coated metals, alumina); also, recent applications of ceramic biomaterials include replacements for the hips, knees, teeth, tendons, and ligaments and repair for periodontal disease, maxillofacial reconstruction, augmentation and stabilization of the jaw bone, spinal fusion, and bone fillers after tumor surgery [12].

Ceramic materials used for biomedical applications are divided into as follows:

i) Inert (Al_2O_3, ZrO_2, TiO_2, and pyrolytic carbon)
ii) Resorbable–bioactive (α-tricalcium phosphate (TCP), β-TCP, tetracalcium phosphate (TetCP), dicalcium phosphate dihydrate (DCPD), dicalcium phosphate anhydrous (DCPA), octacalcium phosphate (OCP), and HA (hydroxyapatite) with low crystallinity)
iii) Bioactive surface (HA sintered, bioactive glasses, bioactive glass-ceramics)

Chemical elements used in the manufacturing of ceramic biomaterials are aluminum, silicon, phosphorus, calcium, carbon, and other elements [9]. The main features of ceramic biomaterials are shown in Figure 8.6. According to this illustration, ceramic biomaterials tolerated by the living body tissues are of the bioactive, inert, and resorbable types. High compression resistance, high humidity degree, high surface tension, stiff (high) Young's modulus, brittle and enhanced cell, tissue adhesion, and low chemical reactivity properties highlight their biocompatibility.

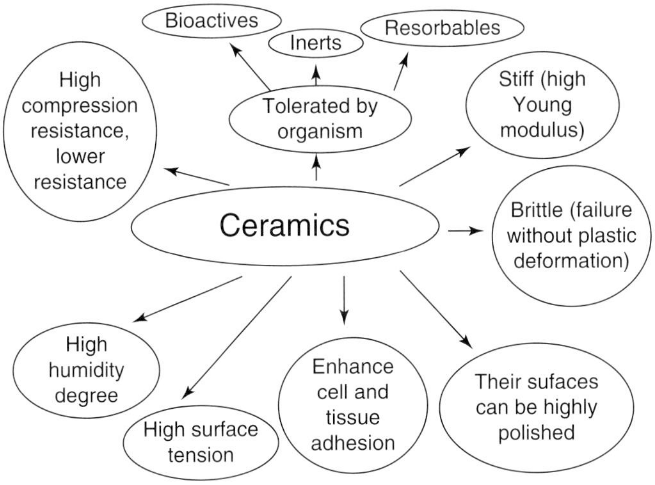

Figure 8.6 Main features of ceramic materials. (Vallet-Regí 2001 [9]. Reproduced with permission of Royal Society of Chemistry.)

Table 8.7 Types of bioceramics–tissue attachment and bioceramic classification.

Type of bioceramic	Type of attachment	Example
1	Dense, nonporous, nearly inert ceramics attach by bone growth into surface irregularities by cementing the device into the tissues or by press fitting into a defect (termed morphological fixation)	Al_2O_3 (single crystal and polycrystalline)
2	For porous inert implants, bone ingrowth occurs, which mechanically attaches the bone to the material (termed biological fixation)	Al_2O_3 (porous polycrystalline) Hydroxyapatite-coated porous metals
3	Dense, nonporous, surface reactive ceramics, glasses, and glass-ceramics attach directly by chemical bonding with the bone (termed bioactive fixation)	Bioactive glasses Bioactive glass-ceramics Hydroxyapatite
4	Dense, nonporous (or porous), resorbable ceramics are designed to be slowly replaced by bone	Calcium sulfate (plaster of Paris) Tricalcium phosphate Calcium phosphate salts

Source: Hench 1991 [12]. Reproduced with permission of John Wiley and Sons.

According to Hench [12], there are several kinds of ceramic biomaterials, classified depending on their attachment with living tissues (Table 8.7), and various kinds of bioactive glasses and glass ceramic materials (Table 8.8).

The main purpose of researchers in those years was to obtain glass ceramic materials combining a maximum strength, comparable with the strength of commonly used bioinert materials (metals and corundum ceramics), and bioactivity. To accomplish this purpose, such well-known techniques as powder technology of glass-ceramics, strengthening additives of zirconium oxide modified by yttrium oxide, and unidirectional growth of wollastonite crystals and chain calcium phosphates were used. In this way it became possible to obtain materials with bending strength of 200–600 MPa, preserving the capacity of intergrowth with adjacent bone [13], as represented in Table 8.9.

For a clearer understanding of the processes occurring in the zone of a material–bone contact, a series of experiments was carried out focusing on the behavior of various materials (silicate and phosphate glasses and glass-ceramics) in artificial media simulating *in vitro* the human physiological medium and blood plasma and experiments *in vivo* in contact with soft and bone tissues tested on animals. The results obtained pointed to numerous simultaneous reactions occurring in the intermediate layer between the bone and the implant with participation of the surface layer of the implant and the ambient physiological medium. As a consequence of studies performed, a scheme of interaction was proposed describing the sequence of processes on the surface of material (Figure 8.7). It should be noted that such scheme of bone structure formation is true for silicate systems, and a prerequisite for successful process is a silica

Table 8.8 Composition of bioactive glasses and glass-ceramics (wt%).

Component	45S5 Bioglass®	45S5, 4F Bioglass®	45B15S5 Bioglass®	KGC Ceravital®	KGS Ceravital®	KGy213 Ceravital®	A/W glass-ceramic	MB glass-ceramic	S45P7
SiO_2	45	45	30	46.2	46	38	34.2	19–52	45
P_2O_5	6	6	6				16.3	4–24	7
CaO	24.5	14.7	24.5	20.2	33	31	44.9	9 to 3	22
$Ca(PO_3)_2$		9.8		25.5	16	13.5			
CaF_2							0.5	5–15	
MgO				2.9			4.6		
MgF_2									
Na_2O	24.5	24.5	24.5	4.8	5	4		3–5	24
K_2O				0.4				3–5	
Al_2O_3						7		12–33	
Ba_2O_3			15						2
Ta_2O_3/TiO_2						6.5			
Structure	Glass and glass ceramic	Glass	Glass	Glass-ceramic	Glass-ceramic	Glass-ceramic	Glass-ceramic	Glass-ceramic	
References	[14]	[14, 56]	[57, 58]	[5]	[5]	[5]	[36]	[32]	[54]

Source: Hench 1991 [12]. Reproduced with permission of John Wiley and Sons.

Table 8.9 Properties and ceramic biomaterial systems.

Material	System	Properties	Published source
Bone	$CaO–P_2O_5$ and small additives	$\sigma_c = 90–170$ MPa $\sigma_b = 120–180$ MPa $E = 15.5–18.0$ GPa	[23]
Materials based on silicate systems			
Bioglass®	$SiO_2–Na_2O–CaO–P_2O_5$	$\sigma_b = 42$ MPa $E = 35$ GPa	[8]
Ceravital®	$CaO–P_2O_5–SiO_2$, additives Na_2O, K_2O, MgO	σ_b up to 150 MPa	[24]
Cerabone®	$CaO–P_2O_5–SiO_2$, additives MgO, CaF_2	$\sigma_b = 178$ MPa $\sigma_{b\ nitr} = 215$ MPa $\sigma_c = 1060$ MPa $E = 117$ GPa $K_{1C} = 2.0$ MPa $m^{1/2}$	[9]
Bioverit®	$Na_2O–MgO–CaO–Al_2O_3–SiO_2$, additives P_2O_5, F_2	$\sigma_b = 178$ MPa $\sigma_{b\ nitr} = 215$ MPa $\sigma_c = 1060$ MPa $E = 117$ GPa $K_{1C} = 2.0$ MPa $m^{1/2}$	[10]
Materials based on phosphate systems			
Aluminum bearing	$CaO–P_2O_5–Al_2O_3$	σ_b up to 100 MPa	[11]
Niobium bearing	$CaO–P_2O_5–Nb_2O_5$, additives Al_2O_3	$\sigma_b = 70–130$ MPa $E = 76$ GPa	[12]
Biositall KF	$CaO–P_2O_5–Al_2O_3$, additives B_2O_3, TiO_2, ZrO_2	$\sigma_b = 100–160$ MPa $E = 75$ GPa	[13]
Materials with increased strength			
Cerabone® strengthened	$CaO–P_2O_5–SiO_2$, additives MgO, $CaF_2 + ZrO_2$, modified I_2O_3 and Al_2O_3	$\sigma_b = 440–480$ MPa $\sigma_{b\ nitr} = 480–550$ MPa $K_{1C} = 2.3–2.8$ MPa $m^{1/2}$	[2007]
Calcium phosphate glass-ceramics	$CaO–P_2O_5$–calcium metaphosphate (oriented crystals)	$\sigma_b = 640$ MPa $E = 85$ GPa Stepwise destruction	[22]
Composite materials			
Composite cellular biomaterial BAK	HC glass, hydroxyapatite powder	Open porosity 10–80% $\sigma_b = 10$ MPa $\sigma_c = 20$ MPa	[25]
Material for transporting medications	Cerabone® + bis-HMA/TEHDMA	$\sigma_c = 68–110$ MPa	[14]

Table 8.9 (Continued)

Material	System	Properties	Published source
Glass ionomer cement with bioactive fibers	$CaO–P_2O_5–SiO_2–Al_2O_3–$ fibers + HY-BOND Glass ionomer CX	Setting duration up to 11 min	[16]
Material for transporting medications	$SiO_2–CaO–P_2O_5$ (glass) + PMMA (matrix)	Rate of exit of medication is equivalent to the rate of ion exchange reaction $Ca^{2+} \leftrightarrow H_3O^+$	[26]
Bioresorptive composite	Bioglass® + polyethyl vinyl alcohol	$\sigma_{tens} = 36.8$ MPa $E = 3.8$ GPa	[25]
Bioverit® with strengthening additives	$Na_2O–MgO–CaO–Al_2O_3–SiO_2–P_2O_5–F_2 + ZrO_2$, pure and modified I_2O_3	$\sigma_b = 50–95$ MPa $\sigma_c = 118–230$ MPa $E = 59–78$ GPa $K_{1C} = 1.7–2.5$ MPa m$^{1/2}$	[21]
Bioactive coatings			
Solid titanium and titanium mesh	Biositall KF (plasma spraying), glass ceramic coating	Thickness 150–300 μm σ_{destr} up to 20 MPa	[18]
Titanium and silicon	$CaO–P_2O_5–SiO_2–MgO$ (magnetron spraying), glass ceramic costing	Thickness 100–700 μm σ_{destr} up to 57 MPa	[19]

Source: Stroganova *et al.* 2003 [13]. Reproduced with permission of Springer.

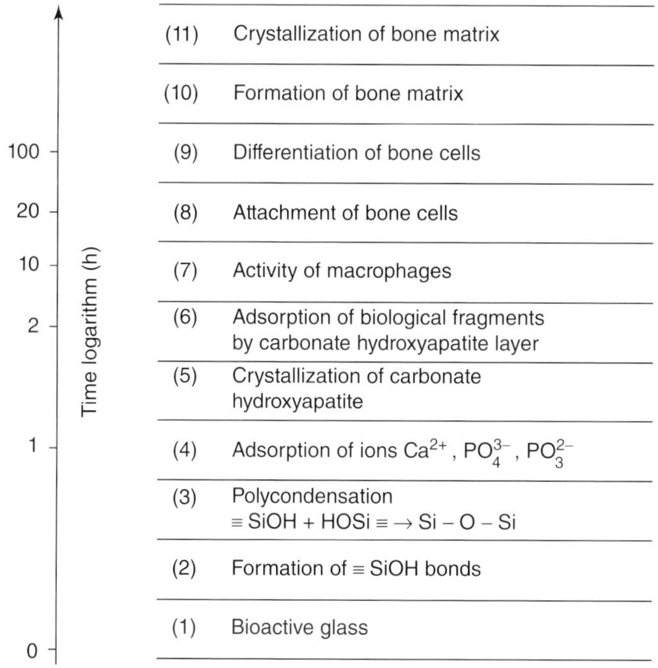

Figure 8.7 Phases of surface reactions. (Stroganova *et al.* 2003 [13]. Reproduced with permission of Springer.)

gel substrate actively absorbing ions of alkali and alkaline earth cations, as well as phosphate and carbonate anions groups, that is, building material for a new bone structure. For phosphate systems, reactions directed to the formation of the apatite structure corresponding to reactions (1)–(6) in Figure 8.7 proceed according to different schemes depending on the composition of the dissolving material. In studying the processes of dissolution for glasses of the $CaO–R_2O–P_2O_5$ system (where R is used for Na and K) in water and in the physiological medium depending on the ratio $CaO:P_2O_5$, the following reactions were registered [13]:

$$CaHPO_4 \rightarrow DefHA \rightarrow HA;$$

$$Ca_2P_2O_7 \rightarrow DefHA \rightarrow HA;$$

$$Ca_8(HPO_4)_2(PO_4)_4{\cdot}5H_2O \rightarrow DefHA \rightarrow HA;$$

A criterion of the bioactivity of glass-based materials can be the rate of formation of an amorphous apatite layer on the surface of the implant in *in vitro* tests. For *in vivo* tests, the bioactivity index is used, $I_b = 100/\tau_{0.566}$ ($\tau_{0.566}$ is the time in which half of the surface area of the implant becomes bonded to the adjacent bone), and the class of bioactivity reflects the capacity of a material to react with different types of tissues. In accordance with these notions, the phase diagram of the $CaO–SiO_2–P_2O_5$ system indicates glass-formation areas, in which vitreous and glass ceramic materials with different capacities for contact with soft and bone tissues can be obtained [13], as represented in Figure 8.8.

The morphology of bioglass particle and bone-derived HAp (hydroxyapatite) ceramic biomaterials [14, 15] revealed after scanning electron microscopy is reproduced in Figures 8.9 and 8.10, respectively. For bioactive glass particles, heterogeneous surfaces consisting of random-sized particles with sharp edges can be seen (Figure 8.9). The bone-derived HAp materials after grinding and sieving (<50 μm) the resultant particles were microporous, as demonstrated subsequently by their high specific surface area, and consisted of crystal agglomerations. Particle dispersion stability by zeta potential measurement and surface area and theoretical particle size by gas adsorption (BET method) analyses were calculated by using Eqs. (8.1) and (8.2).

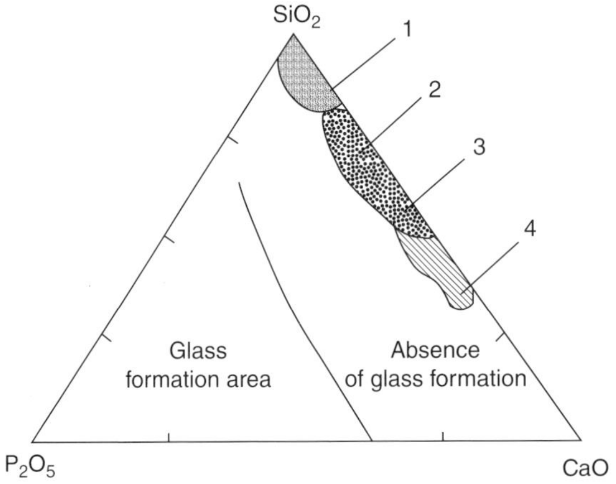

Figure 8.8 Classification of bioactive glasses: (1, 3, and 4) formation of apatite layer on gel glasses after 7–20 days (class B), 1–3 days (class A) and 7 days (class B), respectively; (2) bioresorption in the process of bone regeneration (class A). Phases of surface reactions. (Stroganova *et al.* 2003 [13]. Reproduced with permission of Springer.)

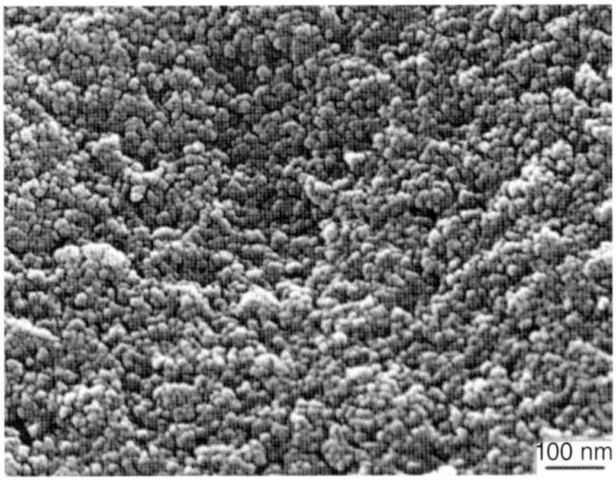

Figure 8.9 SEM micrographs of the bioglass particles. (Doostmohammadi *et al.* 2011 [15]. Reproduced with permission of Elsevier.)

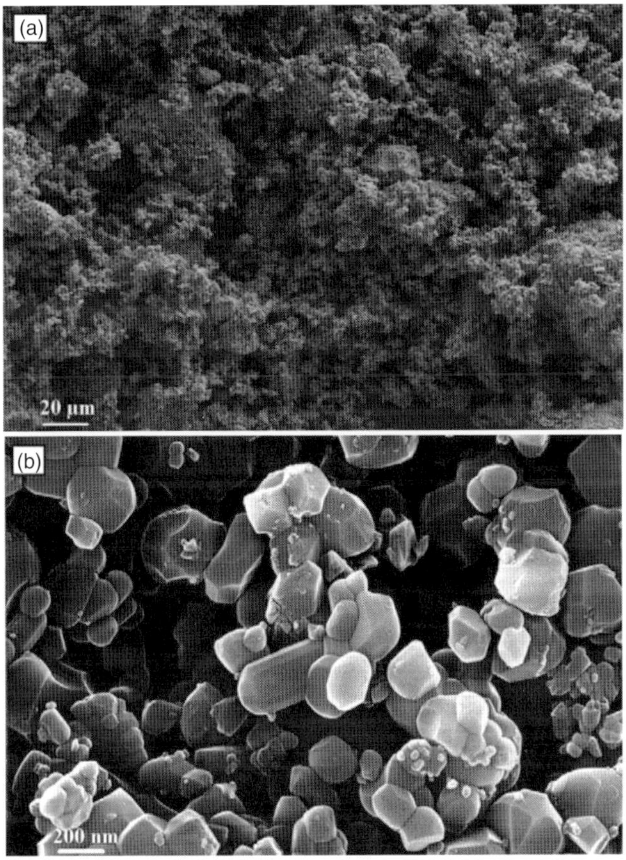

Figure 8.10 SEM photographs of hydroxyapatite particles showing the porous structure (a) and variety in crystal shape and size within the particles (b). (Doostmohammadi *et al.* 2011 [15]. Reproduced with permission of Elsevier.)

The zeta potential of the particles was measured for six times with a laser Doppler electrophoresis (LDE) instrument (each measurement with an average of 40 runs), and the mean values and standard deviations were calculated. The instrument automatically calculated electrophoretic mobility (U) and zeta potential [15] according to Smoluchowski's equation:

$$\zeta = \frac{U\eta}{\varepsilon} \tag{8.1}$$

where ζ is the zeta potential, U is the electrophoretic mobility, η is the medium viscosity, and ε is the dielectric constant.

A theoretical particle size can be calculated from these adsorption data by assuming that the measured surface area for a unit mass of particles is that of a collection of spherical particles of identical size [14]. It can be shown that the resulting theoretical particle diameter, D (in micrometer), is given by

$$D = 6/S_{sp}\rho_a \tag{8.2}$$

where S_{sp} is the specific surface area per unit mass of the sample and ρ_a is the theoretical density of the solid material.

8.3.2 Polymer Biomaterials

Polymeric biomaterials have several important uses in addition to tissue reconstruction. Examples include poly(methyl methacrylate), bone cement, poly(glycolic acid) (PGA), degradable sutures, poly(glycolic-*co*-lactic acid), bone screws, and poly(vinyl siloxane) dental impression materials. Polymers such as PEG are often used to extend the circulation half-life of some drugs. Poly(hydroxyethyl methacrylate) is used to create soft contact lenses. Figure 8.11 illustrates how some of these factors integrate into the appropriate design of new materials. The chemical structures of many natural and synthetic polymers used in medicine are reproduced in Figure 8.12. Polymers with similar chemical characteristics behave differently in certain situations. For example, polyethylene and ultrahigh molecular weight polyethylene behave differently as orthopedic biomaterials for knee and hip replacement. Ultrahigh molecular weight polyethylene exhibits reduced wearing and debris formation compared with polyethylene. *Nondegradable polymers*: Poly(vinyl alcohol) (PVA) was one of the first synthetic polymers tested as an artificial cartilage. PVA is a hydrogel and contains water content similar to that of cartilage; however, like many hydrogels, it lacks sufficient mechanical stability for use as a cartilage replacement in its unmodified form. It does offer several beneficial properties as an artificial cartilage. It is relatively biocompatible, can swell to accommodate high water content, can be sterilized, and can be molded into desired shapes. Polyacrylates: Attempting to improve the quality of neocartilage, Sawtell *et al.* proposed a poly(ethyl methacrylate)/tetrahydrofurfuryl methacrylate (PEMA/THFMA) system. Although they do not biodegrade, these polymer networks provide beneficial properties for mechanical uniformity and implantation. The polymeric properties of PEMA/THFMA are conducive to implantation and *in situ*

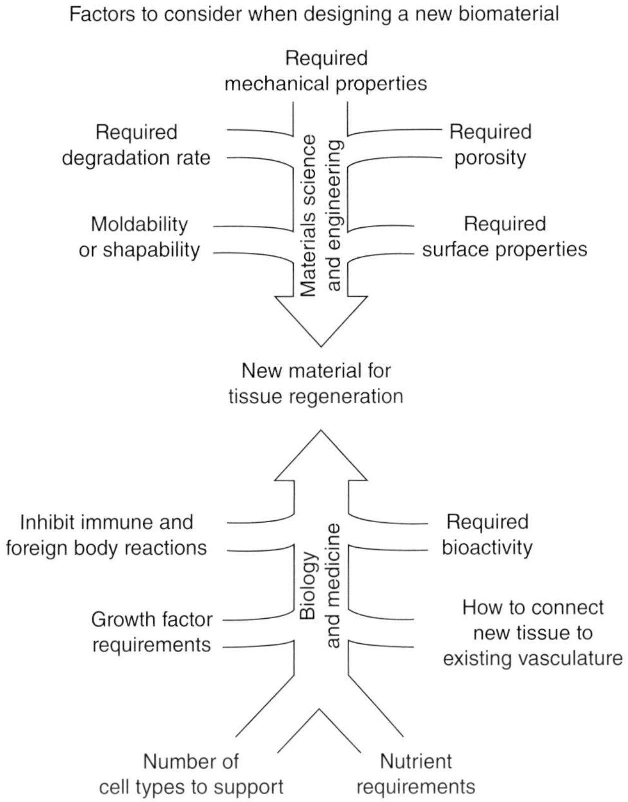

Figure 8.11 Illustration of how some material, biological, medical, and engineering properties must be integrated to achieve successful biomaterials for tissue regeneration. (Seal *et al.* 2001 [16]. Reproduced with permission of Elsevier.)

polymerization. Poly(*N*-isopropylacrylamide) (pNIPAAm): pNIPAAm is an injectable hydrogel for cartilage tissue applications. Since it has a lower critical solution temperature (LCST) of 32 °C, an aqueous solution of pNIPAAm can be injected *in situ* directly into a cartilage defect. As the polymer solution temperature increases to 37 °C, a reversible hydrogel will form. The authors created loosely cross-linked polymers of pNIPAAm and a copolymer of pNIPAAm and acrylic acid (pNIPAAm-*co*-AAc). These polymers had LCSTs of around 32 and 34 °C, respectively. Polyethylene: This polymer had a compressive behavior similar to that of natural cartilage. Regarding its articular surface, the polyethylene material did induce a significantly greater amount of cartilage formation; however, only 15% of the fabric surface was actually covered by cartilage from weeks 8 to 24. *Synthetic degradable polymers*: Polyesters are one of the earliest and most widely investigated groups of materials studied for cartilage repair including the synthetic degradable poly(α-hydroxy acids).

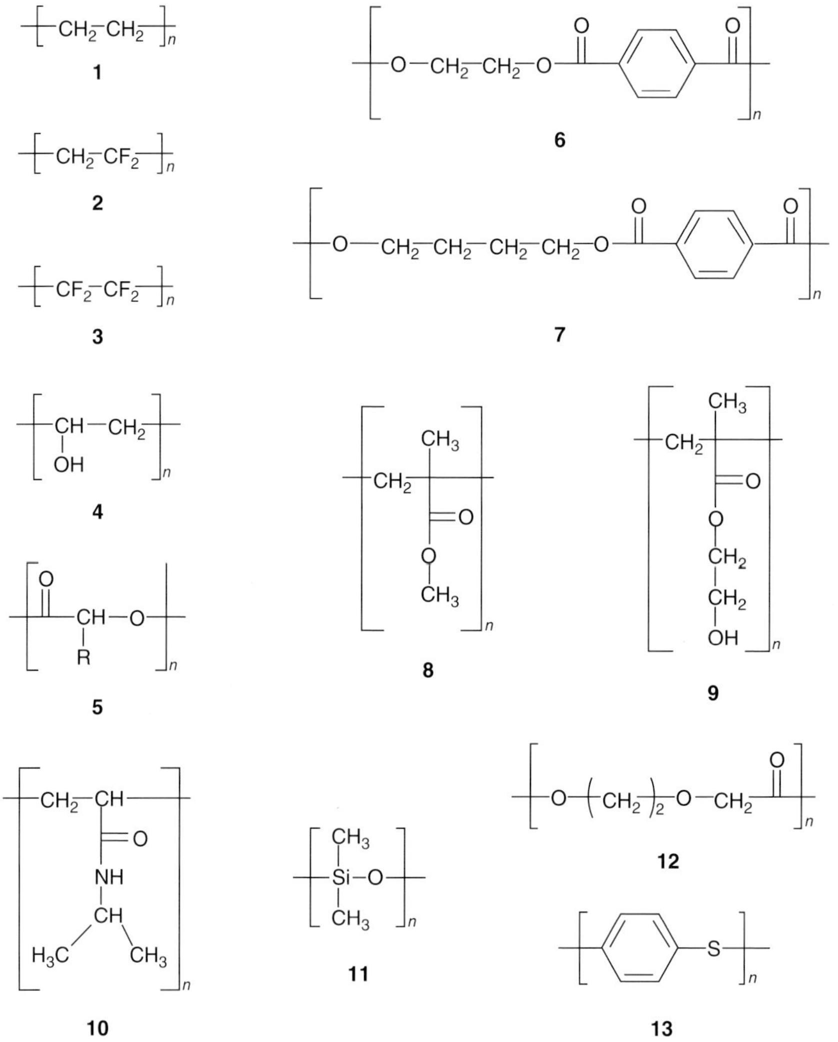

Figure 8.12 Chemical structures of some commonly used nondegradable polymers in tissue engineering. These polymers include (**1**) polyethylene, (**2**) poly(vinylidene fluoride), (**3**) poly(tetrafluoroethylene), (**4**) poly(vinyl alcohol), (**5**) poly(hydroxyalkanoate), (**6**) poly(ethylene terephthalate), (**7**) poly(butylene terephthalate), (**8**) poly(methyl methacrylate), (**9**) poly(hydroxyethyl methacrylate) (**10**) poly(*N*-isopropylacrylamide), (**11**) poly(dimethylsiloxane), (**12**) polydioxanone, and (**13**) polypyrrole. (Seal *et al.* 2001 [16]. Reproduced with permission of Elsevier.)

The two most well known of these polymeric biomaterials include PGA and poly(lactic acid) (PLA). Due to its chiral structure, PLA can exist in two forms: D-PLA and L-PLA. However, L-PLA has experienced more widespread use as a biomaterial since L-lactic acid occurs naturally. Polyethylene oxide (PEO): Both the location and varied geometries of most chondral defects cause difficulties when trying to design a less invasive polymeric device for cartilage repair. Unlike alginate and PEMA, PEO can readily degrade hydrolytically and can be cleared by the kidneys. *Natural degradable polymers*: Alginate is composed of two repeating monosaccharides: L-guluronic acid and D-mannuronic acid. Repeating strands of these subunits form linear, water-soluble polysaccharides. Once these polysaccharides are exposed to calcium ions, a three-dimensional gel quickly forms. Therefore, various pharmaceuticals, growth factors, or cultured cells can be easily encapsulated. Collagen: Collagen gels have also been investigated as polymeric devices for supporting chondrogenesis. Collagen is present in most types of connective tissue within the body. Although there are 16 different types of collagen, the most abundant kind of collagen is type I; type II collagen is most prevalent in hyaline cartilage. Collagen acts as a very good structural matrix protein. Hyaluronan: One attractive characteristic of polyester materials is the ability to allow biologically compatible hydrolytic degradation. In its natural form, however, hyaluronan lacks several desirable characteristics for use as a polymeric scaffold material. Some properties of HyA that are not conducive for biomaterial applications include high water solubility and fast resorption and tissue clearance times. Fibrin gels: Fibrinogen self-assembles to become fibrin upon injury to a blood vessel. Fibrin plays a major role during wound healing within the body. Physiologically, thrombin also activates a transglutaminase enzyme called factor XIIIa. Factor XIIIa will chemically cross-link lysine and glutamine residues found on the α-, β-, and γ-chains of different fibrin molecules. This enzymatic reaction converts the three-dimensional network into a covalent hydrogel. Chitosan: The biopolymer material of interest to cartilage research is known as chitosan. Chitosan, a polysaccharide derived from chitin, consists of a relatively simple glucosamine monomer. In fact, the chemical structure of chitosan produces properties similar to those of many GAGs (glucosaminoglucans) Table 8.10 [16].

Characterization of Polymeric Biomaterials

A number of methods are available for analyzing and characterizing polymeric biomaterials, such as microscopic methods (scanning electron, transmission electron, scanning tunneling, atomic force (tapping, phase imaging and coated tip modes), and confocal scanning microscopy) and spectroscopic methods (Auger electron spectroscopy (AES), X-ray photon spectroscopy (XPS), secondary ion mass spectrometry (SIMS), and the ATR-FTIR, that is, attenuated total reflection Fourier transform infrared spectroscopy [17].

FTIR spectroscopy has been used to analyze the process of bone regeneration taking place in the presence of surface-modified carbon materials. Two types of carbon implant materials differing in their surface properties have been examined: an oxidized carbon fabric and a carbon fabric coated with a pyrolytic carbon layer. The samples of bone tissue have been retrieved at different times after implantation for spectroscopic study. The ratio of bone components has been calculated from the FTIR spectra of the samples based on the integrated areas of the bands brought about by the vibrations of phosphates and amide groups. The FTIR method is also applied to examine both healthy and pathologically altered bones as well as to study the bone mineralization process. Calcium phosphates, the main inorganic bone constituents, bring about the

Table 8.10 Some bone regeneration polymers and their properties[a)].

Material	Degradable	Compressive strength (MPa)	Modulus (MPa)	Porous (μm)	Support cell adhesion	Processable (moldable)
Cancellous bone	Yes	5	50 [114] (compressive)	Yes	Yes	No
Trabecular bone	Yes	NR	50–100 [114] (Young's)	Yes	Yes	No
PLA	Yes (bulk)	NR	NR	100–500	Yes	Yes
PLGA	Yes (bulk)	60 ± 20	0.5 (tensile) 2.4 [128] (Young's)	150–710	Yes	Yes
Poly(*ortho*-ester)	Yes (surface)	4–16	NR	NR	Yes	NR
Polyphosphazene	Yes (surface)	NR	NR	160–200	Yes	NR
Polyanhydride	Yes (surface)	NR	140–1400 [115] (tensile)	NR	Yes	Yes
PET	No		NR	NR	No	Yes
PET/HA	No	320 ± 60	NR	NR	Yes	Yes
PLGA/Ca phosphate	Yes (bulk)	NR	0.25	100–500	Yes	Yes
PLA/Ca phosphate	Yes (bulk)	NR	5 [116] (Young's)	100–500	Yes	Yes
PLA/HA	Yes (bulk)	6–9	NR	NR	NR	NR
PolyActive™	Yes (bulk)	NR	NR	NR	Yes	Yes
DegraPol™	Yes (bulk)	NR	30–1200 [117] (elastic)	NR	Yes	Yes

a) NR indicates not reported.
Source: Seal *et al*. 2001 [16]. Reproduced with permission of Elsevier.

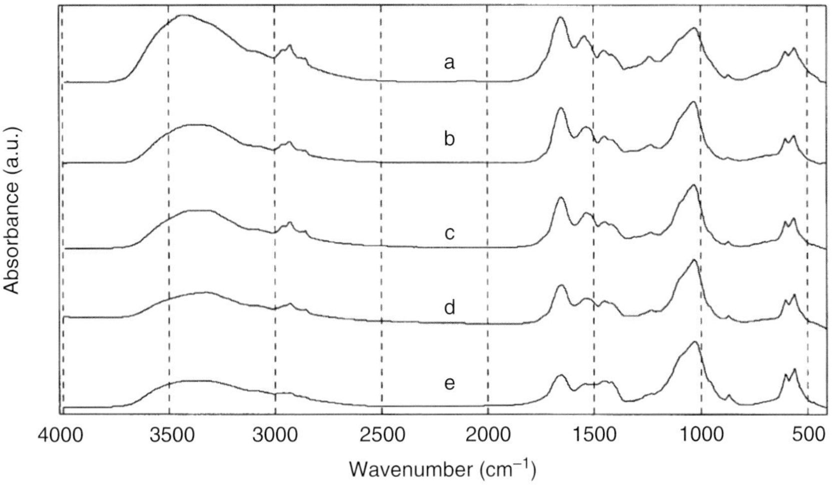

Figure 8.13 FTIR spectra of carbon implant (*I*) surrounded by bone tissue after (a) 1 week; (b) 2 weeks; (c) 3 weeks; (d) 6 weeks of implantation; (e) spectra of rabbit bone. (Blazewicz *et al.* 2001 [18]. Reproduced with permission of Elsevier.)

absorption bands in two ranges: 900–1200 and 550–650 cm^{-1}. The organic matrix is composed mainly of collagen fibers and shows the absorption bands in the range of 1200–1700 cm^{-1}. In order to prepare samples for IR studies, carbon fabrics together with the adjacent tissue were removed from the animal tissue. The samples for the studies were prepared in such a way that only tissue from the internal part of the fibrous implant was examined. Before examination the samples were washed with distilled water, dried at temperatures below 40 °C, and ground. The samples were then mixed with potassium bromide and pressed into the form of pellets. FTIR spectra in the range of 400–4000 cm^{-1} were made using a BIO-RAD FTS-60 device. The IR spectra of carbon implants with the adjacent tissue [18] are shown in Figure 8.13.

Case Study 1: Polymeric Biomaterials Used in Load-Bearing Medical Devices

- Polymeric biomaterials used for load-bearing medical devices were described in ref. [19]. According to this work, examples of polymeric biomaterials used for load-bearing medical implants are presented in Table 8.11.
- Polymers are loaded to a stress value near their yield strength when subjected to the physiological stress state of the implant; this is in contrast to metals and ceramics that typically operate well below their strength levels. Mechanical properties such as relative elastic range of *ceramics*, *metals*, and *polymers* in the realm of applied physiological stress on the implant are reproduced in Figure 8.14.

Table 8.11 Examples of polymers used in load-bearing medical devices.

Application	Devices	Polymers	Performance requirements
Bone	Balloons/catheter grafts	Nylon/polyester/HDPE	Rupture, flexibility, friction compliance, tissue integration
Soft tissues	Suture anchors	PLDLA, PLLA, PEEK	Resilience strength
	Sutures	Polyester, PLLA, PGA	Tensile strength
	Breast implants	Silicone	Burst strength, leak resistance
Dental	Total joint replacement bone cement	UHMWPE	Fracture, wear, fatigue, creep
Orthopedics		PMMA/PS	Interface fracture, fatigue

Source: Pruitt 2009 [19]. Reproduced with permission of Elsevier.

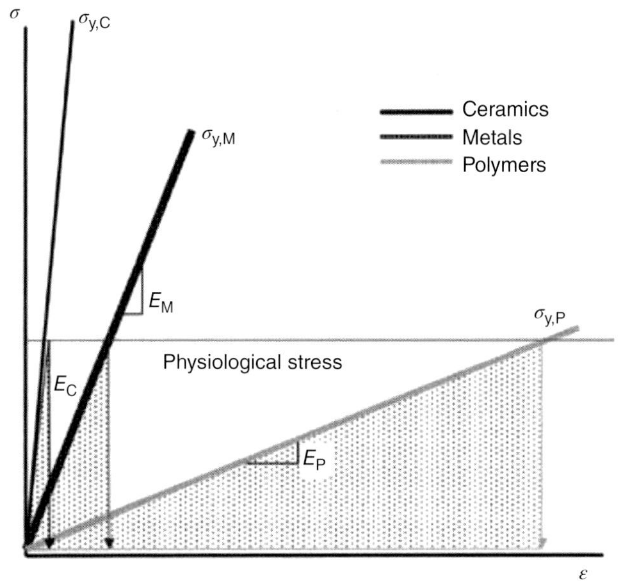

Figure 8.14 Case Study 1: Schematic illustration showing relative elastic range of ceramics, metals, and polymers in the realm of the applied physiological stress on the implant. (Pruitt 2009 [19]. Reproduced with permission of Elsevier.)

Control Questions

1) Describe the mechanical properties of biomaterials and importance of stress shielding, wear resistance, and fatigue in implant fabrication.
2) Determine stiffness, strength, and hardness for biomaterials.
3) Determine the terms of ductility, toughness, and fracture mechanics for biomaterials.
4) Describe and compare the mechanical properties of metallic alloy biomaterials with bone.

5) Determine Young's modulus for metallic biomaterials and its features in implants.
6) Describe the wear resistance of biomaterials used in the living body.
7) Define the techniques for improving the wear resistance of metallic biomaterials.
8) Describe the biological properties of biomaterials and their role in tissue scaffold engineering.
9) What is the difference between *in vivo* and *in vitro* tissue biocompatibility?
10) Determine the biopolymers and proteins and the difference in their mechanical properties.
11) Characterize keratin, elastin, and resilin biomaterials and describe their mechanical properties.
12) Determine biocompatibility and describe the factors that affect biocompatibility in implant design.
13) Describe the chemical properties of biomaterials and the main chemical reactions for biomaterial synthesis.
14) Describe chemical reactivity and the factors that have influence on the chemical reactivity of ceramic biomaterials.
15) Describe the classification of ceramic biomaterials according to L.L. Hench's classification.
16) What kind of metal oxides composes ceramic Bioglass® and Ceravital® bioactive glass and glass ceramic materials?
17) Describe the properties of ceramic biomaterial systems based on Table 8.9.
18) What kind of chemical reactions will take place for building material for a new bone structure?
19) Describe the sequence of chemical processes and reactions occurring on the surface for apatite structure formation.
20) Describe the size determination methods for glass- and hydroxyapatite-based biomaterials.
21) Describe the factors to consider when designing new biomaterials and to integrate to achieve successful biomaterials for tissue regeneration.
22) Describe nondegradable polymeric biomaterials.
23) Describe the degradable polymeric biomaterials.
24) Describe the natural degradable polymers.
25) Describe the polymeric biomaterials for bone regeneration.
26) What kind of methods is used for the characterization of polymeric biomaterials?

References

1 Hussein, M.A., Mohammed, A.S., and Al-Aqeeli, N. (2015) Wear characteristics of metallic biomaterials: review. *Materials*, **8** (5), 2749–2768.

2 Wegst, U.G.K., Bai, H., Saiz, E., Tomisa, A.P., and Ritchie, R.O. (2015) Bioinspired structural materials. *Nat. Mater.*, **16**, 23–36.

3 Niinomi, M.; Nakai, M. Titanium-based biomaterials for preventing stress shielding between implant devices and bone. *Int. J. Biomater.*, (2011) p. 1–10.

4 Liuyun, J. *et al* (2009) Preparation and biological properties of a novel composite scaffold of nano-hydroxyapatite/chitosan/carboxymethyl cellulose for bone tissue engineering. *J. Biomed. Sci.*, **16** (65), 1–10.

5 Chen, P.Y. *et al* (2012) Biological materials: functional adaptations and bioinspired designs. *Prog. Mater Sci.*, **57**, 1492–1704.
6 Tombolato, L., Novitskaya, E.E., Chen, P.-Y., Sheppard, F.A., and McKittrick, J. (2010) Microstructure, elastic properties and deformation mechanisms of horn keratin. *Acta Biomater.*, **6**, 319–330.
7 Singh, R. *et al* (2007) Corrosion degradation and prevention by surface modification of biometallic materials. *J. Mater. Sci. - Mater. Med.*, **18** (5), 725–751.
8 Anseth, K. (2016) Click chemistry in biomaterials, nanomedicine, and drug delivery. *Biomacromolecules*, **17**, 1–3, American Chemical Society © 2016.
9 Vallet-Regí, M. (2001) Ceramics for medical applications. *J. Chem. Soc., Dalton Trans.*, 97–108 DOI: 10.1039/B007852M.
10 Kasemo, B. and Lausmaa, J. (1994) Material-tissue Interfaces: the role of surface properties and processes. *Environ. Health Perspect.*, **102** (5), 41–45.
11 Sáenz, A., Rivera-Muñoz, E., Brostow, W., and Castaño, V.M. (1991) Ceramic biomaterials: an introductory overview. *J. Mater. Educ.*, **21** (5-6), 297–306.
12 Hench, L.L. (1991) Bioceramics: from concept to clinic. *J. Am. Ceram. Soc.*, **74**, 1487–1510.
13 Stroganova, E.E., Mikhailenko, N.Y., and Moroz, O.A. (2003) Glass-based biomaterials: present and future (a review). *Glass Ceram.*, **60**, 315–319.
14 Doostmohammadi, A. *et al* (2012) Preparation, chemistry and physical properties of bone-derived hydroxyapatite particles having a negative zeta potential. *Mater. Chem. Phys.*, **132**, 446–452.
15 Doostmohammadi, A., Monshi, A., Fathi, M.H., and Braissant, O. (2011) A comparative physico-chemical study of bioactive glass and bone-derived hydroxyapatite. *Ceram. Int.*, **37**, 1601–1607.
16 Seal, B.L., Otero, T.C. and Panitch, A. (2001). Polymeric biomaterials for tissue and organ regeneration, *Mater. Sci. Eng.*, **34**, (4–5), 147–230.
17 Merrett, K. *et al* (2002) Surface analysis methods for characterizing polymeric biomaterials. *J. Biomater. Sci., Polym. Ed.*, **13** (6), 593–621.
18 Blazewicz, M. *et al* (2001) Characterization of biomaterials used for bone regeneration by FTIR spectroscopy. *J. Mol. Struct.*, **563-564**, 147–152.
19 Pruitt, L. and Furmanski, J. (2009) Polymeric biomaterials for load-bearing medical devices. *JOM*, **61**, 14.

Further Reading

Huebsch, N. and Mooney, D.J. (2009) Inspiration and application in the evolution of biomaterials. *Nature*, **462**, 26.

Zhou, Y.L., Niinomi, M., Akahori, T., Nakai, M., and Fukui, H. (2007) Comparison of various properties between titanium-tantalum alloy and pure titanium for biomedical applications. *Mater. Trans.*, **48** (3), 380–384.

9

Implants and Artificial Organs

The human body has many secrets, and it does not divulge them to anyone, except those who have learned to wait.

Paul Auster, novelist and poet

9.1 Implants

The term *implant* is defined as "to put an organ, group of cells, or device into the body in a medical operation" (Cambridge Dictionary). "Medical implants fall under the larger category of medical devices, which are defined as products used for medical purposes in patients, in diagnosis and/or treatment" [1]. The *history of implantology* was started long time ago, for example, Albucasis de condue, Arabian ancient era surgeon who had mentioned in his paper about teeth transplants [2]. Application of the gold dental prostheses was also referenced in Ancient Roman literature with information lacking on structure and specific functions of those implants [3]. The history of metal implants application refers back to ancient period of 1875 for pure metals (copper, silver, and gold) applications, and until 1925 for developmental surgery and implantation, then finally, to current period from 1925 for metals and alloys implantation [4]. The structural components of implants used for human body damaged organ replacements are: metals, polymers, ceramics, and composites [5].

9.2 Types of Implants

Figure 9.1 is showing types of implants used for damaged organ replacement, such as: an eye, an ear, brain, heart, joint, inner organs, and the oral cavity.

9.2.1 Intraocular Lenses

Intraocular lenses (IOLs) are defined as "a plastic artificial lens generally inserted into the capsule of the lens after cataract removal" (Mosby's Medical Dictionary,

Nano- and Biomaterials: Compounds, Properties, Characterization, and Applications,
First Edition. Zhypargul Abdullaeva.

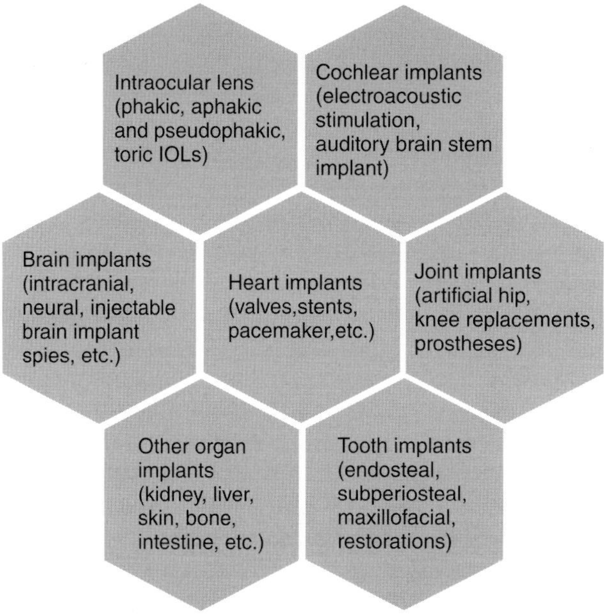

Figure 9.1 Diagram showing some of the implant types.

9th Ed., © 2009, Elsevier). Three types of IOLs have been used in the human body: (i) phakic IOLs were implanted without removal of the patient's original crystalline lens and performed solely to correct refractive error in the presence of a clear crystalline lens; (ii) aphakic IOLs are generally referred to lenses implanted secondarily in an eye already aphakic from previous surgery or trauma; and (iii) pseudophakic IOLs were implanted during cataract surgery, as a sequential step after removal of the cataractous lens [6].

Intraocular refractive procedures offer many potential advantages: a broader range of treatable ametropia, faster visual recovery, more stable refraction, and better visual quality. Refractive lens exchange may increase the risk for retinal detachment and is generally not considered in myopic pre-presbyopic patients who can still accommodate. The risks and benefits of pIOL implantation in appropriate patients may be more favorable than other refractive surgery techniques. The pIOL is removable surgically, with fast visual recovery and preserved accommodation. However, it is important to realize that complications relating to pIOLs can be more disabling than those from keratorefractive surgery. Several generations of both anterior and posterior pIOLs have been introduced in the past few years. For eyes undergoing implantation of posterior chamber pIOLs, the pupil was dilated with mydriatic drops, and the procedure was performed under peribulbar anesthesia. A 3.2-mm temporal clear corneal incision was created, as well as 1 or 2 paracenteses. The anterior chamber was filled with viscoelastic material. The pIOLs were then injected into the anterior chamber, anterior and parallel to the iris plane, and allowed to unfold. Each corner of the footplates was gently tucked beneath the iris. Once the pIOL is well positioned,

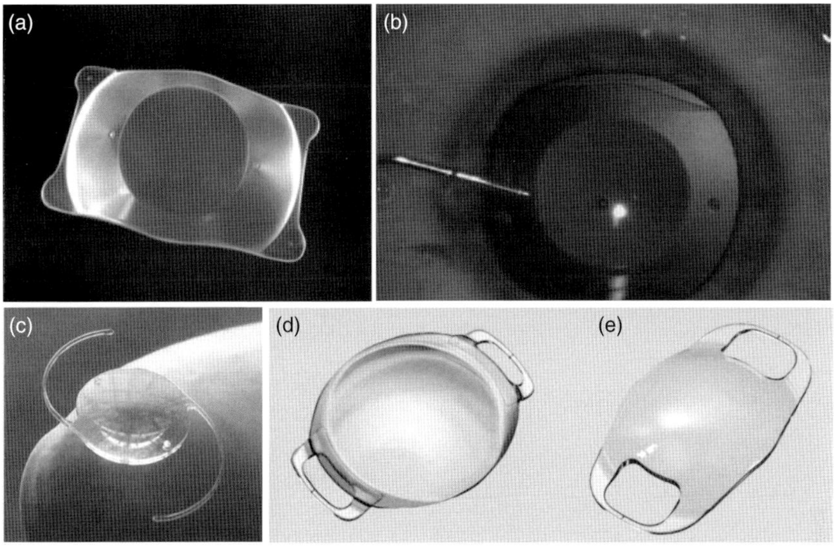

Figure 9.2 (a) Visian implantable collamer lens (ICL) model (reprinted from Wikimedia under CC BY 3.0 license; (b) Visian ICL phakic intraocular lens intraoperative (reprinted by permission from Macmillan Publishers Ltd: Hassaballa *et al.* (2011) [7]); (c) intraocular lenses have been used to treat cataracts since the 1940s (Photo: FLickr/Community Eye Health); (d), (e) modern versions of the iris claw lens (Photo: Ophtec) Copyright World Intellectual Property Organization, 2016.

the viscoelastic material was removed, a peripheral surgical iridotomy was performed, and the corneal wound was checked for integrity. Generally, the procedure on the other eye follows in 1 or 2 as represented in Figure 9.2b [7]. Some examples of eye implants are shown in the Figure 9.2, implantable visian collamer lens, (a) intraocular lens, (b) and modern types of an iris claw lens (d;c) have been used for the treatment of an eye disorders, respectively.

9.2.2 Cochlear Implants

In the past, cochlear implantation was used for patients with otitis media because of the risk of meningitis, tympanic membrane perforation, recurrent cholesteatoma, and extrusion of the electrode in a radical cavity because of breakdown of the thin epithelial lining [8]. Cochlear implants (CIs) have become the standard treatment of prelingual, postlingual, and perilingual deafness and hearing loss in children, and it is a revolutionary yet time-sensitive treatment for deaf children that must be performed within a critical window time for maximum benefit. Also, CIs have enabled a number of severely hearing-impaired individuals to access auditory information and improve speech perception as well as speech production skills. The development of speech perception and speech production in prelingually deafened children was promoted by multichannel cochlear implant [9]. Figure 9.3 shows CI adjusted in a patient (a) and a photograph of the internal part of the CI (b).

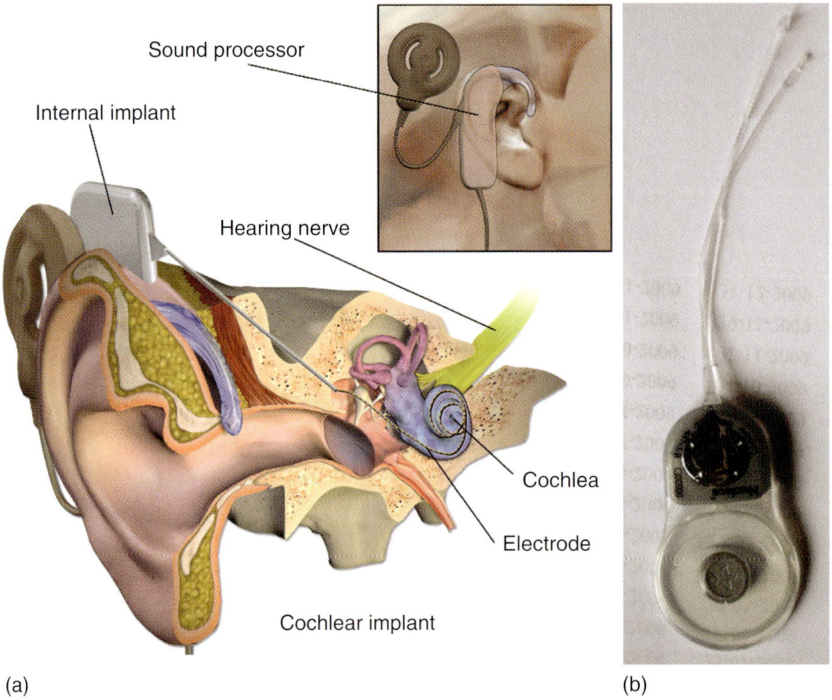

Figure 9.3 Cochlear implant adjusted in the patient (a) and photograph of the internal part of the Cochlear implant (b). (Pauna *et al.* 2014 [9]. http://www.omicsonline.org/open-access/Advanced-Bionics-Cochlear-Implants-in-Patients-2161-119X.1000159.php?aid=24462. Used under: https://creativecommons.org/licenses/by/4.0/.)

As it can be seen from the figure, CI electrode can be inserted into the cochlea (inner ear) of the patient with hearing defect. Sound processor attached to internal implant is connected to an electrode. Hearing nerve will be stimulated with the help of the electrode, thus excluding hearing impairment in the patient.

9.2.3 Brain Implants

Bioresorbable silicon electronic sensors implanted into the rat brain *in vivo* were reported for insulated percutaneous wires connected to an externally mounted, miniaturized wireless potentiostat for data transmission [10]. Multimodal 3D neuroimaging (M3N) pipeline to guide implantation of intracranial EEG (icEEG) electrodes for patients with epilepsy was reported [11]. Injectable brain implant spies on individual neurons hold the potential to unravel the workings of the mammalian brain [12]. Also, deep brain stimulation (DBS) treatment of depression was reported, with target on DBS electrode placement varying significantly based on the treating disorder and the neuroanatomical disorder models, and has shown good efficacy in the treatment of Parkinson's disease, essential tremor, and dystonia [13].

Neural bionic devices aim to electronically substitute damaged nerves or neurons to overcome failed information processing. To achieve distal access of stentrode to vessels equal in size to human cortical veins in the sheep model, an angiography-based coaxial catheter technique effective at delivering a 4F catheter (DAC044, Stryker Neurovascular) was used to the sheep target vessel with a diameter of 2 mm. The catheterization of the cerebral venous system was challenged by irregular venous anatomy including valves, chordae, and arachnoid granulations, and the challenges with specific catheter-over-wire techniques (Online Methods) were overcome. Implanted stentrode into the superior sagittal sinus (SSS) is shown in Figure 9.4 immediately adjacent to the motor area (Online Methods). The lead at the common jugular vein puncture site was sutured in the neck to achieve hemostasis, tunneled subcutaneously to a custom-made hermetic connector secured to the sternocleidomastoid and exited the skin via a flexible percutaneous lead, which terminated in a microcircular plug (Omnetics) [14].

9.2.4 Heart Implants

Pacemakers

Symptoms associated with the need for a pacemaker are fainting, near fainting, dizziness, lack of energy, fatigue, shortness of breath, and exercise intolerance [15].

Modern pacemaker systems stimulate the myocardium ("pace") and sense intrinsic cardiac activity and can record and store a variety of data from intrinsic heart signals and the pacing system, for example, heart rate and lead impedance. The pacemaker consists of a pulse generator ("box") and one or more pacing leads (the leads are sometimes referred to as electrodes). The pulse generator itself is usually made of a titanium shell, containing a lithium iodine cell and complementary metal oxide semiconductor (CMOS) circuits. Traditionally the model and manufacturer of modern devices can be determined by a radio-opaque alphanumeric code (Figure 9.5). All modern pacemakers have some form of communication with an external computer – "the programmer" – via radiofrequency (RF) telemetry. A few older devices still in use do not have this capability. The normal life span of a pacing generator is around 10 years after which the generator can be replaced without changing the leads. Leads have one or more metal alloy conductors encased within a silicone or polyurethane insulation sheath. The tips are specialized to optimize pacing and sensing and have a variety of designs to enable anchorage to the heart. "Passive fixation" endocardial leads have various types of silicone barbs. "Active fixation" leads have small screws at the tip, which are wound into the myocardium. Passive leads have a limited number of stable sites that can be used, while active fixation leads can be positioned at many locations [16].

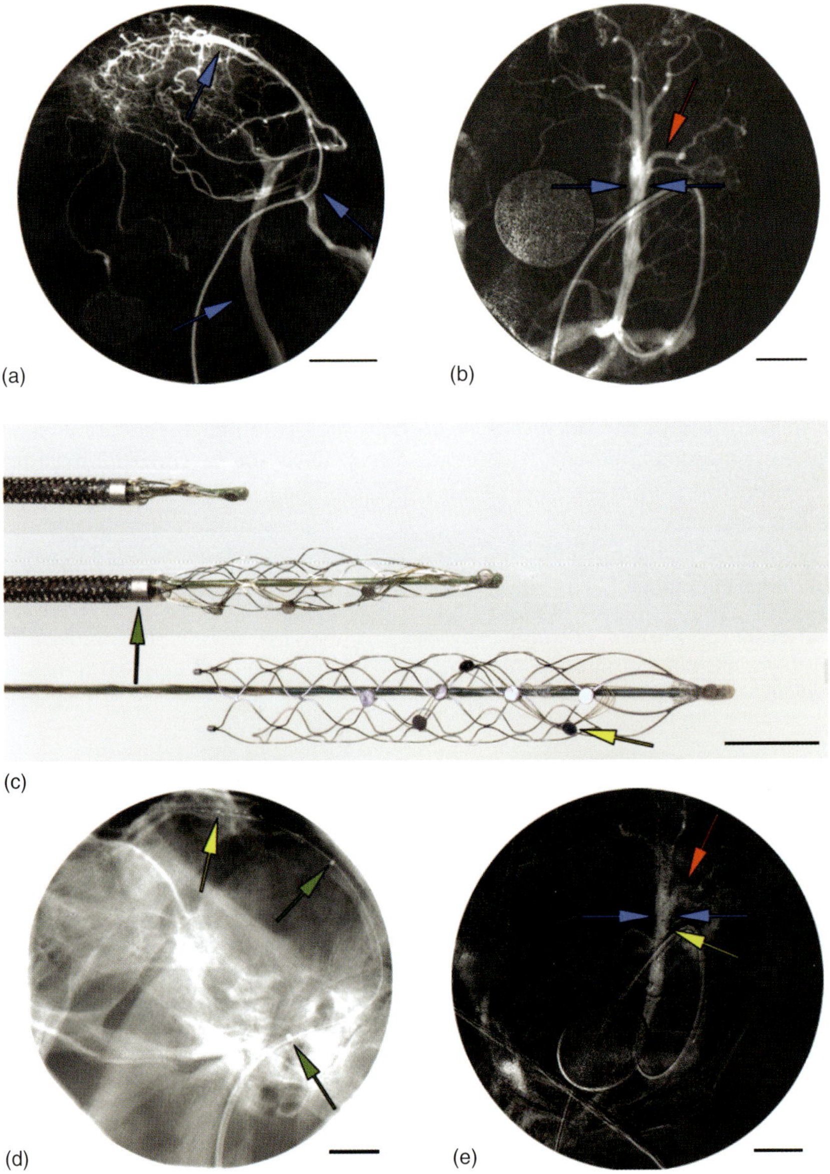

Figure 9.4 Stentrode delivery. (a) Pre-implant lateral projection cerebral venography roadmap of the external jugular vein, confluence of sinuses, and SSS (blue arrows). Scale bar, 20 mm. Circular artifact is a calibration tool. (b) Superior projection of SSS. Lumen diameter (blue arrows) and cortical veins (red arrow) assessed pre- and post-implant. Scale bar, 10 mm. (c) Stentrode with 8 μm × 750 μm electrode discs (yellow arrow) self-expanding during deployment from 4F catheter (green arrow). Scale bar, 3 mm. (d) Post-implantation lateral projection plain X-ray of stentrode in SSS, displaying electrodes (yellow arrow) and delivery catheters (green arrows). Scale bar, 10 mm. (e) Post-implant superior projection contrast study of stentrode (electrodes, yellow arrow). Scale bar, 10 mm. (Oxley *et al*. 2016 [14]. Reproduced with permission of Nature Publishing Group.)

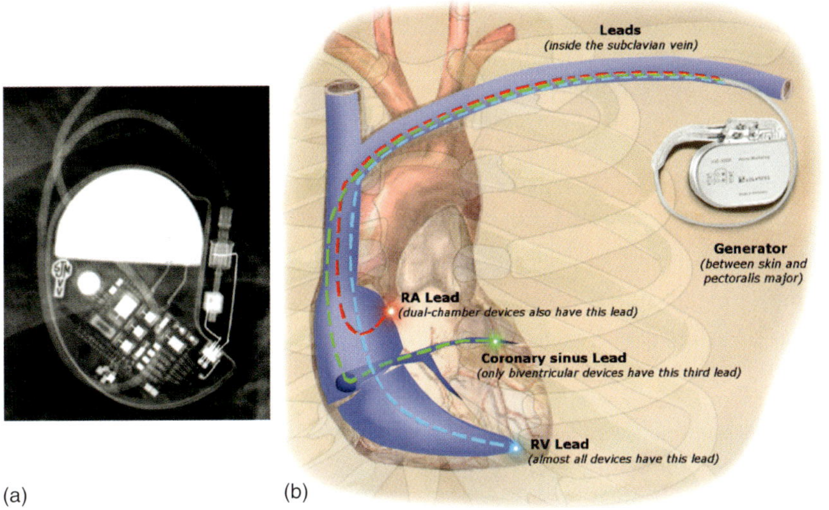

(a) (b)

Figure 9.5 (a) Image showing a permanent pacemaker with the alphanumeric code, the name of the manufacturer, and the lead attachment displayed. (Bruney *et al*. 2004 [16]. Reproduced with permission of Elsevier.) (b) Illustration of implanted cardiac pacemaker showing locations of cardiac pacemaker leads [17]. (https://en.wikipedia.org/wiki/Artificial_cardiac_pacemaker#/media/File:PPM.png. Used under: https://creativecommons.org/licenses/by-sa/4.0/.)

Heart Valves

Transcatheter Valves. The two most widely evaluated catheter implantable valves, the balloon-expandable Edwards SAPIEN valve (successor to the Cribier-Edwards valve; Edwards Lifesciences, Irvine, California) and the self-expanding CoreValve device (CoreValve Inc., Irvine, California), are shown in Figure 9.6a,b. As the procedure has evolved, standard off-the-shelf balloon catheters have been replaced by more complex integrated valve and valve delivery catheter systems. Whereas first-generation delivery systems were large, requiring 24F sheaths

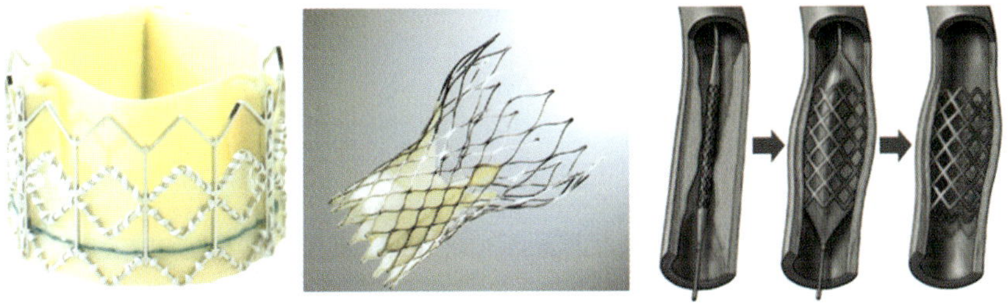

(a) (b) (c)

Figure 9.6 Transcatheter valves: (a) the balloon-expandable Edwards SAPIEN valve incorporates a stainless steel stent, bovine pericardial leaflets, and a fabric sealing cuff; (b) the self-expanding CoreValve device incorporates a nitinol (nickel titanium) alloy stent with leaflets and a sealing cuff constructed of porcine pericardial tissue [18]. (c) A polymer balloon used in the deployment of a coronary stent [19].

(external diameter 9 mm), newer systems are being progressively reduced in profile, moving toward the likely limits of current technology at around 16 to 20F. Multiple other valves and delivery systems with potential advantages in terms of the ability to deliver, deploy, or reposition the prosthesis are under development or in early clinical evaluation [18].

Complications after valve implantation might include thromboembolisms, bleeding complications, and prosthetic valve endocarditis, followed by structural and nonstructural prosthetic valve dysfunctions [20].

Stents

Stents are defined in intracoronary cardiology as expandable tubular devices that can be inserted percutaneously and left within a coronary artery lumen to maintain its patency (McGraw-Hill Concise Dictionary of Modern Medicine). Stents are expanded with the help of polymeric balloon placed inside the implanting stent (Figure 9.6c). Intravascular catheters are widely used in both diagnostic and interventional procedures.

Balloon catheters are probably best known for their clinical success in coronary angioplasty. In such applications the balloon at the distal end of a catheter is inflated to open an occluded blood vessel afflicted with heart disease. Such systems are also used in stent deployment and show a rendition of a catheter balloon used in the deployment of a coronary stent for the repair of an occluded artery. There are a few important functional requirements for the polymeric balloon: its profile must be small enough to be navigated through the coronary arteries; it must provide sufficient radial force to open an occluded vessel and deploy a stent, or in some instances, it may need to exert a radial force on a highly calcified plaque; and it must withstand the inflation pressures necessary for the clinical procedure without rupturing. For these reasons most polymeric catheter balloons are typically made of polyester or nylon due to their tensile strengths and ease of processing [19].

9.2.5 Joint Implants

Primary total *hip arthroplasty* is known as the most successful surgical procedure over the past 50 years and is currently performed worldwide with similar techniques and excellent result [21]. Total hip replacement is a surgical procedure to correct a hip joint damaged by degenerative disease, often arthritis. The head of the femur and the acetabulum are replaced with metal components. The acetabulum is plastic-coated to avoid metal-to-metal articulating surfaces (Mosby's Medical Dictionary, 9th edition). TKA is referred to as *total knee arthroplasty,* and arthroplasty is surgery to relieve pain and restore range of motion by realigning or reconstructing a joint (Gale Encyclopedia of Medicine). The structure of knee replacement is built from elements such as artificial femur, polyethylene artificial tibial tray, and artificial tibial stem [22]. Figure 9.7 shows a reproducing position of a standard hip prosthesis and cement-free hip replacement implant after 16 days of surgery. Based on the requirements on implant materials described in the previous chapters, the satisfactory material combination for manufacturing the implants for joint replacements [23] are shown in Table 9.1.

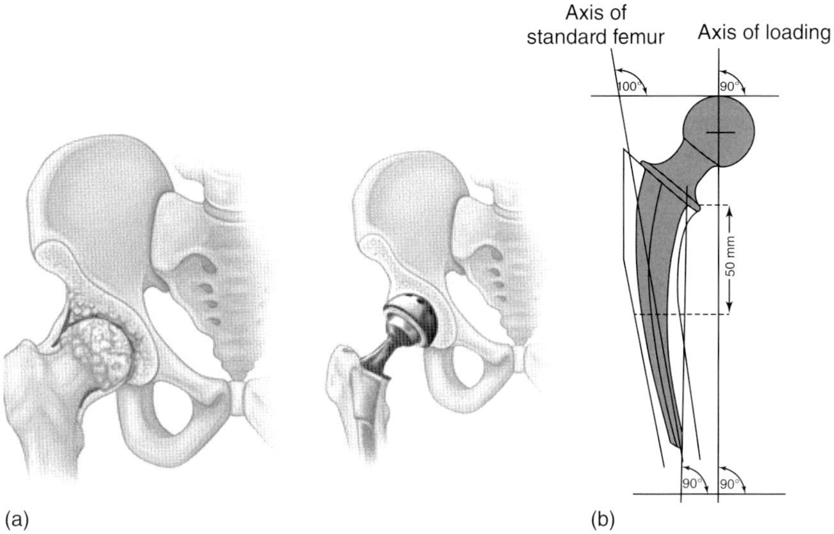

Figure 9.7 (a) (Left) A hip with osteoarthritis. (Right) The head of the femur and the socket have been replaced with an artificial device [24]. (Reproduced with permission of American Academy of Orthopaedic Surgeons.) (b) Position of a standard Muller hip prosthesis, 10.32.20 in the standard femur; uncemented stem length 50 mm. (Semlitsch and Willert 1980 [23]. Reproduced with permission of Springer.)

Table 9.1 Satisfactory material combinations for wear-stressed moving parts of artificial hip joints.

Cup	Head	Pivot	Prosthesis type
Natural	CoCrMo-cast FeCrNiMo-steel 316L CoCrMo-cast Al_2O_3-oxide ceramic	CoCrMo-cast	Thompson, Moore Thompson Weber Weber
CoCrMo-cast UHMWPE-polyethylene	CoCrMo-cast FeCrNiMo-steel 316L CoCrMo-cast CoCrMo-cast Al_2O_3-oxide ceramic	CoCrMo-cast	McKee-Farrar Charnley *et al.* Muller *et al.* Weber Mueller, Weber Christiansen
POM hom.-polyacetal DELRIN Al_2O_3-oxide ceramic	CoCrMo-cast	CoCrMo-cast	Christiansen Boutin *et al.*

Source: Semlitsch and Willert 1980 [23]. Reproduced with permission of Springer.

9.2.6 Other Organ Replacement Implants

Patients with the following symptoms are preferred for *intestine replacement* procedure: presence of PN-associated liver disease, loss of central venous access (loss of three to six central venous access sites in children or two to four central venous access sites in adults), recurrent catheter-related sepsis or a single episode of fungal sepsis, recurrent bouts of severe dehydration, and metabolic abnormalities [25].

Bioartificial Liver Support System

Currently, there are two types of liver support devices such as artificial and bioartificial livers (BALs). The mechanism of artificial liver support systems (LSS) is purification of the blood by albumin dialysis or by plasma separation and filtration to remove accumulating water-soluble and protein-bound toxins during liver failure. Considering the inability of the artificial one to replace synthetic and metabolic functions as well as its limited benefit on patient survival, BAL devices with hepatocytes inside have been developed. The BAL devices are made up of a cell-housing bioreactor and a combination of physical and chemical procedures, which are then connected to the circulation of the patient temporarily. The cell-housing bioreactor is to replace the primary and most important liver functions, such as oxidative detoxification, biotransformation, excretion, and synthesis. Thus, three crucial elements for the functioning of BAL are cell number, cell source, and bioreactor design. The first case report on the successful application of a BAL support system in liver failure was published in 1987, describing survival of a patient receiving two BAL support system treatments, lasting for 5 and 4.5 h each, with no signs of adverse events. Since then, varieties of BAL devices have been produced and undergone clinical investigation, including HepatAssist, extracorporeal liver assist device (ELAD), TECA hybrid artificial liver support system (TECA-HALSS), the bioartificial liver of the Academisch Medisch Centrum (AMC-BAL), the LSS, the bioartificial liver support system (BLSS), the radial flow bioreactor (RFB), modular extracorporeal liver support (MELS), hybrid BAL, and bioartificial hepatic support. Here, a systematic review of the literature was performed to overview and evaluate the current clinical applications and outcomes of extracorporeal BAL support system during the past 15 years [26].

Wearable Artificial Kidney (WAK)

Wearable artificial kidney (WAK) is based on nanoporous biomaterials used in a hemodialysis system, such as charcoal, activated carbon, and zeolite [27]. For years, dialysis has been the standard treatment for uremia. However, regular, long-lasting therapy sessions tethered to an essentially unmovable machine are not ideal for patients. After continuous ambulatory peritoneal dialysis was introduced in the early 1980s, interest has focused on developing a truly wearable or portable dialysis system. Early examples of wearable hemodialysis devices reported in the literature were excessively large and heavy, performed inefficiently, and, most problematic of all, lacked effective safety controls. Only recently have some interesting papers describing innovative and truly wearable devices deservedly spurred interest in the field. Although the idea of a WAK is not new, it is only the advent of nanotechnology and miniaturization that has made the vital qualities of efficiency and safety achievable on a small scale. The reasons for developing a WAK can be categorized as clinical, technical, and/or socioeconomic. The outcomes of patients on chronic renal replacement therapy remain dismal with respect to quality of life, morbidity, and mortality [28].

Damaged skin can be implanted by using *artificial dermis*, for example, MatriDerm®. Artificial dermis (MatriDerm®) was used followed by skin graft for reconstruction in the case of 50-year-old woman with a DFSP in the occipital region. She was referred to us after her first surgery with positive margins. A wide local excision with a 2-cm margin was performed and periosteal tissue was also removed, which led to exposure of the skull. MatriDerm® was placed on the bone surface and dressings were changed every other day. Meanwhile, margins were evaluated by the complete circumferential peripheral and deep margin assessment (CCPDMA) and were positive for DFSP in the superior margin. After 4 weeks the area was completely covered by granulation tissue, and a new resection followed by reconstruction with a skin graft was performed. Dermal substitutes have been widely used in plastic, reconstructive, and burn surgery for many years. MatriDerm® (Dr. Suwelack Skin & Health Care AG, Billerbeck, Germany) – an acellular lyophilized collagen- and elastin-based biomatrix – was introduced several years back, which is a thin (1 or 2 mm) dermal template. It has been successfully used in one-step procedures in combination with split-thickness skin grafts. Although the use of MatriDerm® in burns and trauma surgery has been widely demonstrated, there are only few reports available on its use in surgical oncology, and none has yet reported it for DFSP [29].

The history of *dental implants* has been looked at before, but there have been no documented cases of a functional implant from ancient times [30]. A novel fibrous connected tooth implant using a dental implant and dental follicle stem cells as a bio-hybrid organ was developed. The bio-hybrid implant restored physiological functions, including bone remodeling, regeneration of critical bone defect, and responsiveness to noxious stimulations, through regeneration with periodontal tissues, such as cementum, PDL, and alveolar bone [31].

9.3 Processes between Living Tissue and Implant Interface

Imagine that a cavity were created in bone, soft tissue, or blood without initially perturbing the remaining tissue. If the cavity were filled with a foreign material, an interface would have been created between the native tissue and the foreign material (Figure 9.8). The tissue consists of a variety of molecules such as water,

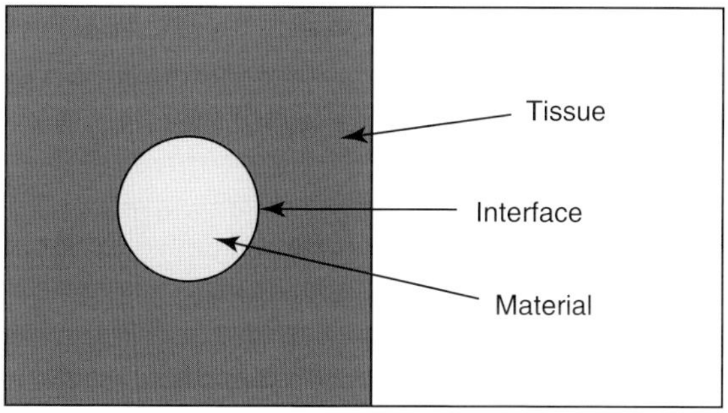

Figure 9.8 The implantation of a foreign material in any tissue will create an interface between the material and the biological system [32].

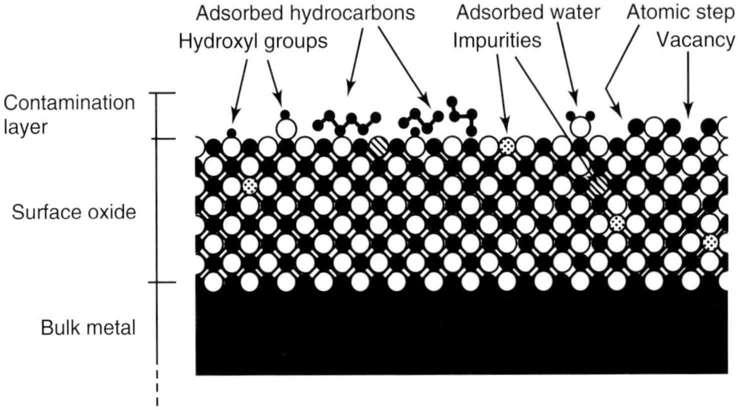

Figure 9.9 Schematic illustration of a "real" metal surface depicting the surface oxide with minor impurities, including surface hydroxyl groups and water, and the adsorbed contamination layer. Structural defects (steps and vacancies) are also indicated [32].

oxygen, negative and positive ions, proteins, and other biomolecules, which may be built up into larger structures such as cells and cell membranes. The foreign material could consist of individual atoms, molecules, or larger polymeric structures. These biological and nonbiological structures meet and interact at the interface.

The chemical constituents and pH, for example, of the biological environment influence the interaction at the surface (Figure 9.9). If the material is a metal, degradation by corrosion may result in the release of metal ions from the oxidized metal surface into solution, which may then migrate throughout the biological system, potentially producing negative systemic effects such as allergic reactions. This has been demonstrated in animal experiments and in humans, with metal ions such as Ni, Cr, Al, and V.

Even if dissolution of ions does not occur, the surface may be attacked by the tissue by an oxidative process if the oxide layer, instead of remaining passive, becomes thicker via anion or cation transport through the oxide layer. This can occur in the presence of oxygen radicals and peroxy species, or certain complex-forming ions in the biological environment, or catalyzing species that accelerate oxidization. If oxide growth occurs *in vivo*, as has been demonstrated experimentally, it may be accompanied by inclusion of ions present in the bioliquid (as indicated for Ca and P in Figure 9.10).

Thus, the surface of the material, and its interface with the tissue, may be very dynamic and may undergo continuous remodeling. Biodegradable materials constitute an extreme and intentional case of this event – the whole material eventually is dissolved. In the other extreme, like bone-anchored devices, the requirement is a stable yet fully tissue-integrated device, which may require an initial or continuous microscopic remodeling of the surface, but at a rate that has a negligible effect on the macroscopic dimensions of the implant (Figure 9.11).

The material surface is, in relation to the tissue, a foreign chemical species that has reactive sites, such as unsaturated chemical bonds, which can be either the

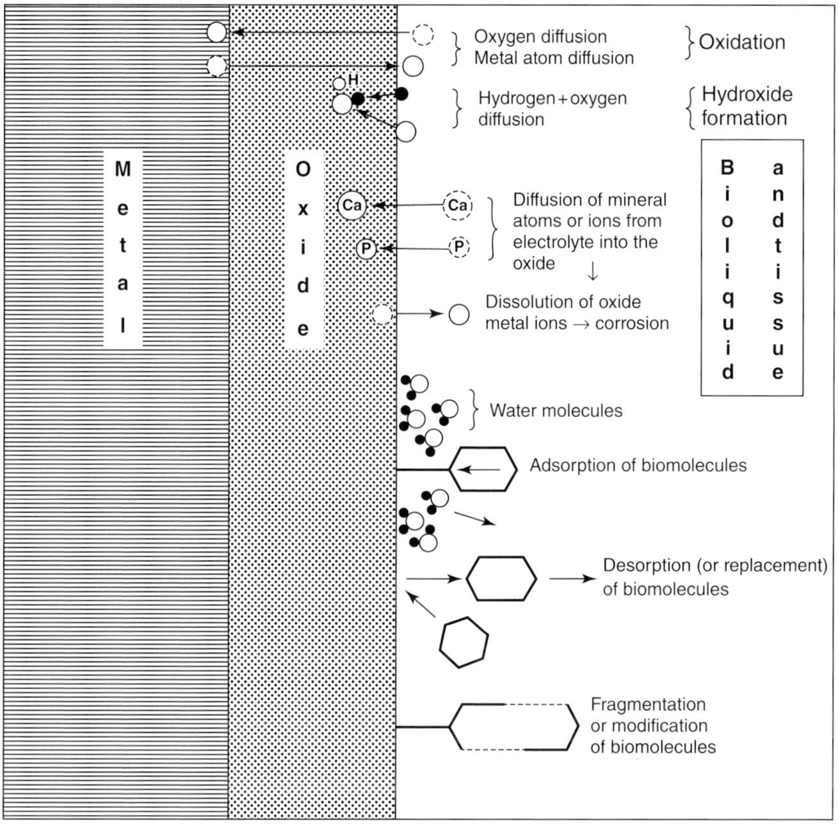

Figure 9.10 Schematic illustration of some molecular processes at the interface between a material and the surrounding biological environment. The top half of the figure shows processes that modify the material; the lower half shows interactions between the surface and biomolecules [32].

main constituents of the surface or impurities that have become incorporated in it. The termination of polymer chains on polymer surfaces also may be reaction sites, which can interact with reactive groups, for example, on protein and carbohydrate molecules. Reactions between a biomolecule and the material surface may lead to a permanent or temporary bond formation, which are either weak, of van der Waals or hydrogen bonding type, or stronger ionic or covalent bonds. In contrast, interactions may be so strong that, for example, proteins are reversibly or irreversibly denatured by formation of multiple bonds with the surface, accompanied by breaking of internal bonds within the protein. Such interaction might lead to total dissociation of the biomolecules, as is frequently seen with smaller molecules like O_2, H_2, H_2O, and hydrocarbons on metal and oxide surfaces. It also may lead to catalytic action that irreversibly modifies the protein conformation and composition, even if it is eventually released from the surface. The molecular events at the material–tissue interface involve small molecules, like water, which can dissociate to –OH groups or bind to the surface by hydrogen bonds. They also

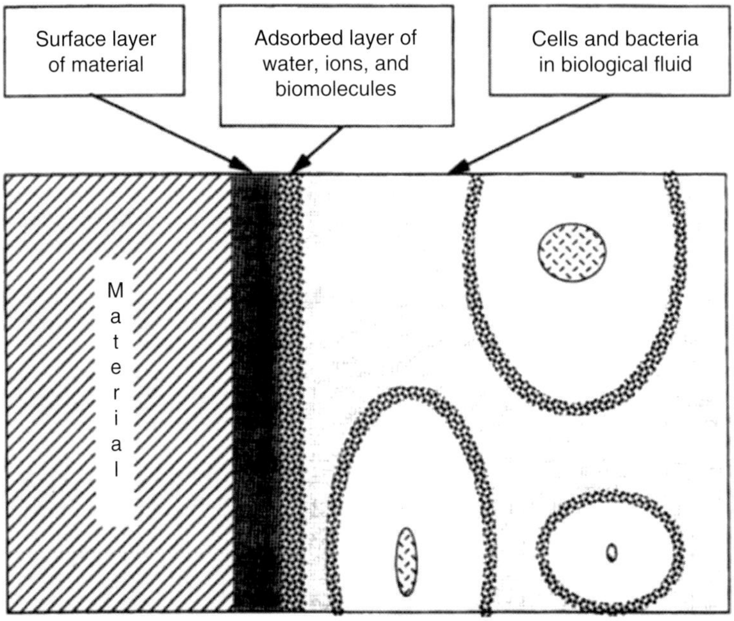

Figure 9.11 Schematic picture of cells close to the material surface, illustrating that the cells interact with the dynamic hydration (water and ions) and protein layers, which cover the material surface in the biological environment [32].

involve larger molecules like proteins, which sometimes denature (Figure 9.12). This hydration and protein layer is dynamic and surface specific since different surfaces will develop very different coatings in the same tissue, because of their different chemical properties. Eventually the larger structures like cells, which have lower mobility, will reach the surface with its organic over layer (Figure 9.12). Since both the cell membrane with its coating of biomolecules and the material surface are dynamic, they can exchange proteins, ions, and other substances and form a complex and dynamic interface. Depending on the nature of the material surface and its organic coating, cells react differently to different biomaterials. They may experience the surface as a serious perturbation and react violently, inducing an inflammatory response; if the surface is experienced as "tissue-like," no reactions or only mild ones may occur.

Case Study 1: Iris-Fixated Phakic Intraocular Lens Implantation after Retinal Detachment Surgery: Long-Term Clinical Results

- Patients having pIOL implantation in both eyes were enrolled [33]. Eyes that had scleral buckling or encircling (RD group) and healthy fellow eyes (non-RD group) were evaluated over a 6-year follow-up. The corrected distance visual acuity (CDVA), endothelial cell density (ECD), intraoperative complications, and long-term complications were safety outcomes.

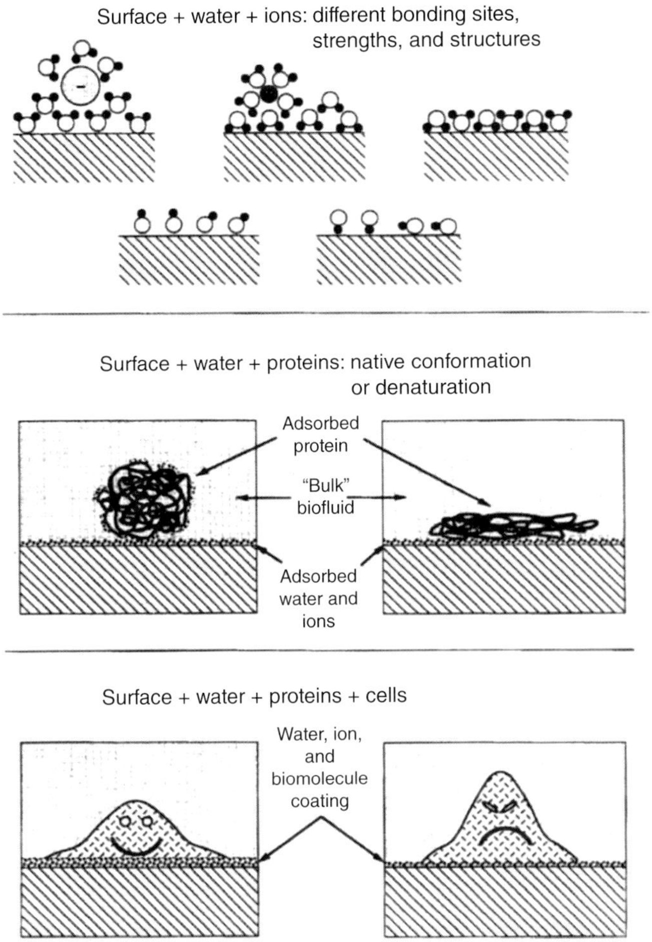

Figure 9.12 Schematic illustration of the material–tissue interaction at different levels. The original surface properties of the material will eventually influence the behavior of the cells and the macroscopic development of the tissue, via interaction with water, ions, and biomolecules such as protein molecules [32].

- The study comprised 34 eyes (17 patients). The mean postoperative CDVA and ECD were not significantly different between groups, and no patient lost CDVA. The rate of transient intraocular pressure spike was significantly higher in the RD group ($P = 0.043$). After 3 years and 6 years, the mean postoperative UDVA was 0.06 log MAR ± 0.09 (SD) and 0.08 ± 0.10 log MAR, respectively, in the RD group and 0.04 ± 0.08 log MAR and 0.04 ± 0.09 log MAR, respectively, in the non-RD group ($P = 0.518$ and $P = 0.478$, respectively).
- Because the biometric results could change after RD surgery and stable refraction could be achieved 6 months after surgery, three consecutive biometric examinations were performed with a 2-week interval at least 6 months after retinal reattachment; consistent data were used for IOL power calculation. The IOL power was calculated by the pIOL manufacturer with the modified van der

Table 9.2 Lines of CDVA gained and lost at 3 years and 6 years by group.

CDVA Lines	Number (%)			
	RD group		Non-RD group	
	3 years	6 years	3 years	6 years
+1	5 (29.4)	3 (25.0)	4 (23.5)	2 (16.7)
0	12 (70.6)	9 (75.0)	13 (76.5)	10 (83.3)

CDVA = corrected distance visual acuity; RD = retinal detachment.
Source: Chung *et al.* 2013 [33]. Reproduced with permission of Elsevier.

Heijde formula using the mean corneal power, subjective spectacle refraction at a 12.0 mm vertex, and ACD. The target refraction was emmetropia in all cases.

- The eyes were divided into two groups. The RD group consisted of eyes that had previous surgery for retinal detachment. The non-RD group comprised the patient's fellow eye that had not had previous ocular surgery.
- After 3 years and 6 years, the mean postoperative CDVA was 0.02 ± 0.08 log MAR and 0.04 ± 0.1 log MAR, respectively, in the RD group and -0.01 ± 0.07 log MAR and 0.01 ± 0.08 log MAR, respectively, in the non-RD group ($P = 0.339$ and $P = 0.376$ between groups at 3 years and 6 years, respectively). No eye in either group gained 2 or more lines or lost lines of CDVA (Table 9.2). The safety index at 3 years was 1.07 in the RD group and 1.05 in the non-RD group and at 6 years, 1.04 and 1.03, respectively [33].

Case Study 2: Cardiac Pacing Systems and Implantable Cardiac Defibrillators (ICDs): A Radiological Perspective of Equipment, Anatomy, and Complications

- *Mode of operation*: Pacemaker systems can operate in many different ways, for example, pacing of the ventricle with sensing in both the ventricle and the atrium [16]. Generic codes have been devised to summarize their mode of operation. The first letter of the code denotes the chamber that is paced, with A indicating the atrium, V the ventricle, and D that both chambers are paced. The second letter of the code designates the chamber(s) sensed; the same letter code is used. The third position denotes the response to sensing, which can be inhibition (I), triggering of a stimulus (T), or both (D). A fourth position is used if the pacemaker has an ability to adjust the pacing rate in response to exercise (R).
- *Single chamber pacing in the ventricle*: The pacemaker is commonly "rate responsive." Rate-responsive pacemakers can automatically increase the pacing rate when the patient exercises. This is achieved by the incorporation of a sensor, which detects a change in a parameter. Available sensors include accelerometers that detect motion and sensors that detect changes in thoracic

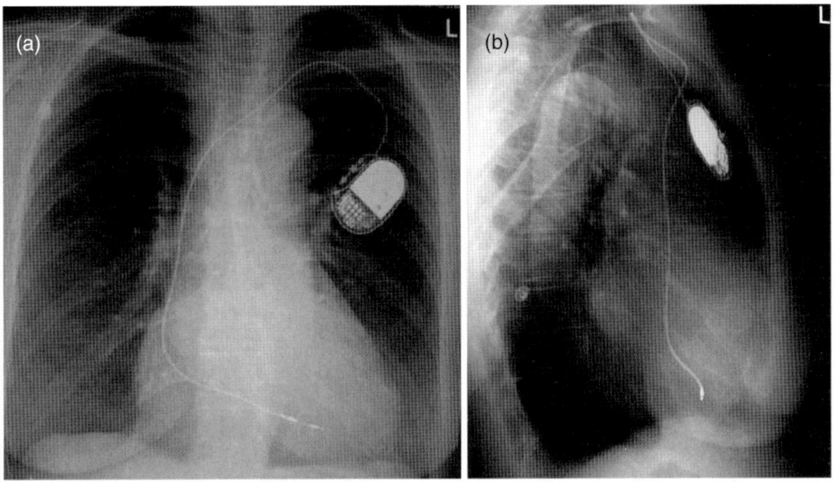

Figure 9.13 Images demonstrating a good ventricular lead position of a passive fixation lead. (a) PA view. (b) Lateral view. (Bruney *et al.* 2004 [16]. Reproduced with permission of Elsevier.)

impedance due to alterations in minute ventilation. The pacing code for this type of pacemaker is VVIR. The usual tip position is at the apex of the right ventricle. Figure 9.13 shows a typical appearance with gentle curves along the lateral wall of the right atrium, a curve as the lead passes through the tricuspid valve, and the tip at the apex directed anteriorly and inferiorly. In the PA view the tip is positioned to the left of the spine.

Control Questions

1) Define the term implant and describe the historical chronology of implantology for the development of implants.
2) Describe the main implant types used for damaged tissue replacement in the living tissue.
3) Describe the types of intraocular lenses (IOLs) and the role of phakic intraocular lenses in the improvement of vision.
4) Determine the cochlear implant and its main components.
5) Discuss brain implants and deep brain stimulation system (DBS).
6) Describe heart implants such as pacemakers, heart valves, and stents used for the replacement of damaged cardiovascular tissues in the living body.
7) Describe the function of balloon catheter in the working of stents.
8) Describe joint replacements and their types, such as total hip and knee replacements.
9) Describe satisfactory material combinations for wear-stressed moving parts of artificial hip joints, based on Table 9.1.
10) Determine other internal organ replacements: intestine and bioartificial liver support system (BALs).

11) Describe the wearable artificial kidney (WAK) as implant for eliminating kidney failure.
12) Describe skin implants and artificial dermis in eliminating skin failure.
13) Describe teeth implants and their types.
14) Determine the main processes between living tissues and implant interface.
15) Describe chemical processes occurring on the surface of metal implant and living tissues, with metal ions such as Ni, Cr, Al, and V.
16) Describe the processes at the interface between a material and the surrounding biological environment.
17) Describe the surface properties of the material that will eventually influence the behavior of the cells and the macroscopic development of the tissue, via interaction with water, ions, and biomolecules such as protein molecules.

References

1 van Eck, C.F., Chen, A.F., Klatt, B.A., D'Antonio, J., and Fu, F. (2009) The classification of implants: class I, II, III. *J. Long Term Eff. Med. Implants*, **19** (3), 185–193.

2 Saini, M., Singh, Y., Arora, P., Arora, V., and Jain, K. (2015) Implant biomaterials: a comprehensive review. *World J Clin Cases*, **3** (1), 52–57, doi: 10.12998/wjcc.v3.i1.52.

3 Becker, M.J. (2000) Ancient "dental implants": a recently proposed example from France evaluated with other spurious example. *Int. J. Oral Maxillofacial Implants*, **14** (1), 19–29.

4 Gray, R.J. (1978) Metallography in failure analysis, in *Failure Analyses of Surgical Implants from the Human Body Can Improve Product and Performance Reliability* (eds J.L. McCall and P.M. French), Springer, pp. 231–256.

5 Patel, N.R. and Gohil, P.P. (2012) A review on biomaterials: scope, applications & human anatomy significance. *Int. J. Emerging Tech. and Adv. Eng.*, **2** (4), 91–101, ISSN 2250-2459.

6 Wikipedia. Intraocular Lens. Text available via, https://en.wikipedia.org/wiki/Wikipedia:Text_of_Creative_Commons_Attribution-ShareAlike_3.0_Unported_License.

7 Hassaballa, M.A. *et al* (2011) Phakic intraocular lenses outcomes and complications: Artisan vs Visian ICL. *Eye*, **25**, 1365–1370.

8 Hellingman, C.A. and Dunnebier, E.A. (2009) Cochlear implantation in patients with acute or chronic middle ear infectious disease: a review of the literature. *Eur. Arch. Otorhinolaryngol.*, **266**, 171.

9 Pauna, H.F. *et al* (2014) Advanced Bionics® cochlear implants in patients with prelingual hearing loss. *Otolaryngology*, **4** (2), 159.

10 Kang, S.K. *et al* (2016) Bioresorbable silicon electronic sensors for the brain. *Nature*, **530**, 71–76.

11 Rodionov, R. *et al* (2013) Feasibility of multimodal 3D neuroimaging to guide implantation of intracranial EEG electrodes. *Epilepsy Res.*, **107** (1–2), 91–100.

12 Gibney, E. (2015) Injectable brain implant spies on individual neurons, understand how the brain works. *Nature*, **522**, 137–138.
13 Delaloye, S. (2014) Deep brain stimulation in the treatment of depression. *Dialogues Clin. Neurosci.*, **16** (1), 83–91.
14 Oxley, T.J. *et al* (2016) Minimally invasive endovascular stent-electrode array for high-fidelity, chronic recordings of cortical neural activity. *Nat. Biotechnol.*, **34** (3), 320–330.
15 Wood, M.A. and Ellenbogen, K.A. (2002) Cardiac pacemakers from the patient's perspective. *Circulation*, **105** (18), 2136–2139.
16 Bruney, K. *et al* (2004) Cardiac pacing systems and implantable cardiac defibrillators (ICDs): a radiological perspective of equipment, anatomy and complications. *Clin. Radiol.*, **59** (8), 699–708.
17 Wikipedia. Implanted Cardiac Pacemaker, https://en.wikipedia.org/wiki/Artificial_cardiac_pacemaker#/media/File:PPM.png (accessed 17 January 2017).
18 Webb, J.G. (2008) Percutaneous aortic valve replacement will become a common treatment for aortic valve disease. *JACC Cardiovasc. Interv.*, **1** (2), 122–126.
19 Pruitt, L. and Furmanski, J. (2009) Polymeric biomaterials for load-bearing medical devices. *JOM*, **61**, 14.
20 Misawa, Y. (2015) Valve-related complications after mechanical heart valve implantation. *Surg. Today*, **45**, 1205–1209.
21 Stephen, R. (2010) Total hip arthroplasty: techniques and results. *Med. J.*, **52** (9), 455–464.
22 Alsamah, M.A. (2013) Rationale analysis of human artificial knee replacements. *J. King Saud Univ. Eng. Sci.*, **25** (1), 49–54.
23 Semlitsch, M. and Willert, H.G. (1980) Properties of implant alloys for artificial hip joints. *Med. Biol. Eng. Comput.*, **18**, 511.
24 OrthoInfo. Total Joint Replacement, http://orthoinfo.aaos.org/topic.cfm?topic=a00233 (accessed 17 January 2017).
25 Kubal, C.A., Mangus, R.S., and Tector, A.J. (2015) Intestine and multivisceral transplantation: current status and future directions. *Curr. Gastroenterol. Rep.*, **17**, 5.
26 Gu, J. *et al* (2012) Systematic review: extracorporeal bio-artificial liver-support system for liver failure. *Hepatol. Int.*, **6**, 670–683.
27 Cheah, W.-K., Ishikawa, K., Othman, R. and Yeoh, F-Y. (2015) Nanoporous biomaterials for uremic toxin adsorption in artificial kidney systems: A review. *J Biomed Mater Res Part B*, p. 1–9.
28 Ronco, C., Davenport, A., and Gura, V. (2008) A wearable artificial kidney: dream or reality? *Nat. Clin. Pract. Nephrol.*, **4**, 604–605.
29 Bertolli, E. *et al* (2013) Artificial dermis (Matriderm®) followed by skin graft as an option in dermatofibrosarcoma protuberans with complete circumferential and peripheral deep margin assessment. *Int. Wound J.*, **12**, 545–547.
30 Crubzy, E., Murail, P., Girard, L., and Bernadou, J.P. (1998) False teeth of the Roman world. *Nature*, **391** (29), 29–30.

31 Oshima, M. *et al* (2014) Functional tooth restoration by next-generation bio-hybrid implant as bio-hybrid artificial organ replacement therapy. *Sci. Rep.*, **4**, article No, 6044.
32 Kasemo, B. and Lausmaa, J. (1994) Biomaterial and implant surfaces: the role of surface properties and processes. *Environ. Health Perspect.*, **102** (5), 41–45.
33 Chung, J.K. *et al* (2013) Iris-fixated phakic intraocular lens implantation after retinal detachment surgery: long-term clinical results. *J. Cataract Refract. Surg.*, **39** (10), 1494–1501.

Further Reading

Andriacchi, T.P., Galante, J.O., and Fermier, R.W. (1982) The influence of total knee-replacement design on walking and stair-climbing. *J. Bone Joint Surg. Ser. A*, **64** (9), 1328–1335.

Cambridge Dictionary on-line (2016). http://dictionary.cambridge.org/dictionary/english/implant.

Duraccio, D., Mussano, F., and Faga, M.G. (2015) Biomaterials for dental implants: current and future trends. *J. Mater. Sci.*, **50**, 4779.

Healy, K.E. and Ducheyne, P. (1992) Hydration and preferential molecular adsorption on titanium in vitro. *Biomaterials*, **13** (8), 553–561.

Jurt, U. *et al* (2002) Heart transplant: what to expect, cardiology patient page. *Circulation*, **106**, 1750–1752.

Lee, D.B.N. and Roberts, M. (2008) A peritoneal-based automated wearable artificial kidney. *Clin. Exp. Nephrol.*, **12**, 171.

Nelson, G.D. (1993) A brief history of cardiac pacing. *Tex. Heart Inst. J.*, **20** (1), 12–18; Bakken, E. (1992) Personal communication, November 1992.

Park, I.S., Won, S.Y., Bae, T.S. *et al* (2008) Fatigue characteristics of five types of implant-abutment joint designs. *Met. Mater. Int.*, **14**, 133.

Torres-Ayala, S.C., Santacana-Laffitte, G., and Maldonado, J. (2014) Radiography of cardiac conduction devices: a pictorial review of pacemakers and implantable cardioverter defibrillators. *J. Clin. Imaging Sci.*, **4**, 74.

WIPO. Seeing the World through a Clearer Lens, http://www.wipo.int/ipadvantage/en/articles/article_0149.html (accessed 17 January 2017).

10

Tissue Engineering, Scaffolds, and 3D Bioprinting

I have developed a unique way of looking at the relationship of the human body to health and disease.

David Agus, physician, Professor of Medicine and Engineering

10.1 Definition of Tissue Engineering

Tissue engineering is defined as manufacturing of functioning organs for implantation and use inside the body (Med. Dict., © 2009 Farlex & Partners). Tissue engineering is defined as a multidisciplinary field incorporating to the principles of fundamental science including biology, chemistry, engineering, and medicine to create biological substitutes of native tissues for scientific research or clinical applications [1]. Regulatory considerations for tissue engineering and regenerative medical product are manipulation of cells, cell source application, and scaffold characterization [2]. Despite tremendous advances using biologically derived scaffolds, the development of synthetically derived scaffolds is reasonable from practical, regulatory, and scientific perspectives [3].

10.1.1 Biomaterials Used for Tissue Engineering

The basic types of biomaterials used in tissue engineering can be broadly classified as *synthetic polymers*, which include relatively hydrophobic materials such as α-hydroxy acid [a family that includes poly(lactic-*co*-glycolic) acid (PLGA)], polyanhydrides, and others; *naturally occurring polymers*, such as complex sugars (hyaluronan, chitosan); and inorganics (hydroxyapatite). There are also functional or structural classifications, such as whether they are *hydrogels*, injectable, surface modified, capable of drug delivery, by specific application, and so on. The breadth of materials used in tissue engineering arises from the multiplicity of anatomical locations, cell types, and special applications that apply. For example, relatively strong mechanical properties may be required in situations where the device may be subjected to weight loading or strain or where maintenance of a specific cyto-architecture is needed. In others, looser networks may be needed or even preferable. The type of materials used is also dependent on the anticipated mode of application (open implantation vs injection or minimally invasive

Nano- and Biomaterials: Compounds, Properties, Characterization, and Applications,
First Edition. Zhypargul Abdullaeva.

procedure), the nature of any bioactive molecules that might be released, the need for surface functionalization, the needs of the cell types of interest in terms of porosity, and other issues. Despite this broad spectrum of potential materials, there are certain generic properties that are desirable. For example, a formulation that is biocompatible in subcutaneous tissue might not be so in the nerve or in the peritoneum. Local tissue reaction to the biomaterial of a construct may be harmful to the host and/or the construct, even in the absence of immune-mediated reaction to the nonautologous cellular material. For example, the inflammatory reaction to relatively benign polymers such as α-hydroxy acids, together with the acidosis that results from their breakdown, can lead to bony destruction and development of draining fistulae; here, the absolute mass of the biomaterial may play a role. Conversely, inflammation can lead to invasion of the construct by host cells with untoward consequences for the transplanted cells. Similarly, the material must be neither cytotoxic nor systemically toxic. Therefore, it is important to be aware of the potential toxicity of the materials' breakdown products, as well as of residual unreacted cross-linking agents (e.g., glutaraldehyde), reactive groups on polymers (e.g., aldehydes, amides, hydrazides), and similar issues. Of note, a material's apparent lack of cytotoxicity does not necessarily predict biocompatibility.

10.1.2 Principles of Tissue Engineering

Tissue engineering is a science dealing with manipulation of synthetic compounds into anatomically and/or functionally specific architectures and, when required, may be integrated with biologically active agents and/or living cells, resulting in properties suitable for support of specific cell life assigned for recipient tissues [5]. Principles of tissue engineering are based on historically used empirical methods intending to devise reparative strategies for optimizing the repair of skeletal tissue defects obtained or established in embryogenesis [6].

10.1.3 Components of Tissue Engineered Constructs

Cells and Scaffolds

Cells used in the tissue engineering are mainly attributed to the stem cells, which have been classified into: (i) Embryonic stem cells (ES) cells used for production of type-matched tissues for each patient, either through stem cell banking or by the use of therapeutic cloning; (ii) bone-marrow-derived mesenchymal stem cells are used for bone and cartilage repair; and (iii) cord-derived mesenchymal stem cells that can undergo multilineage differentiation [7].

Scaffolds affect cell response and must be engineered to support cell adhesion, proliferation, and differentiation, also act as an interim synthetic extracellular matrix (ECM) that cells interact with prior to forming a new tissue [8].

Biomaterial scaffolds can be made from coral, ceramics, hydrogel, fibrous and composite materials, hydroxyapatite (Hap), bioglass, protein (silk, collagen, fibrin), and polysaccharide (agarose, hyaluronan, chitosan) based materials [9, 10].

Approaches in scaffold design must be able to create hierarchical porous structures to attain desired mechanical function and mass-transport (i.e., permeability and diffusion) properties and to produce these structures within arbitrary and complex three-dimensional (3D) anatomical shapes. Hierarchical refers to the fact that features at scales from the nanometer to millimeter level will determine how well the scaffold meets conflicting mechanical function and mass-transport needs. Material chemistry together with processing determines the maximum functional properties that a scaffold can achieve, as well as how cells interact with the scaffold. However, mass-transport requirements for cell nutrition, porous channels for cell migration, and surface features for cell attachment necessitate a porous scaffold structure. This porous structure dictates that achievable scaffold properties will fall between the theoretical maximum set by the material and the theoretical minimum of zero predicted by composite theories. The critical issue for design is then to compute the precise value of mechanical as well as mass-transport properties at a given scale based on more microscopic properties and structure. One way to achieve hierarchical design is to create libraries of unit cells (a mathematical entity not to be confused with a biological cell) at different physical scales that can be assembled to form scaffold architectures. Such libraries may be created either using image-based design approaches or using approaches based on computer-aided design (CAD). Homogenization theory, which uses asymptotic expansion of relevant physical variables to generate multiscale equilibrium equations, can then be used to compute effective properties based on these unit-cell designs. By solving unit-cell deformation under six local strain states, the effective stiffness at a more macroscopic level C_{ijlk}^{macro} is computed from the stiffness at a more microscopic level C_{ijpm}^{macro} and the 3D spatial arrangement of the microscopic level as given by the strain localization tensor M_{pmkl} and the volume of the unit cell [11] ($V_{\text{unit cell}}$):

$$C_{ijkl}^{\text{macro}} = \frac{1}{|V_{\text{unit cell}}|}\int_V C_{ijkl}^{\text{macro}} M_{pmkl}\, dV_{\text{unit cell}} \tag{10.1}$$

Porosity degree of composite incorporated with polymeric material scaffolds can be determined by the following equation [12]:

$$\text{Porosity}\,(\%) = 1 - [(\text{weight}/\text{volume})/\rho\,\text{polymer}] \times 100 \tag{10.2}$$

For designing of hydrogel tissue-engineering scaffolds with appropriate properties, determination of an average molecular weight number between cross-links (Mc) and the network mesh size (ξ) can be achieved by the following equations [13]:

$$M_c = M_0/2X \tag{10.3}$$

$$\xi = \upsilon_{2,s}^{-1/3}(\gamma_0^2)^{1/2} = Q_v^{1/3}(\gamma_0^2)^{1/2} \tag{10.4}$$

where, M_0 is molecular weight of the polymer unit, X is cross-linking degree; $(\gamma_0^2)^{1/2}$ is the root-mean-square end-to-end distance of network chains between two adjacent cross-links in the equilibrium state.

Table 10.1 Functions of extracellular matrix (ECM) in native tissues and of scaffolds in engineered tissues.

Functions of ECM in native tissues	Analogous functions of scaffolds in engineered tissues	Architectural, biological, and mechanical features of scaffolds
Provides structural support for cells to reside	Provides structural support for exogenously applied cells to attach, grow, migrate, and differentiate *in vitro* and *in vivo*	Biomaterials with binding sites for cells; porous structure with interconnectivity for cell migration and for nutrients diffusion temporary resistance to biodegradation upon implantation
Contributes to the mechanical properties of tissues	Provides the shape and mechanical stability to the tissue defect and gives the rigidity and stiffness to the engineered tissues	Biomaterials with sufficient mechanical properties filling up the void space of the defect and simulating that of the native tissue
Provides bioactive cues for cells to respond to their microenvironment	Interacts with cells actively to facilitate activities such as proliferation and differentiation	Biological cues such as cell-adhesive binding sites; physical cues such as surface topography
Acts as the reservoirs of growth factors and potentiates their actions	Serves as delivery vehicle and reservoir for exogenously applied growth-stimulating factors	Microstructures and other matrix factors retaining bioactive agents in scaffold
Provides a flexible physical environment to allow remodeling in response to tissue dynamic processes such as wound healing	Provides a void volume for vascularization and new tissue formation during remodeling	Porous microstructures for nutrients and metabolites diffusion; matrix design with controllable degradation mechanisms and rates; biomaterials and their degraded products with acceptable tissue compatibility

Source: Chan *et al.* 2008 [14]. Reproduced with permission of Springer.

10.2 Scaffolds and Scaffolding

Scaffolds, typically made of polymeric biomaterials, provide the structural support for cell attachment and subsequent tissue development [14]. The term *scaffold* is determined as support, either natural or artificial, that maintains tissue contour (Mosby's Dental Dictionary, 2nd edition, ©2008 Elsevier). The term *scaffolding* refers to providing with scaffold for support or platform. Various functions of scaffolds in engineered tissues are listed in Table 10.1.

10.2.1 Scaffolds for Bone Tissue Engineering

Primarily three biomaterials (metals, polymers, and ceramics) have been used in bone tissue engineering. *Titanium* is a traditional inert biomaterial for implants and is characterized by a minimal immune response, which is the biggest advantage of this material. Some studies have shown that titanium fiber meshes or titanium with zinc-containing hydroxyapatite enhances the osteogenic activity or the proliferation of seeded cells. However, the difficulty in performing histological analyses is a serious drawback in further investigating the biological activity of this material. *Biodegradable synthetic polymers* applied to bone tissue engineering include poly(lactic acid) (PLA), poly(glycolic acid) (PGA), poly(caprolactone), and poly(lactic-*co*-glycolide) (PLGA) copolymers. Although poly(ϵ-caprolactone) carries biocompatibility and processability, it is less suitable for long-term applications because of its high hydrophobicity and low degradability *in vivo.* Among *natural polymers,* bovine type I collagen has been used as a promising biomaterial. Several type I collagen-based materials are commercially available including CollapatII® (Biomet Inc.), Healos® (DePuy Spine Inc.), Collagraft® (Nuecoll Inc., Zimmer Inc.), and Biostite (Vebas S.r.l.). Given that collagens are dominant and an important matrix component in bone tissues, it makes sense that the scaffold has biocompatibility as well as activity to facilitate osteogenesis or cell proliferation.

Hydroxyapatite- and β-tricalcium phosphate-based scaffolds are widely used in bone tissue engineering, and several different bioceramics have been developed in order to improve their properties. In particular, calcium phosphates are the most popular materials for artificial bones. As approximately 70% of bone in the body is made up of calcium phosphates, their biocompatibility and biosafety were, in a sense, already tested in the living body. Calcium phosphates are naturally osteoconductive and metabolized and degraded by the endogenous system for bone remodeling, although the speed of degradation varies depending on particle size and form [15].

As an example, metallic scaffolds for bone tissue engineering are reproduced in Figure 10.1. These scaffolds can act as carriers, restricting the movement of

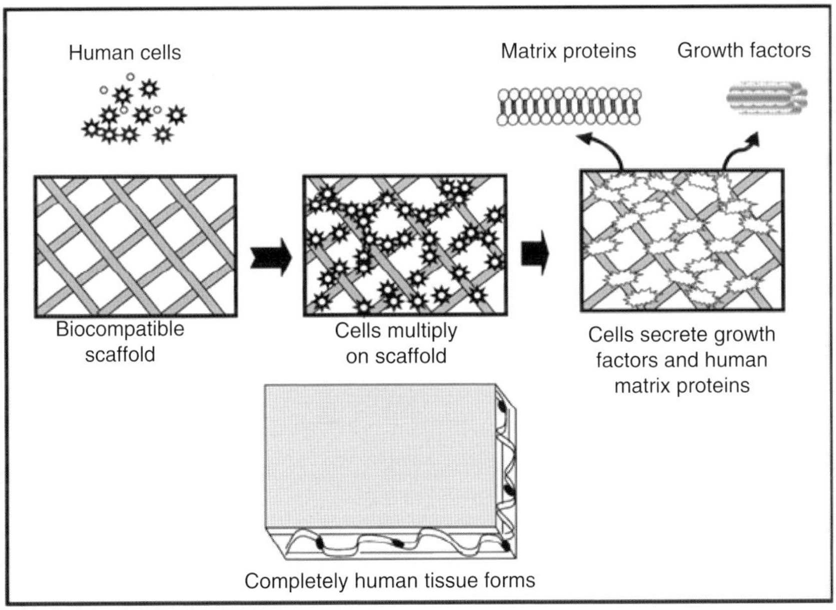

Figure 10.1 Cell-based tissue regeneration approach for the repair of bone defects [16]. (http://www.mdpi.com/1996-1944/2/3/790/htm. Used under: https://creativecommons.org/licenses/by/3.0/.)

mesenchymal stem cells (MSCs) away from the implantation site, and provide support for new bone formation. The osteogenic cells lay down bone extracellular matrix (ECM) in the surface of the scaffold as woven immature bone. Over time, a mature bone structure will form inside and in the exterior part of the scaffold allowing the regeneration of the tissue [16].

10.2.2 Tissue Engineering of Heart Valves

Tissue-engineered heart valve is abbreviated as TEHV. Tissue engineering of heart valves from decellularized valve scaffolds was reported [17]. Tissue engineering of heart valves investigates the possibility to construct and design a fully compatible and biomimetic graft, which is able to provide host cell repopulation like the native living valve [18]. The fundamental principles of tissue engineering applicable to heart valves were examined based on three approaches to achieving the goal of an engineered tissue heart valve: (i) cell seeding of biodegradable synthetic scaffolds, (ii) cell seeding of processed tissue scaffolds, and (iii) *in vivo* repopulation by circulating endogenous cells of implanted substrates without prior *in vitro* cell seeding [19].

Valve replacement has significantly improved the life prospect of patients with severe valve disease, receiving optimum medical treatment; for example, without surgical treatment, a 60-year-old man with severe aortic stenosis has approximately 4 years to live; after aortic valve replacement, his life expectancy increases to 13 years [20]. To avoid and exclude the sacrifice of healthy human vascular structures and circumvent additional surgical interventions, several different stem cell sources have been investigated with regard to their use in cardiovascular tissue engineering, in particular for heart valves [21]. Bioreactors have significant role in successful development of TEHV replacements, at the research stage, as well as in commercial platforms. Their ability to mimic the chemical and physiological conditions of the body has allowed researchers to study *in vitro* cellular responses, and this has helped in the fabrication of better and more efficient tissues *in vivo* [22]. Figure 10.2 shows cultured decellularized tissue-engineered heart valve (DTEHV) and its geometry control [23].

Original design of heart valve was based on the mathematical description [24] with the parameters $R_b = R_c = 13.5$ mm, $H = 19.15$ mm, $H_s = 3.15$ mm, and $\beta = 0°$ without any coaptation. The improved valve geometry was described [25] with the parameters $a = b = 3.1$ mm, $H = 18$ mm, and $R = 13.5$ mm with 5 mm coaptation. All values were obtained as described in [26], and both designs used the experimentally measured tissue thickness of 0.58 mm. The total stress in the tissue was given by the stress in the collagen fibers (with volume fraction ϕ_f) and the isotropic matrix components (with volume fraction $1 - \phi_f$):

$$\sigma = \sigma_m + \sigma_f \tag{10.5}$$

The isotropic matrix stress is equal to

$$\sigma_m = (1 - \phi_f)\left(k\frac{\mathrm{In}J}{J}I + \frac{G}{J}\left(B - J^{\frac{2}{3}}I\right)\right) \tag{10.6}$$

with $B = F \cdot F^T$ the left Cauchy–Green tensor, F the deformation gradient tensor, and $J = \det(F)$ the volumetric change ratio. The tissue was modeled as almost

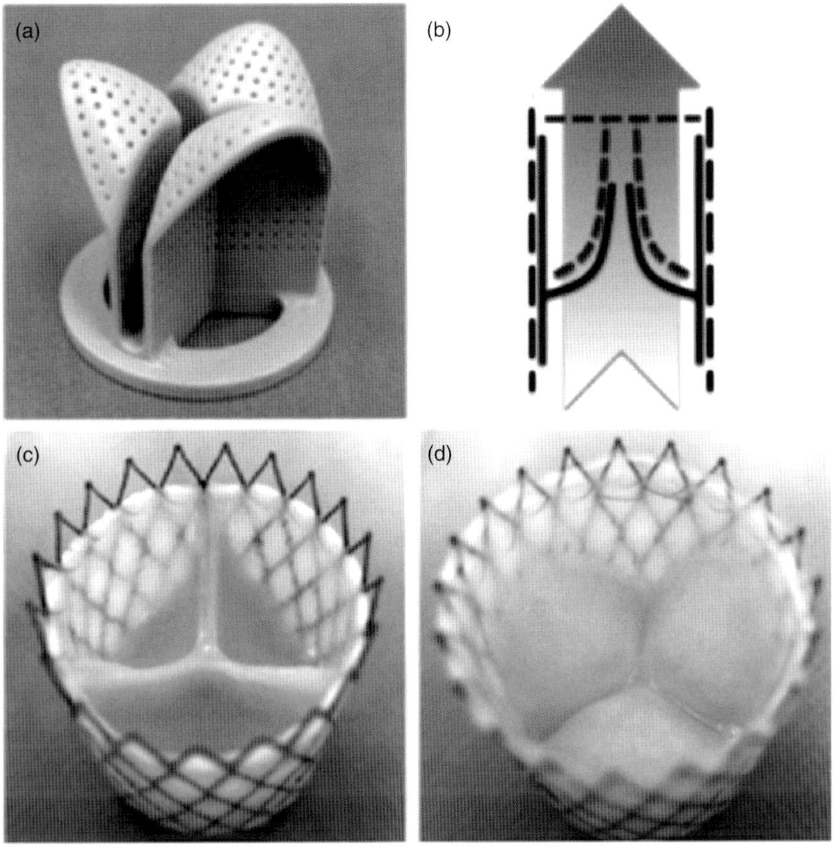

Figure 10.2 Bioreactor insert and representative DTEHV results. The developed bioreactor insert used to impose and control the heart valve geometry during culture (a). A schematic representation of the positioning of the insert depicted in green, inside the bioreactor setup with the heart valve indicated in red, the nitinol stent in black, and the pulsatile medium flow as a blue arrow (b). Two representative pictures of a human cell-based DTEHVs cultivated by using the insert, from a top (c) and bottom view (d), showing large coaptation areas and an profound belly curvature, matching the shape of the bioreactor insert [23]. (http://link.springer.com/article/10.1007/s10439-015-1386-4. Used under: https://creativecommons.org/licenses/by/4.0/.)

incompressible ($\upsilon = 0.498$), and the shear modulus G was set to 10 kPa to prevent numerical instabilities. The compression modulus is defined as

$$k = \frac{2G(1+\upsilon)}{3(1-2\upsilon)} \tag{10.7}$$

The improved heart valve geometry as suggested by the computational simulations was successfully translated into a physical rigid object (Figure 10.2a), matching the exact same geometry. The surface of the insert was smooth and the holes were equally distributed over the entire surface to enable sufficient nutrient exchange to the scaffold. There was sufficient space between the individual posts to prevent leaflet fusion during culture. The insert fitted nicely into the

DPD bioreactor system without obstructing the pulsating flow passing by the ventricular side toward the arterial side (Figure 10.2b). During the 4 weeks of culturing, the leaflets of the TEHVs compacted tightly around the insert, adapting to the imposed geometry. After decellularization, the valves maintained their shape, and there was no leaflet retraction visible upon removal of the insert. The coaptation area was approximately 5 mm in length (Figure 10.2c), and the belly region of the DTEHVs maintained the imposed curvature (Figure 10.2d). The tissue was uniformly distributed throughout the leaflets, without any damage or other macroscopically detectable irregularities [23].

The three basic types and the general overview of scaffolds used for heart valve tissue engineering are shown in Table 10.2 (Table 10.3).

10.3 3D Bioprinting

3D bioprinting was originated from biofabrication, which can be defined as the production of complex living and nonliving biological products from raw materials such as living cells, molecules, ECM, and biomaterials. By combination of accomplishments in the cell with developmental biology, materials science, and mechanical engineering, biofabrication was born [28]. *3D bioprinting* can be defined as the use of a technology or technique for the purpose of precise positioning of layers of cells and biological materials to support them in a 3D fashion in order to resemble or replicate a functional tissue or organ [29]. 3D bioprinting can be generalized into three main categories based on the technique being used, namely, (i) extrusion-based bioprinting techniques using mechanical forces to extrude the material through an orifice, (ii) inkjet-based techniques that eject picoliter droplets of the material onto a substrate, and (iii) laser-based techniques where laser is used to cure photopolymers or to induce material jetting [30]. The skin bioprinter is able to deliver two different types of skin cells and biomaterials directly on target locations and cover skin defects, and delivery of autologous cells facilitates wound healing and repair of skin defects [31].

3D bioprinting is based on three central approaches: biomimicry, autonomous self-assembly, and mini-tissue building blocks.

Biomimicry: Biologically inspired engineering has been applied to many technological problems, including flight, materials research, cell culture methods, and nanotechnology. Its application to 3D bioprinting involves the manufacture of identical reproductions of the cellular and extracellular components of a tissue or organ. This can be achieved by reproducing specific cellular functional components of tissues, for example, mimicking the branching patterns of the vascular tree or manufacturing physiologically accurate biomaterial types and gradients. *Autonomous self-assembly*: Another approach to replicating biological tissues is to use embryonic organ development as a guide. The early cellular components of a developing tissue produce their own ECM components, appropriate cell signaling, and autonomous organization and patterning to yield the desired biological micro-architecture and function. *Mini-tissues*: The concept of mini-tissues is relevant to both of the aforementioned strategies for 3D bioprinting. Organs and

Table 10.2 General overview of types of scaffolds.

Construct	Source	Adjuvant	Advantages	Disadvantages	Side effects	Type of study	References
Bioscaffold	Porcine	Anionic sodium dodecyl sulfate, Triton X-100, Tween family agents, the nonionic BigCHAP and the zwitterionic CHAPS and CHAPSO	Nontoxic tissue results at detergent concentration ($50\ mg\ l^{-1}$)	ECM structure damage compromising reseeding, histological deviations, cost	Inflammation, fibrosis, degradation, damage	*In vitro*, *in vivo*, clinical trials	[7,8]
Synthetic scaffolds	NDGA, POSSPCU, and others	Cross-linking NDGA with collagen	Mechanical properties, tear strength, tensile strength (best results with POSS-PCU)	*In vitro* studies –none	Not known	*In vitro*, *in vivo* (sheep)	[8–10]
Cell entrapment	Collagen gel	Cell source, 3D form	Plasticity	Unpredictable structure and density	Functionality concerns	*In vitro*	[16]

Source: Rippel *et al*. 2012 [27]. Reproduced with permission of Springer.

Table 10.3 Synthetic scaffolds used for heart valve.

Year	Trade name	Material/polymer	Description	Type of study	Outcome	References
1967	Biomer, Elastane	Polyether urethanes	HMDI, MDI, PTMEG, BD, EDA, and DAMCH	Bovine	1. Better hydrolytic stability 2. Oxidative degradation of the soft segment 3. Environmental stress cracking	[14, 15, 20]
1980	Thoralon	Silicone in backbone of polyether urethane	MDI, PTMEG, PDMS, EDA	Rat	1. Siloxane end groups: (a) Give protection to the polyether soft segment (b) Provide low strength	[21]
1990	ChronoFlex, Bionate	Silicone end groups and midblocks with polyether or polycarbonate urethane	MDI, PTMEG and PDMS, PC and PDMS, PHECD and PDMS, BD, EDA, DMACH	*In vitro* and in rabbit	1. Increased resistance to oxidation	[53, 66, 67]
1991	Persil, Cab-O-Sil	Silicone end groups and midblocks with polyether or polycarbonate urethane	MDI, PTMEG and PDMS, PC and PDMS, PHECD and PDMS, BD, EDA, DMACH	Rabbit	1. More stable than PEU 2. Crack resistant 3. Susceptible to hydrolysis	[22, 23, 53, 65]
1996	Elast-Eon	Silicone midblocks and polyether urethanes	MDI, PTMEG and PDMS, PDMS and PHMO, BD	*In vitro* and in sheep model	1. Good biostability	[53, 67, 68]
1997	ChronoFlex C	Silicone midblocks and polycarbonate urethanes	MDI, PC and PDMS, BD	*In vitro*	1. High strength 2. Hydrolytically and proteolytically stable	[69]
2007	Glassy polymeric carbon (GPC)	Liquid resol $C_7H_8O_2$	GPC silver deposition	*In vitro*	1. Less cell adhesions (embolization) compared with pure GPC	[70]
2005	Seifalian	Polyhedral oligomeric silsesquioxane integrated poly(carbonate urea) urethane	MDI, PC, EDA-POSS	*In vitro*	1. High strength, elasticity at high levels of stress 2. Resistance to degradation 3. Reduced calcification 4. Reduced platelet adhesion	[71–73]
2010	Nordihydroguaiaretic acid (NDGA)	Natural with two ortho-catechols	Porcine scaffold NDGA coating cross-linked	*In vitro*	1. Good porous micro-architecture 2. Good tensile strength	[7]

tissues comprise smaller functional building blocks or mini-tissues. These can be defined as the smallest structural and functional component of a tissue, such as a kidney nephron. *Imaging and digital design:* An essential requirement for reproducing the complex, heterogeneous architecture of functional tissues and organs is a comprehensive understanding of the composition and organization of their components. *Tissue bioprinting strategies*: The main technologies used for deposition and patterning of biological materials are *inkjet, microextrusion,* and *laser-assisted printing* [32]. A comparison of bioprinters is reproduced in Table 10.4.

The principal concept of building large diameter, intermediate diameter, and microvascular segments of a vascular tree or *roadmap for organ printing* is demonstrated in Figure 10.3. The microvascular networks can be self-assembled either from single cells placed into hydrogel by vacuole accumulation or from endothelial tissue spheroids. Biofabrication of microvascularized histotypical tissue spheroids is also a reality. It is already proven that essential parts or segments of a vascular tree can be engineered at least separately. Moreover, it has been shown that small isolated fragments of the microvascular tree can be reunited by self-assembly *in vitro* and *in vivo.* Thus, we can argue that building

Table 10.4 Comparison of bioprinter types.

Bioprinter type				
	Inkjet	**Microextrusion**	**Laser assisted**	**References**
Material viscosities	3.5–12 mPa s^{-1}	30 to >6 × 10^7 mPa s^{-1}	1–300 mPa s^{-1}	[48, 63, 78, 107]
Gelation methods	Chemical, photo-cross-linking	Chemical, photo-cross-linking, sheer thinning, temperature	Chemical, photo-cross-linking	[64, 85, 106, 110]
Preparation time	Low	Low to medium	Medium to high	[2016, 64, 94, 107]
Print speed	Fast (1–10 000 droplets per second)	Slow (10–50 μm s^{-1})	Medium-fast (200–1600 mm s^{-1})	[49, 58, 76, 90]
Resolution or droplet size	<1 to >300 pl droplets, 50 μm wide	5 μm to millimeters wide	Microscale resolution	[49, 68, 69, 76]
Cell viability	>85%	40–80%	>95%	[2006, 54, 80, 104]
Cell densities	Low, <106 cells ml^{-1}	High, cell spheroids	Medium, 108 cells ml^{-1}	[2006, 49, 88, 89]
Printer cost	Low	Medium	High	[77]

Source: Murphy *et al.* 2014 [32]. Reproduced with permission of Nature Publishing Group.

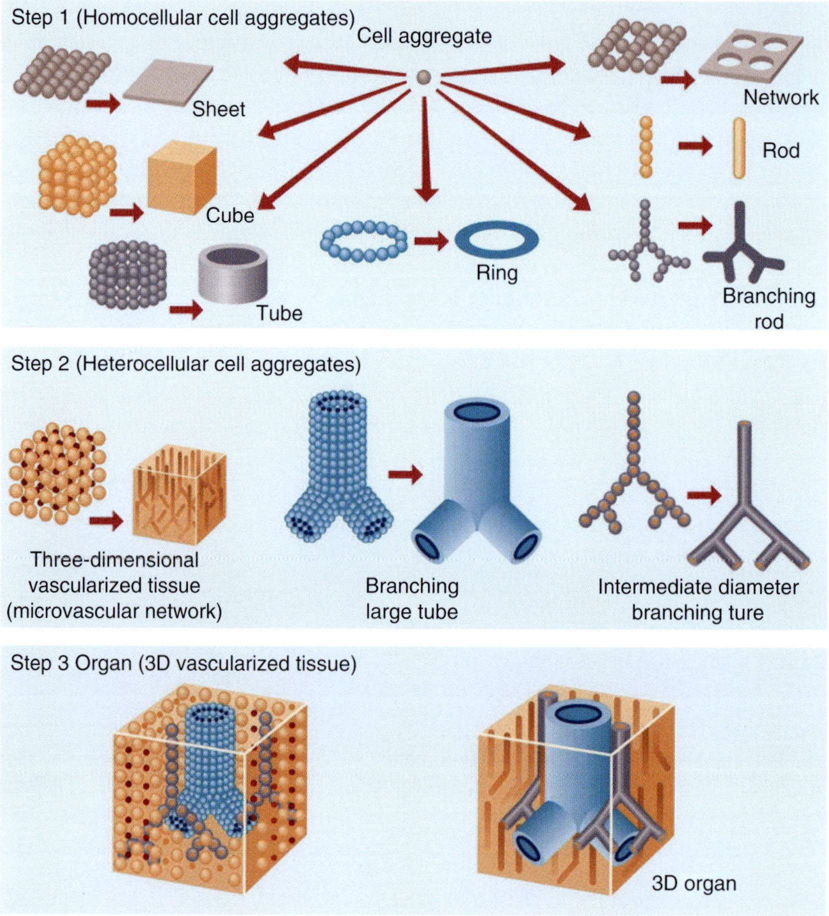

Figure 10.3 Roadmap for organ printing. (Mironov *et al.* 2009 [28]. Reproduced with permission of Elsevier.)

a complete intraorgan branched vascular tree with 10–12 orders of branching is technologically feasible. The proposed concept of bioengineering a natural-like intraorgan branched vascular tree from three types of self-assembled vascular tissue spheroids is specially designed for organ-printing technology. It is important to mention that the layers of vascular tissue spheroids for bioassembly of the vascular tree will be placed simultaneously with the layers of microvascularized organo-specific tissue spheroids. Thus, after finishing bioprinting, post-printed tissue fusion, and accelerated tissue maturation, the bioengineered vascular tree will be suitable for perfusion and integrated into 3D tissue or organ constructs [28].

Bioengineering a natural-like hierarchically branched intraorgan vascular tree that can be "built in" a bioprinted 3D tissue construct represents an enormous challenge, but it is obvious that without bioengineering perfusable intraorgan branched vascular tree, it is practically impossible to print viable human organ constructs. The biomimetic concept of accelerated tissue maturation in microtissue-based approaches implies that the desirable material and biomechanical properties of engineered constructs could be rapidly achieved without using supporting biodegradable solid scaffolds. In order to achieve specified biomechanical properties of tissue-engineered constructs, it is essential to know in advance not only the material properties of mature adult human tissues and organs but also the developmental kinetics of tissue and organ maturation, as well as the structural determinants of material properties of specific tissues or organs at different stages of development. Traditional relatively slow physical, chemical, and genetic approaches for tissue maturation – typical for biodegradable solid scaffold-based tissue engineering – are not well suited for requirements of rapid tissue maturation in a scaffold-free mini-tissue self-assembly-based approach [32].

10.4 Foreign Body Reaction

Foreign body reaction (FBR) is determined as a granulomatous *inflammatory response* evoked by the presence of a *foreign body* in the tissues; a characteristic feature of this is the formation of foreign body giant cells (see giant cell) (Miller-Keane Encyclopedia and Dictionary of Medicine, Nursing, and Allied Health, Seventh Edition. © 2003). From the implantation view, FBR can be determined as a localized inflammatory response elicited by any material (e.g., a splinter or a suture) that would not normally be found within the body (Medical Dictionary, © 2009 Farlex and Partners). Correlations of size, shape, and composition of particles to cell response at both histological and ultrastructural levels were done and reported during the FBR in total hip arthroplasties using the light microscopy, SEM, and TEM studies [33].

Modern healthcare offers a plethora of implantable medical devices to improve quality of life, from cardiac pacemakers and hernia meshes to newer technologies such as continuous glucose monitors, brain-stimulating electrodes, and drug delivery systems. Yet the intended function of these devices is often compromised by the host's foreign body response, which encapsulates the implant in a fibrotic membrane. In the presence of an implanted material, a tissue's normal process of wound healing becomes prolonged and aberrant, producing after several weeks a distinct, avascular collagenous sheath around the implant. The foreign body response (Figure 10.4) begins with instantaneous adsorption of many various host proteins to the implant surface, rapid neutrophil infiltration, and neutrophil activation by the implant surface and neutrophil release of soluble factors. Tissue-resident macrophages and circulating monocyte precursor cells then enter the site; their phagocytic activities are impeded by an inability to digest and remove the foreign body. In addition to fusing with each other to form foreign body giant cells at the implant surface, the macrophages secrete factors that recruit and activate fibroblasts, which produce matrix collagens. The resulting collagenous fibrotic capsule, up to several hundred micrometers thick, physically and physiologically separates the device from the host tissue. Lacking vasculature,

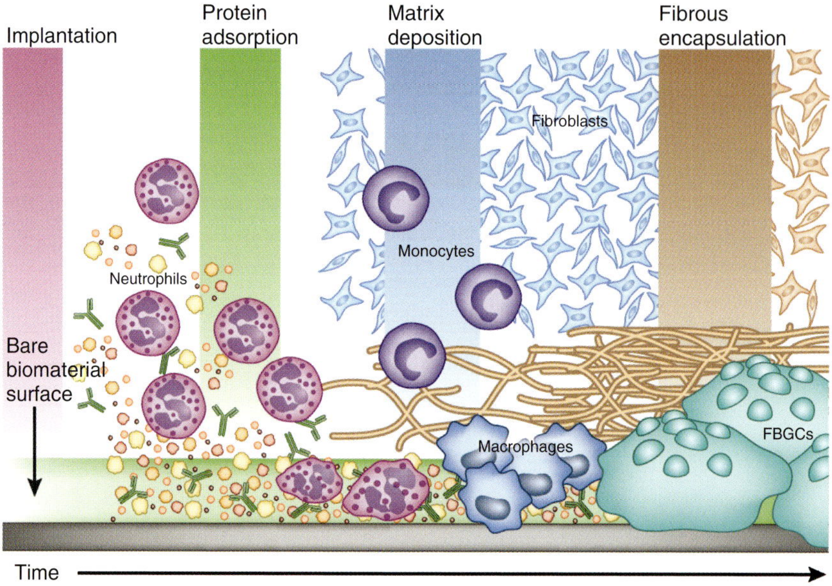

Figure 10.4 Temporal representation of the host response leading to the encapsulation of an implanted material. The process initiates immediately upon implant contact with host fluids (e.g., blood, lymph, wound fluids) by spontaneous uncontrolled adsorption of host proteins to the implant surface. The resulting protein-conditioned surface is coated with diverse protein species in various conformations and adsorbed states. Host cells responsible for normal wound healing encounter this unusual adsorbed protein layer. Within hours, neutrophils enter the implant tissue site and react by producing cytokines, chemokines, reactive oxygen species, and other enzymes. In the next several days, these neutrophil products recruit tissue resident macrophages and undifferentiated monocytes to the wound site, concomitant with the exit of neutrophils. Macrophages respond to the implant by producing their own set of signaling molecules, which attract fibroblasts. Fibroblasts produce excess collagen. Their presence correlates with formation of foreign body giant cells (FBGCs), whose role in the foreign body response is poorly understood. With time, a dense collagenous fibrotic capsule is created around the implant, isolating it physically and physiologically from the host tissue. (Grainger 2013 [34]. Reproduced with permission of Nature Publishing Group.)

the capsule can be impermeable to cells and can hinder metabolite transport, slow healing, resist device-tissue integration and create niches susceptible to infection. Substantial efforts have been devoted to improving implant "biocompatibility," a much abused term with no widely accepted definition. Various modifications to the material's surface properties or to its bulk chemistry, geometry, porosity, mechanical modulus, and other properties are often reported to diminish cellular reactions *in vitro* and short-term inflammatory responses *in vivo.* In general, however, any beneficial effects on the acute host response are eventually attenuated during chronic phase tissue remodeling. Another approach has been to design implants that release anti-fibrotic, anti-inflammatory, or pro-angiogenic drugs; such devices can reduce foreign body cellular responses at implant sites, but only until the last bit of the drug is released [34].

10.4.1 Inflammatory Response Following Material Implantation

Host reactions following implantation of biomaterials include injury, blood–material interactions, provisional matrix formation, acute inflammation, chronic inflammation, granulation tissue development, FBR, and fibrosis/fibrous capsule development (Figure 10.5). In the very early process of implantation, blood–material interactions occur with protein adsorption to the biomaterial surface and development of a blood-based transient provisional matrix that forms on and around the biomaterial. The injury to vascularized connective tissue not only initiates the inflammatory responses (innate immunity) but also leads to thrombus formation involving activation of the extrinsic and intrinsic coagulation systems, the complement system, the fibrinolytic system, the kinin-generating system, and the platelets. These protein cascades may be intimately involved in the dynamic phenomenon of protein adsorption and desorption that is known as the

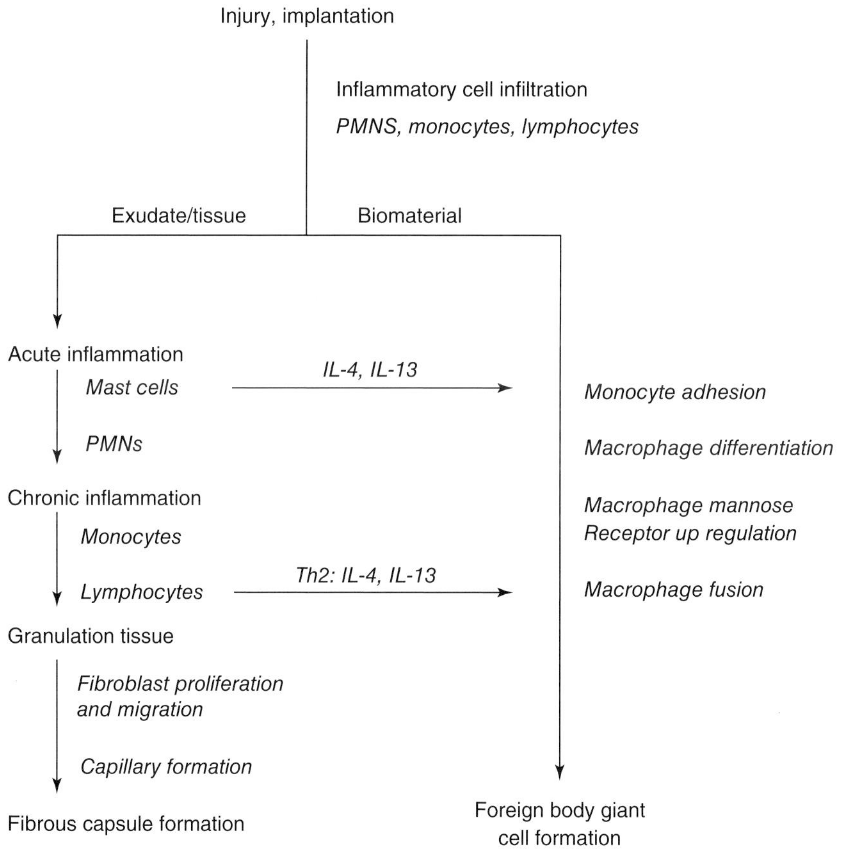

Figure 10.5 Sequence of events involved in inflammatory and wound healing responses leading to foreign body giant cell formation. This shows the potential importance of mast cells in the acute inflammatory phase and Th2 lymphocytes in the transient chronic inflammatory phase with the production of IL-4 and IL-13, which can induce monocyte–macrophage fusion to form foreign body giant cells. (Anderson *et al.* 2008 [35]. Reproduced with permission of Elsevier.)

Vroman effect. From a wound healing perspective, blood protein deposition on a biomaterial surface is described as provisional matrix formation. The provisional matrix furnishes structural, biochemical, and cellular components to the processes of wound healing and FBR. The presence of mitogens, chemoattractants, cytokines, growth factors, and other bioactive agents within the provisional matrix provides for a rich milieu of activating and inhibiting substances capable of modulating macrophage activity, along with the proliferation and activation of other cell populations in the inflammatory and wound healing responses [35].

10.4.2 Monocytes, Macrophages, and Foreign Body Giant Cells

Adsorption of Plasma Proteins

Biomaterials and medical devices immediately and spontaneously acquire a layer of host proteins prior to interacting with host cells. Thus, it is highly probable that the types, levels, and surface conformations of the adsorbed proteins are critical determinants of the tissue reaction to such implants.

Complement Activation

Subsequent reactions have been identified as causing adverse side effects when blood–material interactions occur with devices such as hemodialyzers, oxygenators, catheters, prostheses, stents, vascular grafts, and other devices and materials.

Macrophage Adhesion

Following blood–material interactions, platelets and the clot release chemoattractants, such as transforming growth factor (TGF-β), platelet-derived growth factor (PDGF), CXCL4 (platelet factor, PF4), leukotriene (LTB4), and interleukin (IL-1), that can direct macrophages to the wound site. Some of these products have the potential to recruit additional macrophages to the biomaterial–tissue interface. Once at the implant site or biomaterial surface, the macrophages can then adhere and engage in the subsequent events of the FBR (Figure 10.6).

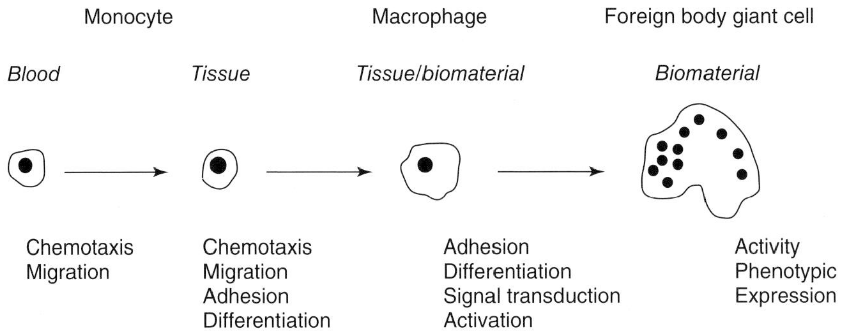

Figure 10.6 *In vivo* transition from blood-borne monocyte to biomaterial adherent monocyte/macrophage to foreign body giant cell at the tissue–biomaterial interface. There is ongoing research to elucidate the biological mechanisms that are considered to play important roles in the transition to foreign-body giant cell development. (Anderson *et al.* 2008 [35]. Reproduced with permission of Elsevier.)

Mediators of Degradation

Biomaterial surfaces in this privileged microenvironment are thus susceptible to high concentrations of these degradative agents. Therefore, the chemistry of the biomaterial surface will dictate its susceptibility to biodegradation. For example, addition polymers such as polyethylene used in artificial joints or polypropylene used as a suture material may undergo surface oxidation by the ROIs. Medical devices and prostheses composed of addition polymers usually contain small amounts of antioxidants to inhibit this oxidative process [35].

10.5 Wound Healing

Wound healing is defined as the process to restore to a state of soundness any injury that results in an interruption in the continuity of external surfaces of the body. It is also called wound repair (Mosby's Medical Dictionary, 9th edition. © 2009, Elsevier). Normal wound healing process is consisted of phases, characterized by cellular and bio-physiologic events, such as (i) *hemostasis* (vascular constriction; platelet aggregation, degranulation, and fibrin formation (thrombus)), (ii) *inflammation* (neutrophil infiltration, monocyte infiltration and differentiation to macrophage, lymphocyte infiltration), (iii) *proliferation* (reepithelialization, angiogenesis, collagen synthesis, ECM formation), and (iv) *remodeling* such as collagen remodeling, vascular maturation and regression [36].

Case Study 1: Bioactive Glass and Glass–Ceramic Scaffolds for Bone Tissue Engineering

- A wide range of materials have been used for orthopedics and dentistry such as: metals, alloys, ceramics, polymers, bioactive glass systems, and hybrid composites, which are holding importance in knowledge about performances of these materials in clinical practice, *in vitro* and *in vivo* tests [37]. Firstly, scaffolds need to encourage cell attachment, differentiation, and proliferation, which are cell functions highly dependent on substrate material properties, which are related to the property of *osteoconductivity* (*the growth of bony tissue into the structure of an implant or graft* (Saunders Comprehensive Veterinary Dictionary, 3 ed. © 2007 Elsevier)), which is important not only to avoid the formation of encapsulating tissue but also to induce a strong bond between the scaffold and host bone.
- In 1969, Hench and his colleagues have discovered chemical bond between the rat bone and certain silicate-based glass compositions. Later, this glass was termed as "bioactive," which means a material that exhibits specific biological response to the material surface, thus resulting in the formation of tissue-material bond [38].
- Figure 10.7 is representing porous 63s glass scaffolds with 10 wt% HANw (a) isometric view; (b) top view; (c) side view.

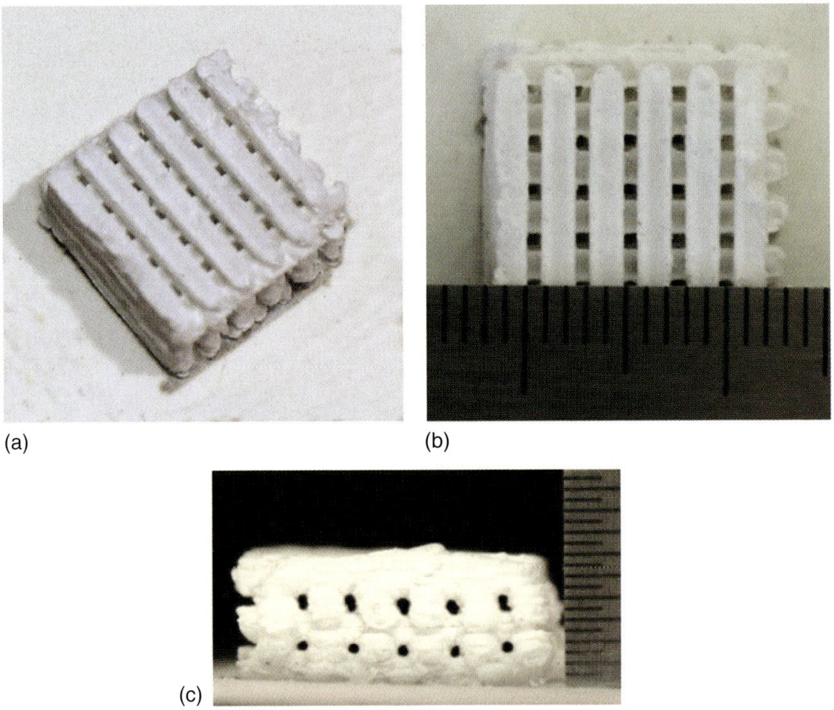

Figure 10.7 The porous 63s glass scaffolds with 10 wt.% HANw (a) isometric view; (b) top view; (c) side view (Shuai *et al.* 2015 [39], https://creativecommons.org/licenses/by/3.0/.)

Case Study 2: Regulatory Considerations in the Design and Manufacturing of Implantable 3D Printed Medical Devices

- 3D printing, or additive manufacturing, technology has rapidly penetrated the medical device industry over the past several years, and innovative groups have harnessed it to create devices with unique composition, structure, and customizability. These distinctive capabilities afforded by 3D printing have introduced new regulatory challenges.
- The customizability of 3D printed devices introduces new complexities when drafting a design control model for FDA consideration of market approval. The customizability and unique build processes of 3D printed medical devices pose unique challenges in meeting regulatory standards related to the manufacturing quality assurance.
- Consistent material powder properties and optimal printing parameters such as build orientation and laser power must be addressed and communicated to the FDA to ensure a quality build.
- Tracheobronchomalacia (TBM) is a pediatric condition of excessive dynamic collapse of the primary airways during respiration. In rare severe cases, standard therapies fail with high rates of treatment-associated and disease-associated morbidity and mortality.

Table 10.5 Definitions of design control model.

Term	Definition
User needs	Qualitative requirements deemed necessary for successful treatment of an illness or condition
Design input	Requirements of a device that are used as a basis for device design. Typically grouped into functional requirements, performance requirements, and interface requirements
Functional requirements	What the device does, focusing on the operational capabilities
Performance requirements	How much or how well the device must perform, addressing issues such as speed, strength, response times, accuracy, limits of operation, etc.
Interface requirements	Characteristics of the device, which are critical to compatibility with external systems
Design process	The process of translating a design concept into a functioning prototype
Design output	The results of a design effort at each phase of the design process and at the end of the total design effort
Verification	The process of checking at each stage of the design process whether the design output meets input requirements. If the data from the output is within the acceptable range established by the design input, then the design concept is verified
Validation	Establishing by objective evidence that final device specifications meet user needs and intended use

Source: Morrison *et al.* 2015 [40]. Reproduced with permission of John Wiley and Sons.

- Patient-specific devices are designed by imaging-based CAD and manufactured from a bioresorbable material using a 3D printer. Each device is designed using patient anatomy for design input, a design process that is consistent with the philosophy of personalized medicine and a hallmark feature of 3D printed medical devices.
- Preparing consideration including design control. *Design control* is a system of device development that promotes identification of potential design flaws, creation of multiple design concepts, and verification and validation of design efficacy via repeated design review. Definitions of design control model are shown in Table 10.5.
- User needs were subsequently translated into *distinct design input requirements* (Table 10.6, A). In a traditional model, device designs are created to set specifications, and a design process is developed to fulfill the specifications. If multiple design variations exist, design processes equal to the number of variants are typically created and validated.
- Standardizing the design process for 3D printed devices is uniquely challenging in that these devices allow many design parameters to be customized based on user needs, resulting in a potentially infinite number of design variants. As such, it becomes necessary to incorporate design verification and design validation steps into the overall design and manufacturing process for personalized 3D printed devices [40].

Table 10.6 Design control process for the 3D printed tracheobronchial splint.

A. User needs and requirements for TBS

Clinical user needs

1) Must maintain support for a critical 24-month duration and subsequently degrade
2) Must predictably and effectively exert a balanced radial force in the axial plane restoring the native lumen size and resisting external compression yet allowing for internal expansion during growth and transverse plane movement during cervical motion
3) Must be placed external to airway to leave mucociliary architecture unaltered
4) Must be straightforward to place the device onto the affected airway segment (i.e., low user complexity)

Performance requirements

1) Must be customized to the patient's specific defect size and location to 0.5 mm accuracy

Functional requirements

1) Must exhibit maximum displacement of less than 10% of initial splint diameter under 50 N compressive load
2) Must exhibit displacement greater than 20% of initial splint diameter, but less than 50% of initial splint diameter under 50 N three-point bending load
3) Must exhibit a displacement greater than 20% of initial splint diameter under 15 N opening angle load

Biomaterial requirements

1) Must not cause tissue reaction or remodeling (i.e., non-erosive), local or systemic toxicity
2) Must exhibit a degradation profile that ensures structural integrity for a critical 24-month duration and be fully bioresorbable

B. Design process for TBS

Generating design inputs

1) Thin-cut computed tomography (CT) images of patient's airway are obtained in inspiration and expiration
2) DICOM images of CT scan are input into mimics and used to generate 3D model of patient's airway using threshold function
3) Centerline function is performed on airway model and measurements performed to generate TBS design inputs
4) Design inputs: X diameter, Y diameter, wall thickness, bellow height, bellow wave shape, bellow periodicity, suture hole thickness, open wedge angle, length, spiral to open wedge angle

C. Device validation for TBS

Clinical validation

1) Manufactured device based on design output alleviates symptoms of TBM in preclinical animal model
2) Manufactured device based on design output does not demonstrate airway growth restriction in preclinical animal model

Mechanical validation

1) Bench mechanical testing of manufactured device based on design output in compression, three-point bending, and open angle displacement meets user needs criteria

Biomaterial validation

1) Device manufacture material composition meets ISO 10993 standards
2) Manufactured device-based produces no adverse tissue reaction in preclinical animal model

Source: Morrison *et al.* 2015 [40]. Reproduced with permission of John Wiley and Sons.

Control Questions

1) Determine tissue engineering and its goals.
2) Describe the types of biomaterials used for tissue engineering.
3) What kind of properties should possess biomaterials considered for tissue engineering applications?
4) Describe the principles of tissue engineering and its main factors.
5) Describe the components of tissue engineering building blocks.
6) Describe the difference between cells and biomaterial scaffolds used for tissue engineering.
7) Determine the patterning of scaffold chemistry and main approaches in the scaffold design.
8) Describe homogenization theory approach in scaffold design.
9) Determine porosity as an important factor in scaffold design.
10) Describe the approaches in the brain scaffold design based on homological features and network design.
11) Determine the terms for scaffold and scaffolding.
12) Describe about scaffolds for bone tissue engineering.
13) Describe tissue engineering of heart valves.
14) Determine the functions of extracellular matrix (ECM) in native tissues and of scaffolds in engineered tissues based on Table 10.1.
15) Describe the cell-based tissue regeneration approach for the repair of bone defects.
16) Describe the general overview of scaffold types.
17) Describe the synthetic scaffolds used for heart valve.
18) Determine 3D bioprinting and its features.
19) Describe the central approaches in 3D bioprinting: biomimicry, autonomous self-assembly, and mini-tissue building blocks.
20) Describe the roadmap for organ printing and its main steps.
21) Determine the FBR occurring after biomaterial implantation in the living body.
22) Describe the main stages of FBR and the host response leading to encapsulation of an implanted material.
23) Describe the sequence of events involved in inflammatory and wound healing responses leading to foreign body giant cell formation.
24) Determine wound healing and its feature characteristics.

References

1 Pallua, N. and Suschek, C.V. (eds) (2011) *Tissue Engineering, From Lab to Clinic*, Springer.

2 Lanza, R., Langer, R., and Vacanti, J.P. (2014) *Principles of Tissue Engineering*, 4th edn, Elsevier, ISBN: 978-0-12-398358-9.

3 Elbert, D.L. *et al* (2011) Bottom-up tissue engineering. *Curr. Opin. Biotechnol.*, **2**, 674–680.

4 Hardingham, T., Tew, S., and Murdoch, A. (2002) Tissue engineering: chondrocytes and cartilage. *Arthritis Res.*, **4** (Suppl. 3), S63–S68.
5 Brekke, J.H. and Toth, J.M. (1998) Principles of tissue engineering applied to programmable osteogenesis. *J. Biomed. Mater. Res.*, **43**, 380–398. doi: 10.1002/(SICI)1097-4636(199824)43:4<380::AID-JBM6>3.0.CO;2-D
6 Caplan, A.I. (2003) Embryonic development and the principles of tissue engineering, in *Tissue Engineering of Cartilage and Bone: Novartis Foundation Symposium 249* (eds G. Bock and J. Goode), John Wiley & Sons, Ltd, Chichester, UK. doi: 10.1002/0470867973.ch3
7 Howard, D., Buttery, L.D., Shakesheff, K.M., and Roberts, S.J. (2008) Tissue engineering: strategies, stem cells and scaffolds. *J. Anat.*, **213**, 66–72. doi: 10.1111/j.1469-7580.2008.00878.x
8 Smith, I.O., Liu, X.H., Smith, L.A., and Ma, P.X. (2009) Nanostructured polymer scaffolds for tissue engineering and regenerative medicine. *WIREs Nanomed. Nanobiotechnol.*, **1**, 226–236. doi: 10.1002/wnan.26
9 Hutmacher, D.W., Schantz, J.T., Lam, C.X.F., Tan, K.C., and Lim, T.C. (2007) State of the art and future directions of scaffold-based bone engineering from a biomaterials perspective. *J. Tissue Eng. Regen. Med.*, **1**, 245–260.
10 Alaribe, F.N., Manoto, S.L. and Motaung, S.C.K.M. (2016). *Scaffolds from biomaterials: advantages and limitations in bone and tissue engineering, Biologia* **71**/4: 353–366, Section Cellular and Molecular Biology, doi: 10.1515/biolog-2016-0056.
11 Hollister, S.J. (2005) Porous scaffold design for tissue engineering, *Nat. Mater.*, **4**, 7, 518–590.
12 Guarino, V., Causa, F., Taddei, P., Foggia, M., Ciapetti, G., Martini, D. *et al.* (2008) Polylactic acid fibre-reinforced polycaprolactone scaffolds for bone tissue engineering. *Biomaterials*, **29** (27), 3662–3670.
13 Zhu, J. and Marchant, R.E. (2011) Design properties of hydrogel tissue-engineering scaffolds. *Expert Rev. Med. Devices*, **8** (5), 607–626. doi: 10.1586/erd.11.27
14 Chan, B.P. and Leong, K.W. (2008) Scaffolding in tissue engineering: general approaches and tissue-specific considerations. *Eur. Spine J.*, **17**, 467. doi: 10.1007/s00586-008-0745-3
15 Ohba, S. *et al* (2009) Tissue engineering of bone and cartilage. *IBMS BoneKEy*, **6** (11), 405–419.
16 Alvarez, K. and Nakajima, H. (2009) Metallic scaffolds for bone regeneration. *Materials*, **2** (3), 790–832.
17 Hopkins, R.A. (2005) Tissue engineering of heart valves. *Circulation*, **111**, 2712–2714.
18 Gallo, M. *et al* (2013) Tissue-engineered heart valves: intra-operative protocol. *J. Cardiovasc. Transl. Res.*, **6**, 660–661.
19 Mendelson, K. *et al* (2006) Heart valve tissue engineering: concepts, approaches, progress, and challenges. *Ann. Biomed. Eng.*, **34** (12), 1799–1819.
20 Yacoub, M.H. and Takkenberg, J.J.M. (2005) Will heart valve tissue engineering change the world? *Nat. Clin. Pract. Cardiovasc. Med.*, **2**, 60–61.
21 Weber, B. *et al* (2012) Stem cells for heart valve regeneration. *Swiss Med. Wkly.*, **142**, w13622.

22 Amrollah, P. *et al* (2016) Bioreactors for heart valve tissue engineering: a review. *Chem. Technol. Biotechnol.*, **91**, 847–856.
23 Sanders, B. *et al* (2015) Improved geometry of decellularized tissue engineered heart valves to prevent leaflet retraction. *Ann. Biomed. Eng.*, **44** (4), 1061–1071.
24 Thubrikar, M.J. (1989) *The Aortic Valve*, CRC Press, ISBN: 9780849347719.
25 Hamid, M.S., Sabbah, H.N., and Stein, P.D. (1986) Influence of stent height upon stresses on the cusps of closed bioprosthetic valves. *J. Biomech.*, **19**, 759–769.
26 Loerakker, S., Argento, G., Oomens, C.W.J., and Baaijens, F.P.T. (2013) Effects of valve geometry and tissue anisotropy on the radial stretch and coaptation area of tissue-engineered heart valves. *J. Biomech.*, **46**, 1792–1800.
27 Rippel, A.R. *et al* (2012) Tissue-engineered heart valve: future of cardiac surgery. *World J. Surg.*, **36**, 1581–1591.
28 Mironov, V., Visconti, R.P., Kasyanov, V., Forgacs, G., Drake, C.J. and Markwald, R.R. (2009) Organ printing: tissue spheroids as building blocks, *Biomaterials* **30**, **12**, 2164–2174.
29 Munoz-Abraham, A.S. *et al.* (2016) 3D Printing of organs for transplantation: where are we and where are we heading? *Curr. Transplant. Rep.*, **3**, 93–99.
30 Wang, S., Lee, J.M., and Yeong, W.Y. (2015) Smart hydrogels for 3D bioprinting. *Int. J. Bioprinting*, **1** (1), 3–14.
31 Albanna, M.Z. *et al* (2012) In situ bioprinting of skin for reconstruction. *J. Am. Coll. Surg.*, **215** (3), S87.
32 Murphy, S.V. *et al* (2014) 3D bioprinting of tissues and organs. *Nat. Biotechnol.*, **32** (8), 773–785.
33 Pazzaglia, U.E. *et al* (1987) The foreign body reaction in total hip arthroplasties A correlated light-microscopy, SEM, and TEM study. *Arch. Orthop. Trauma Surg.*, **106**, 209–219.
34 Grainger, D.W. (2013) All charged up about implanted biomaterials, a zwitterionic polymer hinders the foreign-body response that leads to fibrotic encapsulation of implants. *Nat. Biotechnol.*, **31** (6), 507–509.
35 Anderson, J.M., Rodriguez, A., and Chang, D.T. (2008) Foreign body reaction to biomaterials. *Semin. Immunol.*, **20** (2), 86–100.
36 Guo, S. *et al* (2010) Factors affecting wound healing. *J. Dent. Res.*, **89** (3), 219–229.
37 Rau, J.V., Antoniac, I., Cama, G., Komlev, V.S. and Ravaglioli, A. (2016). Bioactive materials for bone tissue engineering, *BioMed. Res. Int.*, Volume **2016**, Article ID 3741428, 3 pages, doi: 10.1155/2016/3741428.
38 Hench, L.L. (2006) The story of Bioglass®. *J. Mater. Sci. Mater. Med.*, **17**, 967–978.
39 Shuai, C., Cao, Y., Gao, C., Feng, P., Xiao, T., and Peng, S. (2015) Hydroxyapatite Whisker reinforced 63s glass scaffolds for bone tissue engineering. *BioMed. Res. Int.*, **2015**, Article ID 379294, 8 pages, doi: 10.1155/2015/379294
40 Morrison, R.J., Kashlan, K.N., Flanangan, C.L., Wright, J.K., Green, G.E., Hollister, S.J., and Weatherwax, K.J. (2015) Regulatory considerations in the design and manufacturing of implantable 3D-printed medical devices. *Clin. Transl. Sci.*, **8**, 594–600.

Further Reading

Huebsch, N. and Mooney, D.J. (2009) Inspiration and application in the evolution of biomaterials. *Nature,* **462**: p. 426–432. doi: 10.1038/nature08601

Kim, S.S. *et al* (2006) Tissue engineering of heart valves by recellularization of glutaraldehyde-fixed porcine valves using bone marrow-derived cells. *Exp. Mol. Med.*, **38** (3), 273–283.

Kohane, D.S. and Langer, R. (2008) Polymeric biomaterials in tissue engineering. *Pediatr. Res.*, **63**, 487–491.

Kuzyk, P.R. and Schemitsch, E.H. (2011) The basic science of peri-implant bone healing. *Indian J. Orthop.*, **45**, 108–115.

Li, Z., Ji, S., Wang, Y. *et al* (2013) Silk fibroin-based scaffolds for tissue engineering. *Front. Mater. Sci.*, **7** (3), 237–247.

Miller-Keane Encyclopedia and Dictionary of Medicine, Nursing, and Allied Health (2003), 7th edn. © 2003 by Saunders, an imprint of Elsevier, Inc. All rights reserved.

Mosby's Dental Dictionary (2008), 2nd edn. © 2008 Elsevier, Inc. All rights reserved. http://medical-dictionary.thefreedictionary.com/scaffold; http://medical-dictionary.thefreedictionary.com/wound+healing.

National Institute of Biomedical Imaging and Bioengineering (2016) Tissue Engineering and Regenerative Medicine. https://www.nibib.nih.gov/science-education/science-topics/tissue-engineering-and-regenerative-medicine (accessed 13 January 2017).

Saunders Comprehensive Veterinary Dictionary (2007), 3rd edn. © 2007 Elsevier, Inc. All rights reserved. http://medical-dictionary.thefreedictionary.com/osteoconduction.

Shachar, M. and Cohen, S., Cardiac tissue engineering, ex-vivo: design principles in biomaterials and bioreactors, *Heart Fail. Rev.* (2003) **8**: 271. I

Index

a

achiral tubular nanoclusters 51–52
aerosols 28
agglomerate 28
aggregates 28
Ag nanomaterial 65
alginate 233
arc discharge method 21
armchair type carbon nanoclusters 51
artificial biomaterials 192
artificial dermis 249
atomic force microscope (AFM) 177–178
autonomous self-assembly 266

b

bioactive glasses and glass-ceramics 275–276
bio artificial liver support system 248
bioceramics-tissue attachment and bioceramic classification. 224
biocompatibility 220
biological constituents 217
biological properties of biomaterials 215–220
biomaterials 1
  body systems 191–192
  ceramic biomaterials 222–230
  composite 199
  general requirements for 190–191
  goals of 189
  main problems of 189
  mechanical properties 203
  metallic 193–199
  nanostructured CaP composites 200–203
  polymeric biomaterials 230–235
  purpose 189
biomimicry 266
biopolymers 217
bone cements and tissue interface formation 203
bone tissue engineering 262–264
brain implants 242–243
BSCCO/$SrTiO_3$ 105

c

carbon fiber (CF) composite materials 202–203
carbon nanotubes
  mechanical properties and physical parameters 52–53
  structural characteristics 54
  types and classification 49–52
carbon tubular nanoclusters 49
carboxymethyl cellulose (CMC) 215
cardiac pacing systems 254
  and implantable cardiac defibrillators 254
catalysis 160–163
cavitation-hydrodynamic method 8
centered (double-layered) fullerenes 43
centrifugal mill 3
centrifugal spraying 10
ceramic biomaterials 222–230
characterization tools in nanotechnology 172

Nano- and Biomaterials: Compounds, Properties, Characterization, and Applications,
First Edition. Zhypargul Abdullaeva.

chemical dispersion methods 14
chemical properties
of biomaterials 220–235
of nanomaterials
catalysis 160–163
oxidation process 153–157
pyrophoricity 157–160
size effects 151–153
spontaneous combustion temperature 158
chitosan 233
clusters 30
coagulation 82
coagulative mechanism 81
coalescence 81
cobalt oxide nanoparticles 61
cochlear implants 241–242
coherent region size distribution 86
collagen 233
colloidal solutions 28
colloidal system 28
combined plasma 11
composite biomaterials 199–200
comprehensive forging 6
Co nanoparticle lattice parameter 63
condensation of steam in the inert gas 12
copper-based nanomaterials 105
co-precipitating 15–16
crystal lattice defects 65–66
Curie temperature 115

d

Debye temperature 121–122
defective grain structure 166
dental implants 249
diffraction methods 173–174
diffusion
definition 133
mechanism 81
nanopowders 133–136
diffusionless mechanism 81
dispersion characteristics
grain boundaries 91–92
morphology 92–94
size distribution 80–89
specific surface area 79–80
surface, boundaries and morphology 89–91
dispersity 31
dispersive systems
aggregation state 27–28
definition 27
dimension 31–32
size 28–31
dynamic pressing 71

e

elastin 217
electrical arc melting 12
electrical conductivity 97–99
electrical detonation of semiconductors 12
electrical precipitation 20
electrochemical synthesis method 21
electro flotation 20
electron work function 99–101
equichannel angular pressing 6
evaporation-condensation methods 10–13
evaporative thermal decomposition method 16
extinction
by dielectric nanoparticles 125–128
in metallic nanoparticles 128–131
extrusion 73

f

Fe and Mo nanopowders 154
Fe_2O_3 nanoparticles 173
ferromagnetic characteristics
size dependence of
coercive force 112–114
saturation magnetization 114–15
substance in single domain condition 109–111
superparamagnetism 111–112
fibrin gels 233
fibrous composite materials 199
foreign body reaction (FBR) 271–275
Fourier transform infrared spectroscopy (FTIR) 181
fullerene
carbon materials 33

history 34
icosahedral 42–47
physical properties 47–49
tetrahedral fullerenes 34–42

g

gas phase chemical reactions method 18
gas static pressing 69
gels 28
gold nanoparticles 151
grain boundaries 91–92
slipping theory 169
granules 28
graphene
characterizations 142–145
electronic properties 138
physical properties and ionization potential 139–141
synthesis 141–142
topology 138–139
grinding in vortex mills 3

h

hardness 163–166
heart implants 243–246
heart valves 245
heat conductivity
crystal lattice 120–121
size dependence 116–120
hemostasis 275
heterodiffusion 136
heterophase interaction method 15
high temperature sintering 71
hip arthroplasty 246
hooves 219
hot pressing 72
HRTEM characterization of nanomaterials 177
hyaluronan 233
hydrogels 259

i

icosahedral fullerenes
classification 42–45
description 42
image force 99
implantable cardiac defibrillators 254
implantable 3D-printed medical devices 276–278
implants
bio artificial liver support system 248
brain 242–243
cochlear 241–242
definition 239
intestine replacement 247
intraocular lenses 239–241
iris-fixated phakic intraocular lens implantation 252–254
joint implants 246–247
living tissue and 249–252
wearable artificial kidney 248–249
inflammation 275
inflammatory response following material implantation 273
intensive plastic deformation methods 5–7
interrelation of nanomaterials size characteristics 87
intraocular lenses (IOLs) 239–241
in vivo tissue biocompatibility 215–220
iris-fixated phakic intraocular lens implantation 252–254
iron nanopowder 156
isostatic shaping 69

j

joint implants 246

k

keratins 217

l

laser heating 12
length of free electron path 95–96
Lennard–Jones potential 44
light scattering 123–125
liquid-like coalescence 81
liquid metal cathode 21
liquid spraying method 9–10
load-bearing medical devices, polymeric biomaterials 235–236

m

magneto-impulse pressing 71
Matriderm® 249
mechanical characteristics of nanomaterials
  hardness 164–166
  plasticity 166–170
  superplasticity 170–172
mechanical milling 3
mechanical properties of biomaterials
  ductility 209
  hardness 209
  high wear resistance 209
  long fatigue life 209
  stiffness 209
  strength 209
  stress shielding 209
  titanium alloy with self-adjustable Young's modulus 211–212
  toughness 210
  wear resistance 212–215
  Young's modulus 210
mechanochemical method 4–5
metallic biomaterials
  CoCr alloys 195–196
  FeMn alloys 194–195
  Tiadyne 1610 199
  Ti and Ti alloys 196
  TIMETAL® 21SRx 198
  Ti-15Mo alloy 199
  Ti-13Nb-13Zr alloy 198
  TMZF™ alloy 196–198
metallothermic method 17
metal salts hydrolysis 20
microdistorsions 66–68
microscopical characterization of nanomaterials
  AFM characterization 177–178
  HRTEM 177
  SEM characterization 178–181
  transmission electron microscopy 174–177
mini-tissues 266
monocytes, macrophages, and foreign body giant cells 274
mouthpiece pressing 74

n

nanocomposite materials
  applications 74–75
  consolidation of nano-sized powders 68–74
  crystal lattice defects 65–66
  definition 57
  melting temperature changes 61–62
  microdistorsions 66–68
  phase equilibrium changes 60–61
  size dependence 57–58
  structure 62–64
  thermodynamical features 58–59
nanocrystal 31
nanomaterials
  arc discharge method 21
  cavitation-hydrodynamic method 8
  centrifugal spraying 10
  chemical dispersion methods 14
  chemical flame in gas mixture method 21
  combined plasma 11
  comprehensive forging 6
  condensation of steam in the inert gas 12
  co-precipitating 15–16
  definition 1
  electrical arc melting 12
  electrical detonation of semiconductors 12
  electrical precipitation 20
  electrochemical synthesis method 21
  electro flotation 20
  environmental safety considerations 22–23
  evaporation-condensation methods 10–13
  evaporative thermal decomposition method 16
  gas phase chemical reactions method 18–19
  grinding in vortex mills 3
  heterophase interaction method 15
  history of applications 1
  intensive plastic deformation methods 5–7

interaction between metal oxides and gases 17
laser beams 21
laser heating 12
liquid metal cathode 21
liquid spraying method 9–10
mechanical milling 3
mechanochemical method 4–5
metallothermic method 17
metal salts hydrolysis 20
plasma method 21
plasma technology 11
precipitation method and process 15, 20
property control 23
radiation 21
reduction of metal oxides and other solid compounds 17
reduction methods 16
salt melts electrolysis 21
shock wave loading 22
sol-gel method 16
solid phase transformations 14
solid spraying method 9
solvent evaporation 16
spinning 10
sublimated drying 16
synthesis process in vacuum 12
thermal dissociation/pyrolysis 19–20
vacuum-sublimation technology 13–14
vibrational method 8–9
nanoparticles
of C20@C240 46
of C60@C540 46
nanosized catalysts 162
nanostructured calcium phosphate cement (CPC) 199
nanostructured CaP composites 200–203
natural biomaterials 192
natural degradable polymers 233
naturally occurring polymers 259
n-HA/CS/CMC composite 216
Ni and Pd nanoparticles 161
nondegradable polymers
polyacrylates 230
poly(N-isopropylacrylamide) 231
poly(vinyl alcohol) 230

o

one-dimensional materials 32
optical characteristics of nanomediums 122
extinction by dielectric nanoparticles 125–128
extinction in metallic nanoparticles 128–131
light scattering 123–125
morphology and polydispersity 131–133
oxidation
of Fe nanoparticles 182–183
process 153–157

p

pacemakers 243
phonon gas 120
plasma chemical process 84
plasma method 21
plasma technology 11
plasticity 166–170
polyacrylates 230
polyesters 231
polyethylene 231
polyethylene oxide 232
polymeric biomaterials 230–235
poly(N-isopropylacrylamide) 231
polystyrene sphere emulsions 128
poly(vinyl alcohol) (PVA) 230
porous biomaterials 199
powders 28
precipitation method 15, 20
pressing 69
in elastic shells 70
proteins 217
pure metal oxide mesocrystals 58
pyrophoricity 157–160

r

reduction methods 16
reduction of metal oxides and other solid compounds 17
resilin 217

s

salt melts electrolysis 21
scaffolding 262
  bone tissue engineering 262
  functions of extracellular matrix 262
  tissue engineering of heart valves 264–266
scanning electron microscopy (SEM) 178–181
self-diffusion 136
shock wave loading 22
sintering 72
SiO_2 particles 180
size dependence
  of coercive force 112–114
  on Curie temperature 115
  of saturation magnetization 114–115
sol-gel method 16
solid phase transformations 14
solid spraying method 9
solvent evaporation 16
specific surface area 79–80
spectroscopical characterization methods
  FTIR spectroscopy 181
  hierarchical schematics 181
spherical aluminum nanoparticles 128
spinning 10
spontaneous combustion temperature 158
static single-axial pressing 69
stents 246
strength in nanomaterials 184
sublimated drying 16
superconductivity phenomenon 101–105
superparamagnetism 111–112
superplasticity 170–172
surface diffusion 135
synthetic degradable polymers 231
synthetic polymers 259

t

tetrahedral fullerenes
  classification 34
  description 34
  topological models 39
thermal dissociation/pyrolysis 19–20
3D bioprinting 266–271
three-dimensional nano systems 32
tissue bioprinting strategies 269
tissue engineering
  biomaterials 259
  definition 259
  of heart valves 264–266
  principles 260
total knee arthroplasty 246
tracheobronchomalacia (TBM) 276
transmission electron microscopy (TEM) 174–177
two-dimensional dispersive systems 32

v

vacuum-sublimation technology 13–14
vibrational interaction 72
vibrational method 8–9
visian implantable collamer lens (ICL) model 241

w

wave number 117
wave vector 117
wearable artificial kidney (WAK) 248–249
work function 99
wound healing 275

z

zero-dimensional dispersive systems 31
zigzag type tubular carbon nanoclusters 49–51